THIRD EDITION

THE COMPLETE MAKE-UP ARTIST

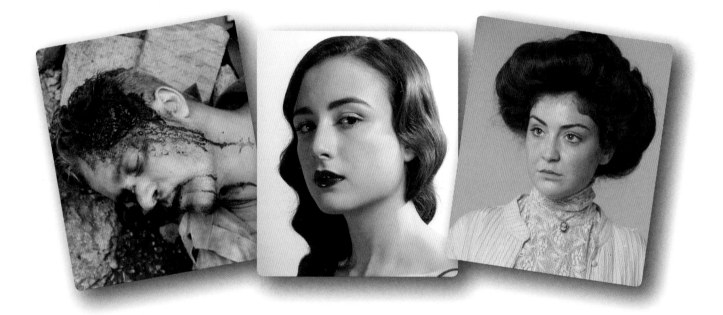

PENNY DELAMAR

with contributions from Leda Shawyer, Jo Frost,
Gideon Shawyer and Heather Jones

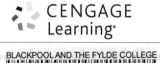
CENGAGE
Learning·

Australia • Brazil • Japan • Korea • Mexico • Singapore • Spain • United Kingdom • United States

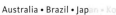

The Complete Make-up Artist: Working in Film, Fashion, Television and Theatre, 3rd Edition
Penny Delamar

Publisher: Virginia Thorp

Development Editor: Claire Napoli

Content Project Manager: Melissa Beavis

Manufacturing Buyer: Elaine Bevan

Marketing Manager: Vicky Fielding

Typesetter: MPS Limited

Cover design: HCT Creative

Text design: Design Deluxe Ltd

For product information and technology assistance,
contact **emea.info@cengage.com**.

For permission to use material from this text or product,
and for permission queries,
email **emea.permissions@cengage.com**.

British Library Cataloguing-in-Publication Data
A catalogue record for this book is available from the British Library.

ISBN: 978-1-4737-0371-1

Cengage Learning EMEA
Cheriton House, North Way, Andover,
Hampshire, SP10 5BE
United Kingdom

Cengage Learning products are represented in Canada by Nelson Education Ltd.

For your lifelong learning solutions, visit **www.cengage.co.uk**

Purchase your next print book, e-book or e-chapter at
www.cengagebrain.com

Printed in China by RR Donnelley
Print Number: 01   Print Year: 2015

HABIA SERIES LIST

Hairdressing

Student textbooks

Hairdressing and Barbering The Foundations: The Official Guide to Hairdressing and Barbering to Level 2 REVISED 7e *Leo Palladino & Martin Green*

Begin Hairdressing & Barbering: The Official Guide to Level 1 3e *Martin Green*

Professional Hairdressing: The Official Guide to Level 3 7e *Martin Green and Leo Palladino*

The Pocket Guide to Key Terms for Hairdressing *Martin Green*

The Official Guide to the City & Guilds Certificate in Salon Service 1e *John Armstrong with Anita Crosland, Martin Green and Lorraine Nordmann*

The Colour Book: The Official Guide to Colour for NVQ Levels 2 & 3 1e *Tracey Lloyd with Christine McMillan-Bodell*

eXtensions: The Official Guide to Hair Extensions 1e *Theresa Bullock*

Salon Management *Martin Green*

Men's Hairdressing: Traditional and Modern Barbering 3e *Maurice Lister*

Hairdressing for African & curly hair types from a Cross-Cultural Perspective 3e

The World of Hair Colour 1e *John Gray*

The Cutting Book: The Official Guide to Cutting at S/NVQ Levels 2 and 3 *Jane Goldsbro and Elaine White*

Professional Hairdressing titles

Trevor Sorbie: The Bridal Hair Book 1e *Trevor Sorbie and Jacki Wadeson*

The Art of Dressing Long Hair 1e *Guy Kremer and Jacki Wadeson*

Patrick Cameron: Dressing Long Hair 1e *Patrick Cameron and Jacki Wadeson*

Patrick Cameron: Dressing Long Hair 2 1e *Patrick Cameron and Jacki Wadeson*

Bridal Hair 1e *Pat Dixon and Jacki Wadeson*

Professional Men's Hairdressing: The Art of Cutting and Styling 1e *Guy Kremer and Jacki Wadeson*

Essensuals, the Next Generation Toni and Guy: Step by Step 1e *Sacha Mascolo, Christian Mascolo and Stuart Wesson*

Mahogany Hairdressing: Step to Cutting, Colouring and Finishing Hair 1e *Martin Gannon and Richard Thompson*

Mahogany Hairdressing: Advanced Looks 1e *Martin Gannon and Richard Thompson*

The Total Look: The Style Guide for Hair and Make-up Professional 1e *Ian Mistlin*

Trevor Sorbie: Visions in Hair 1e *Trevor Sorbie, Kris Sorbie and Jacki Wadeson*

The Art of Hair Colouring 1e *David Adams and Jacki Wadeson*

Beauty therapy

Beauty Basics: The Official Guide to Level 1 REVISED 3e *Lorraine Nordmann*

Beauty Therapy – The Foundations: The Official Guide to Level 2 VRQ 6e *Lorraine Nordmann*

Beauty Therapy – The Foundations: The Official Guide to Level 2 6e *Lorraine Nordmann*

Professional Beauty Therapy – The Official Guide to Level 3 REVISED 4e *Lorraine Nordmann*

The Pocket Guide to Key Terms for Beauty Therapy *Lorraine Nordmann and Marian Newman*

The Official Guide to the City & Guilds Certificate in Salon Services 1e *John Armstrong with Anita Crosland, Martin Green and Lorraine Nordmann*

The Complete Make-up Artist: Working in Film, Fashion, Television and Theatre 3e *Penny Delamar*

The Complete Guide to Make-Up 1e *Suzanne Le Quesne*

The Encyclopedia of Nails 1e *Jacqui Jefford and Anne Swain*

The Art of Nails: A Comprehensive Style Guide to Nail Treatments and Nail Art 1e *Jacqui Jefford*

Nail Artistry 1e *Jacqui Jefford*

The Complete Nail Technician 3e *Marian Newman*

Manicure, Pedicure and Advanced Nail Techniques 1e *Elaine Almond*

The Official Guide to Body Massage 2e *Adele O'Keefe*

An Holistic Guide to Massage 1e *Tina Parsons*

Indian Head Massage 2e *Muriel Burnham-Airey and Adele O'Keefe*

Aromatherapy for the Beauty Therapist 1e *Valerie Worwood*

An Holistic Guide to Reflexology 1e *Tina Parsons*

An Holistic Guide to Anatomy and Physiology 1e *Tina Parsons*

The Essential Guide to Holistic and Complementary Therapy 1e *Helen Beckmann and Suzanne Le Quesne*

The Spa Book 1e *Jane Crebbin-Bailey, Dr John Harcup, and John Harrington*

SPA: The Official Guide to Spa Therapy at Levels 2 and 3, *Joan Scott and Andrea Harrison*

Nutrition: A Practical Approach 1e *Suzanne Le Quesne*

Hands on Sports Therapy 1e *Keith Ward*

Encyclopedia of Hair Removal: A Complete Reference to Methods, Techniques and Career Opportunities, *Gill Morris and Janice Brown*

The Anatomy and Physiology Workbook: For Beauty and Holistic Therapies Levels 1–3. *Tina Parsons*

The Anatomy and Physiology CD-Rom

Beautiful Selling: The Complete Guide to Sales Success in the Salon *Rath Langley*

The Official Guide to the Diploma in Hair and Beauty Studies at Foundation Level 1e *Jane Goldsbro and Elaine White*

The Official Guide to the Diploma in Hair and Beauty Studies at Higher Level 1e *Jane Goldsbro and Elaine White*

The Official Guide to Foundation Learning in Hair and Beauty 1e *Jane Goldsbro and Elaine White*

Contents

Endorsers

About Habia

Habia, the Hair and Beauty Industry Authority, is appointed by government to represent employers in the Hair and Beauty Sector. Habia's main role is to manage the development of the National Occupational Standards (NOS) for hairdressing, barbering, beauty therapy, nails and spa. They are developed by industry for industry and represent best practice for achieving skills and knowledge in a particular job role. The NOS are used as the building blocks for the development of all qualifications that are developed by awarding organisations and by Cengage to develop textbooks and support products for learners.

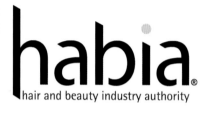

Habia is also responsible for the development and implementation of Apprenticeship Frameworks and issuing the apprenticeship certificates. Alongside providing information to employers on government initiatives that may affect the hair and beauty industry, be it educational, environmental or financial. A central point of contact for information, Habia provides guidance on careers, business development, legislation, salon health and safety.

Habia is part of SkillsActive, the Sector Skills Council that covers Hair & Beauty, Sports and the Active Leisure Sector.

About VTCT

The Vocational Traning Charitable Trust (VTCT) is a government approved specialist awarding organisation responsible for qualifications in the beauty therapy, complementary therapy, hairdressing, sports, fitness, hospitality and catering sectors. VTCT has been in existence for over 50 years, and in fact it was VTCT that originally coined the phrase *Beauty Therapy*. VTCT has remained at the forefront of developing the vocational system of qualifications in the UK and internationally. VTCT is the main sponsor and organiser of Worldskills UK (beauty therapy competitions) and VTCT also fund the development of the European and British Standard for Beauty Salon Services.

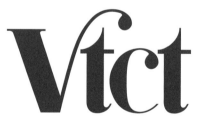

VTCT has the widest and most diverse range of qualifications in the beauty industry and is leading on many new initiatives in education, including online assessment and registration, e-portfolio and e-resources.

Foreword

It is with pleasure that I write the foreword for Penny Delamar's textbook. I have known Penny both as a colleague working on films and running the Delamar Academy of Make-up and Hair and have always been impressed by her passion and dedication to the craft.

Perhaps I should introduce myself and explain why I would undertake to write the foreword. I have worked primarily in the film industry as a make-up artist for more than 30 years, having had the good fortune to head the make-up department on some marvellous projects with a wide range of looks. Some of these films you may be familiar with, *Saving Private Ryan*, *The Fifth Element*, *The Princess Bride*, *Lincoln*, *War Horse*, *Almost Famous*, to name a few. So, I have been around the block a few times . . .

When I first began to yearn to be a make-up artist there were very few schools to train at, in fact two: the BBC and the London School of Fashion. I did not, back then, have the desire to learn hairdressing, this was needed and taught in both of these schools. I wanted to work in film and was very clear about that. Film work then was divided into make-up OR hair, not make-up AND hair, you could not do both on a film set. So I did not attend either school but began to seek experience hoping to be taken under a film make-up artist's wing as a trainee. This was tricky to say the least as, other than making up my friends and family and experimenting on my own, the 'how to' achieve certain looks with technical competence was challenging, if not impossible. There was not a 'how to' manual to hand, to make me into a useful trainee for someone to take on board.

Without contacts in the film industry, and minus formal training in make-up I would have given my worldly goods, such as they were at the time, to have access to such a textbook as this one you hold in your hands right now. Which is why I'm pleased to write the foreword.

Nothing can replace experience or give talent where there is none, neither a school nor a textbook, but what it can do is show the way to begin the journey of the lifetime of learning it takes to be a make-up artist. Offering methods of achieving looks in a safe and practical way, giving pointers for you, the individual, to expand upon with your own style and creativity. The rest is up to you.

Good luck and enjoy the work. That actually is the most important essence that makes a career a success, far more than accolades, love of the work for the sake of creating and contribution to the storytelling process.

Lois Burwell

About the Delamar Academy

Delamar Academy is based at Ealing Film Studios, in West London, where it provides world-class tuition by leading freelance make-up artists, nurturing and guiding students for entry into the TV, film, fashion and theatre industries.

Accredited by BAC, with university validation, Delamar Academy continues to maintain its standards of excellence, training the next generation of successful make-up artists.

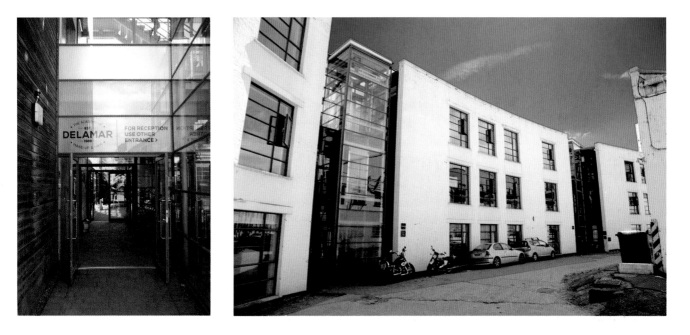

About the author

Penny Delamar is Founder and Principal of Delamar Academy, the most successful media training provider in the UK. She has trained a generation of top class professional make-up artists and counts Oscar and Bafta winners among her graduates and fellow teachers. She is a member of Bafta and has served on the judging panel for 'Best Make-up and Hair'. Penny has also been chair of the working party for National Vocational Qualifications for Make-up and Hair in Broadcast, Film and Video for Skillset.

Penny has a unique breadth of experience having spent ten years at the BBC where her numerous credits include successful series like *Dad's Army*, *Steptoe and Son*, *The Two Ronnies*, *The Morecombe and Wise Show*, *The Likely Lads* and *Z-Cars,* dramas such as *David Copperfield* and *A Midsummer Night's Dream* and The Beatles on *Top of the Pops*. This was followed by freelancing for 20 years on pop promos such as The Rolling Stones' '*Too Much Blood*', commercials and photographic shoots. Penny also worked on numerous feature films including *Chariots of Fire*, *Return to Oz*, *Robin Hood Prince of Thieves*, *Indiana Jones and the Last Crusade* and *High Spirits*. She was personal make-up artist to Dudley Moore on *Santa Claus – The Movie* and to Nastassja Kinski on *Revolution*.

She has made up Prime Ministers for over 30 years, from Sir Edward Heath to Sir John Major.

Now living in Devon, Penny still maintains a strong interest in Delamar Academy, and now finds time to paint, read and write.

Penny hopes this book will encourage the next generation in building their careers, and that it will help to ensure future growth and skills in the UK media industry.

Contributors

Leda Shawyer

Leda trained at Delamar Academy in 1986, having gained a 2.1 BA in English Literature and Greek and Roman Studies at Exeter University. She worked as a make-up artist for over ten years on films such as *Sleepy Hollow* and *Topsy Turvey*, and on television productions such as *Band of Brothers*, *Murder City*, *Wire in the Blood* and *Eastenders*. Leda has worked as Managing Director at Delamar Academy for the last seven years, overseeing the expansion of the Academy and securing its reputation as the most prestigious make-up training establishment in the UK.

Jo Frost

Jo Frost is a London-based make-up artist working internationally who trained in 1998. Sydney born but Devon raised, Jo is influenced by her early years travelling and experiences of foreign cultures, coupled with her innate passion for nature, art and literature. She is known for her high-end aesthetic, specialising in both beauty and fashion. In 2012 Jo joined CLM Hair and Make-up agency; she has worked on editorials for magazines such as *Dansk*, *Wonderland*, *iD, CR Fashion*, *Dazed & Confused*, *Vanity Fair*, *Jalouse*, *Glamour*, *Amica, Bon*, *Crash*, *Harpers Bazaar*, *Porter*, *Elle* and *Vogue*.

Jo has collaborated with photographers Boo George, Aitken Jolly, Marco Grob, Joachim Müller-Ruchholtz, Jem Mitchell, Thomas Lohr, Laurence Ellis, Scott Trindle, Simon Emmett, Michael Sanders, Benjamin Vnuk, Nick Dorey, Stefan Zschernitz, Emma Summerton, Sebastian Mader, John Balsom and Lee Broomfield.

Her client roster includes Erdem, Nicole Farhi, Antoni & Alison, Teatum Jones, Lara Bohinc, Twenty8Twelve, Markus Lupfer, Paul Smith, Vivienne Westwood, Preen, Joseph, Liberty, Saks, M&S Beauty, and Julien MacDonald. Celebrity clients include Natalie Dormer, Karolina Kurkova, Alexa Chung and Kaya Scodelario in addition to musicians and bands such as Jess Glynne, Lily Allen, Muse, Plan B, Jessie Ware, Banks and Florence Welch.

Gideon Shawyer

Gideon qualified as a chartered accountant at Deloitte in 2006, having gained a 2.1 BA in Economics at Newcastle University. He joined Delamar Academy as the Finance Director in 2011 having been Commercial Finance Manager at TalkTalk.

In the three years since Gideon joined, he has developed the academy's use of social media to help students network with each other when looking for work. He has interviewed tutors and graduates from Delamar Academy to pass on advice to future make-up artists. He also discusses book-keeping, tax, the use of social media and relevant business skills both during the course and afterwards.

Heather Jones

Heather has contributed to this book through mapping the teaching material to the qualification criteria. She has 20 years' experience in the hair and beauty industry: working as a beauty therapist, make-up artist, retail assistant and lecturer. After 10 years in the industry, Heather gained her teaching qualification. She also holds A1 & V1 awards. Heather is course leader for the Level 3 hair and media make-up course at Burton & South Derbyshire College and has taught over a variety of different levels from junior beauty, KS4 Level 1, 2, 3 and hair and media make-up. Working with the awarding bodies' City & Guilds and VTCT, Heather has worked as a make-up artist for Sky Live television, BBC period dramas, ITV National Soap awards, photo shoots, weddings and private clients. She is a judge for VTCT WorldSkills body art and media make-up and achieved 2nd place in the National Make-up Artist Award at the NEC May 2014.

Acknowledgements

*T*he Complete Make-up Artist 3rd edition is the result of many creative people freely sharing their knowledge and experience to bring this book together. My grateful thanks to the professional experts for their generous contribution as guest writers, case profiles and giving us photographs of their work. Their collaboration has made it possible to give our readers a deeper insight into the profession.

A big thank you to the brilliant make-up artists who, on the hottest days of the year, gave their time to work tirelessly on the photo shoot. The step-by-step pictures, book cover and other photos throughout the text are due to their collaboration. Thank you to Nathan Allen, our photographer, for his professionalism and artistry in producing the quality pictures that we wished for.

My grateful thanks to Stephanie Linnell for her computer skills, typing, editing and encouragement from start to finish. Such kind generosity is much appreciated. Also thank you to Peter Linnell and Chris Franklin for their help with our research. Very grateful thanks to Claire Napoli, Development Editor for Cengage Learning for the hard work and firm support all the way through to the final manuscript. Thank you to all at Cengage including Virginia Thorp, for seeing the need for a 3rd edition and making it happen.

Thank you so much Heather Jones for the excellent work in mapping all the techniques to the standards of the Awarding Bodies. Also for clarifying the text, making it an easily accessible format for students to follow.

Very big thanks to Jo Frost for the *Beauty and Fashion* chapter. At the peak of her career in the fashion industry, no one could have been more qualified as a guest writer to do it. I am sure it will provide insight and inspiration for students in the years ahead.

Tremendous thanks to Lois Burwell for writing such a lovely foreword. Lois is an international Oscar-winning make-up designer with many awards and nominations to her name. She is an inspiring role model for every make-up artist and I have always admired her work, so I feel honoured that she gave us such a perfect introduction to this book.

Many thanks to my son, Gideon Shawyer, for Chapter 14 Launching your career, which is full of advice to students on what to do next. As Finance Director at Delamar Academy he is very aware of how important it is for trainee make-up artists to start earning a living.

Finally, heartfelt thanks to my daughter, Leda Shawyer, for doing most of the work, gathering information, checking on make-up artists' availability, organising the photo shoot, matching pictures to text and much more. As Managing Director of the Delamar Academy, with two young children, I don't know how she did it. Thank you for your partnership in this project. And for the laughs along the way.

Penny Delamar

The author would like to thank the following people and organisations for their assistance in producing this book:

For their contribution as case profiles:

Chapter 1 – Jane Richardson, Giorgio Galliero, Louise McCarthy, Namrata Soni

Chapter 2 – Joanne Byrne, Sarah Jagger, Lauren Whitworth

Chapter 3 – Jo Frost

Chapter 4 – Holly Edwards, Hafdis Larusdottir

Chapter 5 – Raphaelle Fieldhouse

Chapter 6 – Caroline O'Connor, Wendy Topping, Stefan Musch, Robin Lough

Chapter 7 – Nikki Hambi, Catherine Scoble, Cate Hall,

Chapter 8 – Laura Solari, Jo Neilsen

Chapter 9 – Sallie Jaye, Stacey Holman, Helen Speyer, Lorraine Hill

Chapter 10 – Sarah Weatherburn, Emma Jones

Chapter 11 – Brian Kinney, Sharon Anniss

Chapter 12 – Andy Deubert, Kristyan Mallett, Adrian Rigby

Chapter 13 – Amanda Warburton, Angie Mudge

Chapter 14 – Oliver Hickey

For their help with the photo shoot:

Nathan Allen Photography, www.nathanallenphotography.com

Make-up artists:

Joanne Byrne	Adrian Rigby
Lorraine Hill	Helen Speyer
Julio Parodi	Amanda Warburton

Models:

Svetlana Chikhireva	Gabor Karkekes
Cliodhna Cremin	Rosanna Nicholls
Bethany Fletcher	Valentina Nesti
Alyson Forbes	Gunnihildur Olafsdottir
Charlotte Gilliland	Erica Procopis
Zyna Goldy	Jacqueline Read
Laura Gutierrez	Amber Snow
Paula Harris	Charlotte White
Pippa-Grace Johnson	

The publisher would like to thank:

The many copyright holders who have kindly granted us permission to reproduce material throughout this text. Every effort has been made to contact all rights holders but in the unlikely event that anything has been overlooked, please contact the publisher directly and we will happily make the necessary arrangements at the earliest opportunity.

Image credit list

Although every effort has been made to contact copyright holders before publication, this has not always been possible. If notified, the publisher will undertake to rectify any errors or omissions at the earliest opportunity.

Photos

The publishers would like to thank the following sources for permission to reproduce their copyright protected images:

Alexa Ravina pp 105, 141, 228, 273; Alexandra Reader pp 106; Amanda Warburton pp 283; Andrew Deubert pp 240, 251, 254; Angela Betta pp 286; Angie Mudge pp 289; Annie Botta pp 210; Balmain Hair pp 94, 98; Brian Kinney pp 225; Cara Louise Logan pp 113; Cate Hall pp 139, 308; Catherine Scoble pp 2, 134, 137, 143; Charles Fox/Kryolan pp 5; Charlotte Jameison pp 236; Cinderella hair pp 97; Diandra Ferreira pp 108; Ella van der Zwart pp i, 264; Emma Jones pp 204; Emma Nash pp 53, 56; Faith Elizabeth Bailey pp 4; Gabor Kerekes pp 91, 187; Georgina L Coverdale glcoverdale@hotmail.co.uk pp 102, 106; Giorgio Galliero pp 127, 156, 182, 184, 212, 286; Goldwell pp 89, 90; Hadia Ahmed pp 19, 279; Hafdis Larusdottir pp 90; Heather-Jay Ross pp i, 182, 211; HSE pp 9; Holly Edwards pp 99; Jane Richardson pp 6; Jo Frost pp 78, 84; Joanne Byrne pp 37; Kett Cosmetics pp 112, 113, 114; Kristyan Mallett pp 234, 238, 239, 244, 249, 253, 262, 281; Laura Solari pp 166; Lauren Whitworth pp 52, 136; Leda Shawyer pp 196, 199, 200, 202, 203, 207, 208, 209, 216, 217, 249, 254, 261; Lisa Cartlidge pp 259; L'Oreal Professional pp 97; Lorraine Hill pp 195; Louise Crouch pp 285; Lucy Arnold pp 185, 188, 272; Make-up by Ella van der Zwart pp 184; Make-up by Ella van der Zwart, model Cliodhna Cremin pp 176, 185; Megan Royle pp i; Milady, a part of Cengage Learning pp 34, 36, 44, 45, 54, 55, 57, 58, 115; Molly Drumm pp 168; Namrata Soni/Elle India pp 41, 47, 293, 294, 295; NARs pp 23,35; Namrata Soni pp 29; Nathan Portlock Allan Photography pp ix, 8, 27, 32, 35, 39, 40, 45, 46, 49, 58, 81, 83, 88, 90, 91, 92, 93, 96, 97, 103, 104, 123, 129, 130, 133, 141, 158, 162, 163, 169, 170, 171, 173, 182, 186, 191, 199, 218, 219, 221, 223, 224, 230, 237, 257, 258, 266, 268, 278, 284, 290; Nikki Hambi pp 154; Oliver Hickey pp 143; Parmjit Barker pp 171; Penny Delamar pp 47, 48, 167, 174, 180, 181, 182, 193, 198; Penny Delamar (illustrations) pp 129, 139, 161, 179, 194, 203, 209, 248; Pippa Johnson pp 100; Raphaelle Fieldhouse pp 108; Robb Crafer pp 219; Ruby Lonsdale pp 226; Sarah Hubbauer pp 107, 127; Sarah Jagger pp 60; Sarah Weatherburn pp 201; Shannon Belle Webster pp 220; Sharon Anniss pp 233; Shutterstock/AlexAnnaButs pp 102; Shutterstock/ ngirl pp 106; Shutterstock/AnnaKostyuk pp 189; Shutterstock/carlo dapino pp 86; Shutterstock/CREATISTA pp 116; Shutterstock/Ermolaev Alexander pp 274; Shutterstock/Hein Nouwens pp 179; Shutterstock/KUCO pp 186; Shutterstock/Max_Wanted_Media pp 178; Shutterstock/Nina Buday pp 106; Shutterstock/Pandorabox pp 5; Shutterstock/Peter Bernik pp 4; Shutterstock/Pressmaster pp 274; Shutterstock/Sergey Rusakov pp 179; Shutterstock/StudioTS pp 299; Shutterstock/Svetlanamiku pp 28; Shutterstock/Tom Grundy pp 210; Shutterstock/White Room pp 406; Sophie Crudgington pp 263; Stacey Holman pp 150; Stefan Musch pp 118, 119, 120; Tom Smith pp 280; Trefor Proud pp 270, 287, 288; Victoria Stride pp 102, 106; Wendy Topping pp 126; Zia Austrin pp 190.

Chapter 3 photos

Page 62 and page 82: Publication: Amica, Photographer: Joachim Müller-Ruchholtz, Stylist: Giulia Bassi, Make-Up: Jo Frost, Hair: Panos Papandrianos, Model: Kelsey Van Mook @ Next

Page 65, page 66 and page 80: Publication: Twenty6 Magazine, Photographer: Rupert Tapper, Make-Up: Jo Frost, Styling: Marie-Louise Von Haselberg, Hair: Philippe Tholimet, Model: Daniela K @ IMG London

Page 66: Publication: Twenty6 Magazine, Photographer: Rupert Tapper, Make-Up: Jo Frost, Stylist: Marie-Louise von Haselberg, Hair: Philippe Tholimet, Nails: Steph Mendiola, Model: Daniela K @ IMG London

Page 67: Publication: Bon, Photographer: Oskar Gyllensvärd, Styling: Marie-Louise von Haselberg, Make-Up: Jo Frost, Hair: Nao Kawakami, Model: Gem @ IMG London

Page 67: Publication: Bon, Photographer: Oskar Gyllensvärd, Stylist: Marie-Louise von Haselberg, Make-up: Jo Frost, Hair: Nao Kawakami, Model: Harriet Taylor @ IMG London

Page 72: Publication: Dansk, Photographer: Markus Pritzi, Stylist: Marie-Louise von Haselberg, Make-up: Jo Frost, Hair: Panos Papandrianos, Model: Stef Van Der Laan @ IMG London

Page 74: Publication: Black Magazine, Photographer: Andy Eaton, Stylist: Sara Dunn, Make-Up: Jo Frost, Model: Naty Chabanenko @ Next

Page 79: Publication: Amica, Photographer: Joachim Müller-Ruchholtz, Stylist: Giulia Bassi, Make-Up: Jo Frost, Hair: Ben Jones, Model: Ehren Dorsey @ Next

Page 82: Publication: Amica, Photographer: Joachim Müller-Ruchholtz, Stylist: Giulia Bassi, Make-Up: Jo Frost, Hair: Naoki Komiya, Model: Filippa Hamilton @ Next

About the book

Throughout this textbook you will find many colourful text boxes designed to aid your learning and understanding as well as highlight key points. Here are examples and descriptions of each:

TOP TIP

Shares the author's experience and provides positive suggestions to improve knowledge and skills.

HEALTH & SAFETY

Draws your attention to related health and safety information essential for each technical skill.

CASE PROFILE

Case profile boxes give you an inspirational glance into the knowledge and experience of a trusted industry expert, helping to motivate and instruct you in your own career.

Tools & equipment

Help you prepare for each practical treatment and show you the tools, materials and products required.

ACTIVITY

Featured in the book to provide additional tasks for you to further your understanding.

Directional arrows point you to other parts of the book that explore similar or related topics, so you can expand your learning.

REVISION QUESTIONS

At the end of each chapter there is a useful revision section which has been specially devised to help you check your learning and prepare for your oral and written assessments. Use these revision sections to test your knowledge as you progress through the course and seek guidance from your supervisor or assessor if you come across any areas that you are unsure of.

Introduction by the author

The make-up artists of today have a much broader role than in the past. Instead of working in a niche area they now move across the board, adjusting their techniques for the different media. Since they are mostly freelance they undertake any work, anywhere in the world. They have acquired new skills to add to their own: in skincare, cosmetology, airbrushing, hairdressing, nails, beauty, character or prosthetics. This has resulted in make-up artists working from the same basic kit box for any medium, adjusting when necessary, to the brief. We now have make-up artists who are successful in their careers because they are well-rounded in their skills. They are what I call complete make-up artists.

The present generation of students, who will be tomorrow's make-up artists, have more need than ever to learn as much as possible. The effect of globalisation and technology has brought not only a more exciting, stimulating industry – but also much more competition. This book is for them.

In these uncertain times, with computers replacing people in many areas of work, we can be confident that machines will never replace make-up artists. Once learned, make-up is a skill that cannot be taken away from you – a worthwhile possession in the changing fortunes of modern times.

Penny Delamar

1 Media make-up as a career

LEARNING OBJECTIVES

This chapter covers the following:

◆ Introduction to a career as a media make-up artist.

◆ Careers within the industry and areas for specialisation for long-term progression.

◆ The make-up room.

◆ Health and hygiene.

◆ Faces and head shapes.

◆ Colour theory.

◆ Skincare.

◆ Student kit.

◆ Lighting.

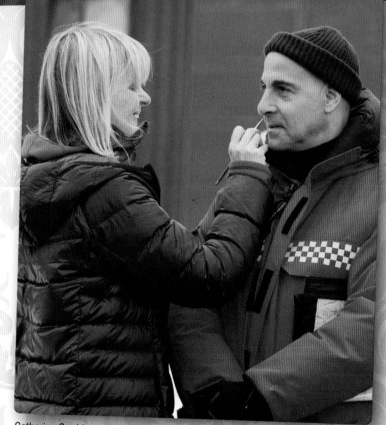

Catherine Scoble making up Stanley Tucci on the set of 'Fortitude'

KEY TERMS

Acetone

Adhesives

Aquacolour

Camouflage make-up

Continuity

False eyelashes

Fantasy make-up

Foundations

Hair lace

Highlighting

Latex

Pencils

Portfolios

Powder brush

Shading

Spirit gum

Swing job

Tongs

Toning down a colour

UNIT TITLE

◆ Co-ordinate the design team and performers

INTRODUCTION

To begin with, young make-up artists are better off accepting every job that comes their way to gain knowledge and experience within a realistic working environment as a professional make-up artist. This may include unpaid work experience as a trainee. It may take up to two years to gain this knowledge and develop the personal skills required of a make-up artist. For example, make-up artists must understand how to conduct themselves when working on set and with other industry professionals, and they must develop interpersonal skills for working with actors, models, etc. Young make-up artists may work in fashion, theatre, television or film. Eventually, either through circumstances or choice, they may settle into a specialised area as a lifestyle choice. This could be because of having a family, not wishing to travel, or maybe not wanting 5 a.m. call times and having to drive to remote locations. There are opportunities in many areas if you work hard and are passionate. Over time you will find an area you excel in and you will be able to develop your skills further to make a successful career.

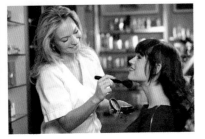

Department store sales and promotion of products for a make-up company

Areas of specialism for long-term progression

Department stores (retail)

Working in a department store on the sales and promotion of products for a make-up company, e.g. Nars, Chanel, MAC, etc.

This type of work involves giving make-up lessons at the counter, giving advice on the product range, plus skill and speed in applying day and evening make-up with realistic expectations for everyday clients to achieve. Department stores sell cosmetic camouflage and natural make-up suitable for all ages and skin types. There is often commission paid on the sale of products. There are also opportunities in the business side of the cosmetic company, such as becoming an area representative or a manager.

Beauty salon

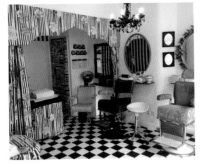

Beauty salon

Providing work in a permanent beauty room along with beauty therapy services such as massage, nails, tanning, etc. This often involves retail sales products. The opportunities are either working for the salon owner or establishing your own business and include day, evening, bridal, promotional and special occasion make-ups.

Wig (postiche) making

Working in a company that makes wigs for television, film and theatre productions. The company might hire out the wigs as well as sell them. The work consists of dressing as well as making wigs, hairpieces and facial hair – plus alterations and fittings on actors. This is a specialist area and a knowledge of period, fantasy and current styles is needed. Knowledge and understanding of maintaining wigs, blocking on, setting and restyling are required.

Facial hair

Working in a company that makes, dresses and fits facial hair for television, film and theatre. The **hair lace** is very fine for television and film, less so for theatre. This is a very specialised area as the work consists of making facial hair to order using hot tongs to style them in the required shape. The worst case scenario would be to damage or burn the hair resulting in problems for **continuity**. Health and safety is very important.

Prosthetic workshops

Working for a company that makes prosthetics to order for television, film or theatre. Includes sculpting, casting, mould making, artworking and inserting hair into prosthetics for a particular production. Some companies also apply the pieces as a separate team alongside the make-up and hair departments on a film.

Camouflage make-up

Working in burns units in hospitals and private clinics for cosmetic surgery, as well as salons or freelance work showing people how to cover scars, birth marks, tattoos, etc.

TOP TIP

Working in a salon gives you an excellent opportunity to build up regular clients. Keep updated with changes in the industry and go on regular training courses so you can offer your clients the latest products and services.

HEALTH & SAFETY

When working with heated equipment ensure it is always in a safe place on a heat resistant surface.

HEALTH & SAFETY

Ensure ventilation meets the required levels when working with chemical products.

Camouflage make-up is a sensitive area of the industry and realistic expectations need to be given to the client. An understanding of products and the colour wheel is required. Trial services will be required for special occasions to gain the perfect outcome.

Bridal make-up

Providing a service in bridal make-up in a salon or as a freelancer. This usually includes a practice (trial) session ahead of the wedding day. The bridal party may include the bride, bridesmaids and mother of the bride. You may be working to a theme. Additional media may be needed such as eyelashes and hairpieces to create the desired look as required by the client.

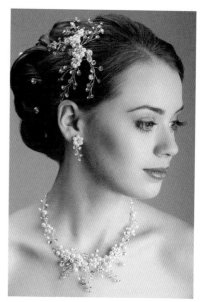

Bridal make-up

Teaching

Many make-up artists enjoy passing on their skills to the next generation. In colleges and state schools they are required to complete a teacher's training course and assessor's award. The awarding body generates the qualification. The standard setting body and sector skills councils set the national occupational standards from which the qualifications are written by the awarding body. There are many employers and specialists within the industry that are involved in the content of the national occupational standards. In private media make-up schools, teachers need a proven track record in the industry as a designer. Many lecturers will also work within the industry to keep their skills current and relevant. Full-time lecturers are required to undertake a minimum of 30 hours continued professional development (CPD) a year to ensure they have the most up-to-date skills within the industry.

Creating a cosmetic brand

Some make-up artists create a cosmetic brand either by themselves or for a large company. Professional media shops sell specialist products manufactured by make-up artists such as ready-made blood, bald caps, small prosthetic pieces and other special effect products.

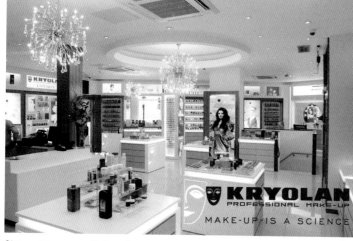

Shop selling cosmetic brand

CASE PROFILE: JANE RICHARDSON, INTERNATIONAL LEAD MAKE-UP ARTIST

One of the many wonderful aspects of my job representing a well-known cosmetic brand is to talk to students about the brand and what I do. I often talk about the incredible mentors that have inspired me in my life, of which Penny Delamar is one.

I originally trained as a beauty therapist and was lucky enough to have an inspirational lecturer who ignited my passion for make-up one day by introducing us to 'casualty' special effects. I held onto this passion and dreamt of becoming a professional make-up artist even as I went on to work as a therapist and, later, a salon owner.

My work as a retail make-up artist started with me accepting a counter manager position in order to 'consult' for three months. This led to my becoming a National Artist, Europe Training Manager and finally the position I hold today, International Lead Stylist. I have worked hard and grabbed any opportunity to learn from the people around me. I have been privileged to see this amazing brand grow from small beginnings and in doing so have gained insight into the various aspects of building a successful brand: marketing, PR, education, sales.

I love my job. Not many people can say that and the moment that you stop loving what you do is the moment to look for other avenues for your artistry. There are so many avenues and each one will show you something new about yourself. Our creativity relies on inspiration, and that comes from collaboration and the sharing of ideas. Let your artistry lead you always, not your ego …

WORKING IN RETAIL

I believe that the strongest quality required for retail is a passion for people. So many artists come to the counter and focus on themselves (the ego) not the person in front of them. They are more concerned with somehow proving that they are the most amazing make-up artist and often get upset when a customer walks away without purchasing. Granted, making people happy isn't always easy but patience and good listening skills help to create a more solid understanding. When you understand you can recommend (sell) and when recommendations are based upon what the customer needs as opposed to what you, the artist, thinks they need you will be more likely to sell. Go a step further and take time to

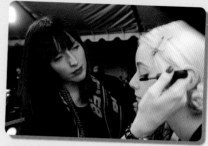

show (educate) your customer on how they can use the products themselves and you start to create a relationship. These relationships (customer loyalty) make a brand, and it's the artists at the counter that create it. I have clients that I still see today that I first met at the counter. They return to me for trusted, honest advice and, more importantly, education. Being able to teach people about the products but also their application doesn't always come easy and is something I've seen artists struggle with often in the training room.

Selling in the right way is a skill and like any skill it takes time to learn. Once learnt, though, like your artistry it is a skill to be proud of. When you see the transformative effect of make-up and understand that you are a part of how it makes women feel, nothing can beat it!

TIPS FOR SUCCESS AT THE COUNTER

- **Understand sales techniques and language** Learn about targets, how you reach them and take every opportunity to practise different approaches. Understand that selling is a key part of your job and you will be expected to reach your targets.

- **Be a good listener** Listen carefully to your customers and only select products that they need. Highlight clearly what the initial takeaways are and never oversell.

- **Have integrity** If you don't know something, find someone that does and keep the customer informed as to what you are doing. Never make claims against a product that aren't true.

- **Be a team player** Be aware of your other artists and help out if necessary, even if it is tidying their station. Work respectfully of others and be open and honest to avoid any misunderstandings.

- **Educate yourself** Keep up-to-date with the latest products, ingredients and brand techniques, and don't be afraid to ask for more training support if you need it. Be an expert!

- **Take pride** Understand that you are representing a brand and as such will have image guidelines to follow. A professional image helps present you to the customer in the right way, and all brands and stores have these expectations.

◆ **Look out for opportunities** There are many roles within a company that will be available to you, if you have the right skill sets. Some artists go on to become national artists, counter managers, area managers, trainers or even take on office-based positions. If you feel that you would like another position, always speak to your line manager first and gain information as to the kind of skills you would need. Be aware that the process may take time but if you are passionate about something it will come to you eventually.

The trainee make-up artist

It is often said that you do not learn to drive until you have passed your driving test. The same could be said of make-up artistry. After gaining your qualification you need to obtain work experience on professional productions. The best way to do this is to contact make-up artists and ask them to take you on for a day, a week or a month. If the tutors on your course are working make-up artists they may take you on a job or be able to place you with a colleague. It is important to get as much work experience as possible in the first year after graduating. Every job, however small, will lead to others. Trainees are paid a minimal amount, but this should be regarded as a continuation of the training process, and done with enthusiasm. Starting from the bottom is how everyone begins their career – by making the coffee, cleaning the make-up stations, checking the stock, or handing pins to the designer. When running errands you meet other people in different departments and begin to understand their roles. When you clean up a senior make-up artist's workstation you will learn about the way the make-up was applied and products used.

Attitude is more important than exam results when you are being considered for work by a designer. There are some attributes that are key to long-term success:

1 The ability to take criticism gracefully.

2 Self-control – the ability to regulate emotions and thoughts.

3 Grit – perseverance in finishing what you start.

Plus, doing everything that you are asked to do with goodwill.

CASE PROFILE: GIORGIO GALLIERO, TRAINEE MAKE-UP ARTIST

How long have you been working in the industry?
Although I started work as a freelance make-up artist in 2010 when I was still living in Italy, I had my first proper work experience in the industry in 2012 while training at the Delamar Academy.

How did you get into the industry?
I decided to move from Italy to London to train, where I met several established make-up artists who gave me the chance to work with them while I was studying. I started with some work experience and **swing jobs** in theatre productions such as *Shrek*, *Wicked* and *Book of Mormon*, I then moved onto television series such as *Poirot* and *Endeavour* and recently on feature films such as *Exodus* and *Macbeth*. All of these gave me the opportunity to create invaluable contacts within the industry and get myself known.

Did you have a lucky break or turning point?
I guess my lucky break was to get on board as a trainee on Ridley Scott's feature film *Exodus*. Working on this production for several months in the UK and in Spain gave me the chance to prove myself on a big production and get to know many brilliant make-up artists who then called me to work on their next projects.

What has been your most significant project?

I guess my answer would always be 'the one I'm working on at the moment'. I like to fully commit to the project I'm working on and I always make sure to get the most from it, trying to make it a bit better than the last one!

What do you enjoy most about the job?

I love the research behind a look, getting to know the background story of characters so that my make-up can help bring them to life and make them believable. I also love the atmosphere of the set where everyone works together to make the magic happen.

What do you enjoy least about the job?

The very early mornings, the very late nights and the travel time on different locations can be a bit of a pain sometimes. And dreadful weather when in an outdoor location certainly doesn't help. But as long as you do the job you love, you don't really feel the tiredness or the aches of your body.

What advice would you give to a new make-up artist starting out?

Always be yourself and be a team player! Always push yourself beyond your limits and improve your skills! Always be up for a challenge, but at the same time try to have fun!

The make-up room

The working area

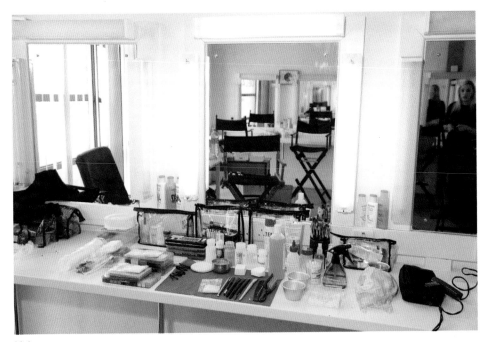

Make-up room

Make-up rooms in film and television studios, beauty salons and theatres are custom-built to provide work surfaces, lighting and storage facilities. On location, low-budget productions and student films, the working area may be uncomfortable, cramped and ill-equipped. In such situations it is the make-up artist's job to establish the working environment. On location you may be working in make-up trailers or buses and you may be travelling from place to place.

◆ **The room** The make-up room allocated should be well-ventilated to meet health and safety regulations.

- ◆ **The facilities** There should be a mirror with lights and a table for each make-up artist.

- ◆ **Electricity points** There must be adequate electricity points which have been checked prior to use.

- ◆ **Washbasin** There should be a washbasin nearby with hot and cold running water.

- ◆ **The environment** The temperature and humidity must be comfortable for working – and stable for the storage of make-up products.

If these basic conditions are not met it is essential to notify the location manager or production office promptly and to state clearly what is required.

Health, safety and hygiene

Once the make-up room has been set up, the make-up artist should maintain a safe, healthy and hygienic working environment to safeguard actors and colleagues from accident and cross-infection. Provided that you take sensible precautions, the make-up room should be kept clean and safe. You must ensure all electrical equipment used meets the legal requirements. If portable electrical equipment is new it is valid for 12 months without a PAT (portable appliance test) although it may be a requirement of the venue for additional electrical equipment safety. Refer to HSE for further guidance on risk assessment. If the required tests are not carried out this could invalidate insurance. It is vital that make-up artists hold relevant insurance. A correct and professional appearance must be followed, suitable for the working environment. This includes suitable clothing and footwear. Risk assessments will need to be carried out due to the nature of the job and the environment.

HEALTH & SAFETY

Ensure the working area is safe at all times. This includes keeping walkways clear and securely replacing the lids on chemical products after use.

Cross-contamination via make-up

Infections, such as scabies, cold sores, styes and other bacterial and viral diseases, can be spread via sponges, powder puffs, **foundations**, creams, lipsticks and so on. Diseases can also be passed on via equipment that has not been sterilised properly. For this reason, and because the pH of your skin could contaminate the make-up, you should not touch make-up products with your hands. Instead, use spatulas and brushes.

HEALTH & SAFETY

Always ensure a complete consultation is performed to ensure the client is suitable for treatment.

Control of Substances Hazardous to Health (COSHH) 1988

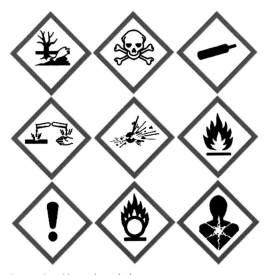

International hazard symbols

The COSHH 1988 regulations provide guidance and lay down rules about the safe storage, disposal and use of potentially dangerous substances. You should be familiar with these regulations. A copy of the COSSH regulations can be obtained from the Health and Safety Executive (HSE) website (www.hse.gov.uk). In particular you should know about correct storage and use of cleaning agents and products such as **acetone**, isopropyl alchohol (IPA) and **adhesives**. It is a manufacturer's legal responsibility to supply a material data sheet for each product. This data sheet provides the required information from which a risk assessment can be performed. The client may require patch testing for certain chemical products prior to application.

Working hygienically

General preparations

- ◆ Make-up products should always be labelled clearly, with full instructions for use. This is to avoid accidents, such as mistaking surgical spirit for skin tonic.

- ◆ Hazardous materials should be kept securely in metal trunks or cabinets with locks.

- ◆ Wraps and towels must always be freshly laundered.

- ◆ Individual kit boxes should be cleaned out regularly.

- ◆ Electrical sockets and plugs must be safe. If any are faulty, they must be labelled and removed from use immediately.

- ◆ Tools must be sterilised. Electrical equipment such as shavers, beard trimmers, tongs, etc. should be cleaned after use with surgical spirit (or according to manufacturer's instructions).

- ◆ Mirrors should be polished regularly.

Before starting the make-up

- ◆ Check that you have clean powder puffs, sponges and brushes to hand.

- ◆ All products required should be ready on the workstation prior to service.

While working

- ◆ When applying lipstick use a spatula to transfer lipstick onto a plastic or stainless steel palette. Then use a clean lipbrush to transfer the lipstick from palette to lips.

- ◆ Disposable foam applicators, mascara wands or foundation sponges are good for using once and throwing away, e.g. for eyeshadows.

- ◆ A paper tissue wrapped around a powder puff is good for powdering crowd artists. Use a new tissue for each face.

When you have finished

- ◆ Brushes should be cleaned in brush-cleaning solvent.

- ◆ Sponges and powder puffs should be washed and sterilised – or thrown away after special effects and heavy character make-up.

- ◆ Dispose of solvent removers in covered bins.

- ◆ Clean work surfaces and mirrors at the end of the working day.

HEALTH & SAFETY

Ensure all spillages are cleaned up immediately and hair on the floor is removed to minimise the risk of someone slipping or falling.

TOP TIP

A ceramic tile makes a good palete.

Professionalism

The make-up artist who behaves professionally will be more successful than the one who does not. The best time to develop this skill is whilst you are training. The make-up room should be calm and relaxing. Actors, models and clients all need a restful atmosphere away from the noise of the studio or set. The make-up artist may be the last person they speak to before going in front of the camera. Being calm and efficient will give the performers confidence in themselves and you.

Efficient working

It will be easier to appear calm and purposeful if you are organised and your working area is clean and tidy. If everything is laid out ready before the actor arrives, it not only inspires confidence but also saves time.

Storing materials

◆ **Kit boxes** Keep separate boxes for beauty make-up, hairdressing and casualty effects.

◆ **Storage** Store materials in such a way that they will not be damaged, crushed, split or broken. Potentially messy products such as artificial blood and dirt should be stored separately.

◆ **Containers** Plastic bottles are often preferable to glass ones for storing non-toxic chemicals, as they do not break. However, some chemicals can melt plastic, so make sure that the product can be safely stored in a plastic container.

Routine checks

◆ **Stock** Check regularly so that you do not run out of products.

◆ **Cleaning** Check that you have sufficient sterilising fluids and cleaners appropriate for the materials you are using.

◆ **Labels** Ensure that the labels on all containers are clear and accurate.

Ordering materials

◆ **Avoiding waste** When purchasing products for a production, take care that they are suitable and economical. Don't use expensive brands for crowd scenes where there are no close-ups.

◆ **Special needs** Make sure the actors, models or clients have the skincare products they need, including sunblock.

◆ **Getting quotes** When ordering facial hair and prosthetics, or when hiring or buying wigs, get quotes from several suppliers. The cheapest may not be the best quality, but at least consider the options.

◆ **Keeping records** Keep clear and accurate records of expenses incurred for the production office.

Working abroad

◆ **Air freight** If you need to have tools and products sent by air freight, arrange this in advance. Pack carefully to avoid breakages and list everything for inspection at airports.

Clothing

◆ **Plan ahead** Be sure to have appropriate clothing for working conditions.

Continuity

◆ **Keeping reference materials** To ensure continuity, make notes, charts and sketches to record your work as well as taking photos. Keep them in a file or pinned to the wall so that you can refer to them whilst working.

Personal appearance

◆ Maintain high standards of personal hygiene. Be discreet with your choice of clothing. It is not a good idea to outshine the leading actress or actor; he or she is the star – not you.

◆ Heavy, theatrical make-up can be off-putting, and low-cut necklines can send the wrong message to a mainly male-based crew.

◆ Wear flat shoes; high heels are dangerous.

◆ Keep nails clean and reasonably short. Actors are often nervous of long nails near their eyes, and long nails make application of make-up difficult.

◆ Keep hair tied back from your face in order to see the mirror clearly while working.

◆ Avoid jangly, noisy jewellery.

TOP TIP

If you wear too much make-up, the actors might think you will apply too much to them.

Working on set

When the make-up is completed and the actor is on the set, your responsibility has not ended. The make-up must be maintained throughout the working day. Whether working inside the studio under hot lights, or outside on location in the rain, it is the make-up artist's responsibility to stand by, ready to repair any damage to the make-up or hair.

◆ All necessary tools and products should be to hand in a set box or bag.

◆ Clear plastic bags are often labelled with the actor's name and contain their individual products.

◆ The make-up is checked between shots, and again after each meal break. Touching up includes adding more lipstick, blotting shine, tidying hair, or re-sticking wig hair laces, facial hair and prosthetics.

HEALTH & SAFETY

Whilst working on set always be aware of the potential hazards identified during the risk assessment.

Teamwork

To an outsider it always looks as if everyone is hanging around on the set, doing nothing. This is because everyone has to wait while someone finishes their work. Lights need adjusting; props are moved; tracks laid down for the camera; costumes, hair and make-up changed – all at different times. There are potential hazards on the set such as trailing wires and cables, which is why flat, rubber-soled shoes should be worn. Any sound made will hold up the shoot – so no mobile phones on set, squeaky shoes or jangling charm bracelets.

The crew work closely together, everyone relying on one another to work well and to be fast and efficient. Since intense pressure is normal on a shoot, and indeed necessary to generate the energy required, the make-up artist must, like everyone else, learn to cope

TOP TIP

Be yourself and do whatever job you see needs doing. This may be tidying the work area or making tea. Make yourself indispensable and you will make valuable contacts.

with stress. This can be difficult to do on a long shoot, lasting months, working long hours. Good stamina, good health and a good sense of humour are key to survival.

Face and head shapes

Both make-up and hair should be designed to suit the actor's head and face shape. There are seven basic head shapes.

The oval face

This face is generally considered to be the perfect shape. It is easy to work with and photographs well.

The round face

This face has a soft shape with no angles. Contouring at the sides of the face, under the cheekbones, will add light and shade for a more interesting shape for the camera. Hair dressed straight down the sides will minimise the jawline. Avoid fullness at the sides when designing the hairstyle, to avoid emphasising the round face shape.

The long face

This face has a high forehead and hairline, with a long chin. By **shading** the chin the face will appear shorter. Blusher can be placed on the apples of the cheeks to give the illusion of a rounder shape. Hair dressed full at the sides will also add width to the shape.

The square face

This face has a straight-across hairline and square-shaped chin. Shading at the jawline will soften the shape. Blusher can be placed high on the cheekbones, defining the shape, and contoured beneath the cheekbones for a slimming effect.

The heart-shaped face

This face is thinner on the bottom half with a broad forehead. Try placing blusher on the round apples of the cheeks. No contouring is necessary, unless at the sides of the forehead, close to the hairline. The shape can be balanced with a hairstyle that is full at the jawline.

The pear-shaped face

This face is broad on the bottom half and narrow at the top of the head. It is the opposite shape to the heart-shaped face. Definition can be added by shading to slim the sides of the face, working from below the cheekbones. The hairstyle should be designed to add width and height at the top of the head.

The rectangular face

This face has no fullness and is an unusual shape being long and square. If you come across it use plenty of contouring, especially under the cheekbones and at the jawline. The hairstyle should be designed to soften the shape with forward hair movement and fullness at the sides of the face.

TOP TIP

To help you determine your client's face shape:

◆ Pull the client's hair away from the forehead and look at the shape.

◆ Look at the length and width of the sides of the face.

◆ Follow the angles of the jawline.

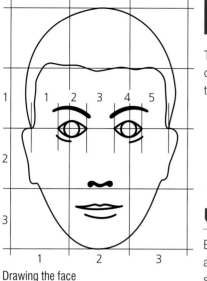

Drawing the face

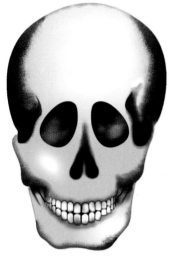

Lighting and shading

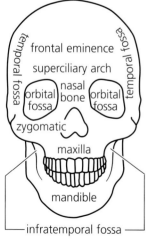

The bones of the face

Face drawing, mapping the spaces

The best way to understand the structure of the face is to draw it on paper. Draw an oval or egg shape for the head. To measure the face, start where the hairline would be at the top. Then divide the face into three horizontal sections:

◆ From the hairline to the centre of the eyes.

◆ From the eyes to the tip of the nose.

◆ From the tip of the nose to bottom of the chin.

Using the eye as units of measurements

Each eye consists of two semicircles, the upper one being slightly wider in diameter and more curved than the lower one. An eye can be used to measure five areas from side-to-side on the face (see the image 'Drawing the face'):

◆ one eye width measures the space between the eyes

◆ the space between the outer corner of the eye to the hairline at the edge of the face

◆ between the eye and the eyebrow, there is roughly an eye's depth of space.

The mouth is three quarters of the way down the face. The top lip is usually wider than the bottom one. The bottom lip is normally fuller than the top one.

In profile, the top of the ears are in line with the eyebrows, and the bottom of the ears in line with the tip of the nose. Shapes and sizes of facial features vary but are placed according to this useful guide, which is used by portrait artists.

Studying the anatomy of the skull, and drawing it several times, is also a quick way to understand facial proportions. Studying the structure of the bones is important for a make-up artist in order to improve or change the appearance of a face.

ACTIVITY

Drawing the human skull

Using a soft lead pencil draw the skull on white paper, noting the darkest and lightest areas.

Draw the skull again without the shading, marking in the technical names of the bones.

ACTIVITY

Understanding facial anatomy

You will need a fellow student to work on, two brushes – one for black, the other for white – two make-up colours – black and white – in cream or water-based products.

1 Using your colleague as a model, feel the prominences and depressions on the entire face.

2 Paint in the hollows of the face with black and the prominent bone areas with white.

At the end, your model's face will resemble the skull you have been studying.

ACTIVITY

Drawing the face

Take pencil and paper and draw the face of a fellow student or look in the mirror and draw yourself. Try to achieve a good likeness.

Measure the proportions by holding your pencil out in front, between your eye and the subject you are sketching. Transfer the measurement to your paper.

Drawing a face from life is the best way to observe facial proportions:

1 Note the shape of the face – round, oval, etc.

2 Consider the character in the face, the expression, the set of the features and the relation of each feature to the others. These aspects determine the person's liveliness, humour, pensiveness, etc.

3 Look out for something unusual or quirky about the face you are drawing; something that makes it interesting – a distinctive nose perhaps, or a prominent jaw, chin or lower lip.

4 Practise this technique on various face shapes to gain knowledge and understanding.

Colour

A real understanding of colour is essential for the make-up artist.

Principles of colour

The colours we see depend on the colour of the light source, the colours of any filters used, and the colour of the objects that then reflect the light.

In the retina at the back of the eye there are two kinds of receptor cells. These respond to light focused on them by the lens of the eye. One type is responsible for colourless vision in dim light and the other for colour perception in bright light.

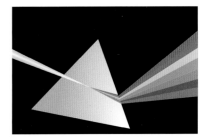

The colour spectrum

White light is a mixture of light of many different wavelengths. If you shine a beam of white light through a glass prism, the rays are bent according to their wavelengths and spread out to form a multicoloured spectrum. The spectrum can be seen if a screen is placed in its path. The order of the colours is always the same – the order that you see in a rainbow: violet, indigo, blue, green, yellow, orange and red.

When white light strikes a white surface most of the light is reflected, which is why the surface looks white. When light strikes a black surface most of it is absorbed. When light strikes a grey or coloured surface some is reflected and some is absorbed. When white light strikes a red surface, for example, the surface appears red because it is reflecting red light, but absorbing light of other colours. When light strikes a transparent surface, most of it simply passes through.

From a technical point of view, make-up and paint pigments have no colour of their own. They seem coloured to us because they absorb light of some wavelengths and reflect light of others. The light reflected produces the particular colour we see.

Classifying colour

Colours are classified in three ways, according to their *hue*, their *brightness* and their *intensity*.

Hue

The hue of a colour represents the difference between pure colours – the name by which we know them – red, blue, yellow, etc.

Brightness

Brightness represents the range from light to dark. From any light colour to any dark colour there is a brightness scale. The scale of greys is simple because there are no hues.

The darkness or lightness of a colour – its position on the range – is called its *value*. A light colour has *high* value while a *dark* colour has a *low* value.

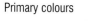

The scale of greys

Intensity

Intensity is the range from any pure hue to a point of the grey scale. A grey-blue, for example, has a blue hue, yet is different from the pure blue of the colour wheel (see following section for more about the colour wheel). Although it is of the same hue (blue) it is lower in intensity. It is nearer to the centre of the wheel and is more grey. The colours on the outside of the wheel are brilliant. Those nearer the centre of the wheel are less brilliant and known as tones.

Intensity scales are of three kinds:

◆ **Tints** Ranging from any pure hue to white.

◆ **Shades** Ranging from any pure hue to black.

◆ **Tones** Ranging from any pure hue to grey.

Each hue can be produced by mixing a combination of the three primary colours: red, yellow and blue. Variations can be made by adding black, white or both. Similarly, you can change make-up foundation colours by mixing them. If a colour is not warm enough, add some red; if it is too dark, add some white. If it looks too bright, add some grey (made by mixing black and white).

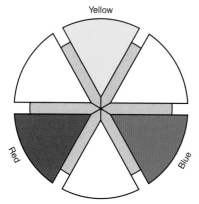

Primary colours

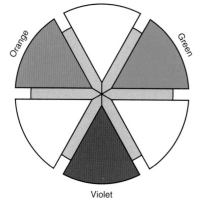

Secondary colours

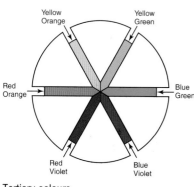

Tertiary colours

The colour wheel

The colour wheel, used by artists and designers for distinguishing colours, can also be applied to make-up colours: which are really paints for the face.

How to use the colour wheel

◆ **Primary colours** Red, blue and yellow when mixed in equal proportions make a muddy, brown colour.

◆ **Secondary colours** Orange, green and violet are each made by mixing two adjacent primary colours.

◆ **In-between colours** Made by mixing more of one colour than another, e.g. bluish green or greenish blue.

◆ **Tints** Made by adding white – this can produce colours such as opal, green and white.

◆ **Shades** Made by adding black – this can produce colours such as emerald green, black and navy blue.

Colour co-ordination

It is important that the make-up artist is careful to select and match products that co-ordinate – that is, colours that relate to one another in the completed make-up.

◆ **Foundation** The foundation should match the skin colour.

◆ **Eyebrows** The eyebrow pencil, powder or wax should match the hair colour, or at least harmonise with it, e.g. people with ash-blonde hair would need their eyebrows defined with taupe, which is a grey-brown. If you used any other shade of brown, such as red-brown, it would look wrong. Use a lighter shade to fill in the eyebrow shape to begin with, it looks more natural.

◆ **Cheeks** In women's make-up, blusher or rouge should be harmonious with the skin tone. It should not be treated as an accessory to match the dress.

◆ **Lips** Lip colour can be considered in relation to the costume as well as in relation to the skin tone and hair.

◆ **Eyes** Eye colour should improve or define the eyes as well as harmonise with the total look and style.

Making the most of colour

There are thousands of colours in the world – however many colours you have in your make-up box, you will almost certainly need to mix some of them in order to create the colour you need.

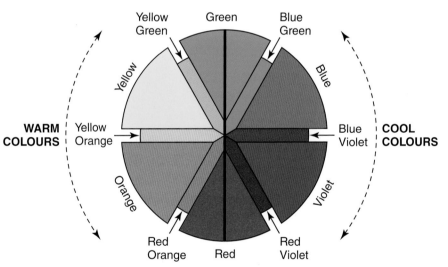

The colour wheel divided to represent both warm and cool colours

Mixing colours

The cleanest, clearest colours come straight from the tube or palette. Mixed with other colours they become muddy. As a general rule, it is best to mix no more than two colours together, although the result can be modified with a spot of another colour.

Primary and secondary colours

The primary colours in make-up are blue, red and yellow.

◆ Blue mixed with yellow gives a series of greens, from bluish-green (more blue than yellow) to a pale, yellowish green (more yellow than blue).

◆ Red mixed with yellow gives a full range of oranges.

◆ Red mixed with blue gives a full range of purples.

The secondary colours are green, orange and purple. The hues of the primary colours from which they are mixed will have a large effect on the result.

Adding white Pastel shades – such as delicate pinks, blues, greens, apricots, creams and lilacs – can be made by adding white to red, blue, green, orange, yellow or purple. If you add too much white the colour will look chalky.

Adding black The addition of black will add a shade of any given colour. It will dull any pigment you mix it with, so should be used with caution. Mixed with yellow ochre it makes a pleasant olive green.

Adding grey Black and white together gives tones of grey. By themselves, these are cold; add a touch of yellow, brown or red to warm the colour.

Complementary and harmonising colours

By taking a colour from the outside of the colour wheel (a pure hue) you can alter the colour by tinting with white, or taking the complementary colour (the opposite colour on the wheel) and shading or tinting it to produce a different effect.

Each colour has a complementary colour opposite it on the colour wheel. When any two complementary colours are placed next to each other they produce a strong contrast, and each of the colours looks more vivid.

Colours that share a pigment, such as blue and green, are called harmonising colours. When placed next to each other they appear to blend.

If you stare long and hard at a particular colour (say, red), and then look hard at a white surface you may see an after-image of the complementary colour (green). This is because the eye has ceased to register the original colour and is now registering the remaining colours in the mixture that makes up white light. This explains why it is so hard to match colours. After comparing many different samples for a long time, your brain ceases to register the correct colour. Complementary colours can be used in make-up in these ways:

◆ A colour can be neutralised by adding a little of the complementary colour. So a red which is too bright can be neutralised by adding a touch of green.

◆ Any colour can be neutralised by adding a small quantity of its opposite colour on the colour wheel, i.e. the complementary colour.

Neutral or earth colours

These are blacks, greys and browns. You will make an earth colour if you mix together:

◆ the three primary colours

◆ any two secondary colours

◆ all the primary and secondary colours.

Mixing colours for skin tones

Every skin tone is a mixture of red, yellow, white and brown. All foundation colours can be changed by mixing in these colours to find the exact skin tone required, e.g. white with a touch of red makes pink – add yellow for a warmer tone. Brown skin tones are made

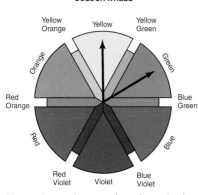

COLOUR WHEEL

Harmonious colours on the colour wheel

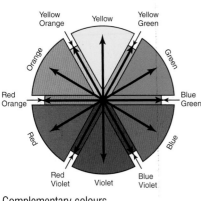

COLOUR WHEEL

Complementary colours

warmer with a touch of orange by adding red and yellow mixed together. Students should experiment to understand colour effects.

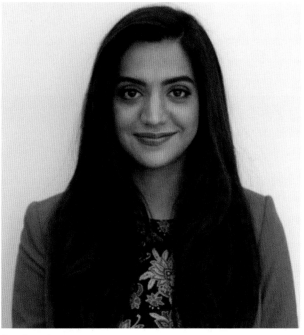

Beauty make-up

Colours used in special effects

◆ **Orange red** Gives a warm glow to golden skin, and is also used by make-up artists to show casualty effects such as sun damage.

◆ **Red** Used to neutralise grey or blue such as blocking tattoos before adding the skin tone. Also for painting rashes, bruises and using on the eyelids to portray a weeping effect. Red is used for creating a first-degree burn effect.

◆ **Blue** Used to convey illness and death, plus bruising and frozen effects.

◆ **Yellow** Complementary to blue and adds warmth to skin tones, but is also used to show old bruises and deteriorating effects such as infected scars etc.

◆ **Green** Used to neutralise redness, and mixed with yellow goes well with warm golden skin tones for eyeshadow colour.

◆ **Orange** Made by mixing red and yellow and is a good colour for **highlighting** dark skin tones. It is useful as a concealer to kill the blue/black under-eye shadows sometimes seen on older people from countries such as India and Pakistan. It can also be used on tattoos to block the blue ink colour, which is hard to cover. If a dark skin foundation is not vibrant enough, orange will 'lift' the colour, giving it warmth.

◆ **Pink** Red with a touch of white. It can look cool with a touch of blue, or warm with a touch of yellow. This colour is used a lot on white skin tones, and used extensively on the cheeks and lips.

◆ **White** Used to lighten a colour for highlighting or to lighten a foundation colour. Add a touch of yellow if it is not warm enough.

◆ **Black** Used to create a shade of any given colour by darkening it. Used for added drama in strong make-up effects, for eyeliners and eyebrows etc. However, it will also dull the colour you mix with it, and is not as natural looking as dark browns.

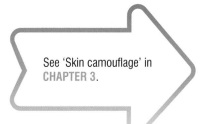

See 'Skin camouflage' in
CHAPTER 3.

ACTIVITY

Matching colours

Equipment required – primary colours, palette, spatula to mix

◆ Working from a basic palette of primary colours, experiment in matching a colour.

◆ Aim to mix a particular tint, shade or tone.

◆ Make notes on the proportions of colours used.

◆ Make another batch to match the first one.

Colour

Colour is important to make-up artists because every job they work on involves decision-making in the choice of colours used. Foundations, blushers, lipsticks, eyeshadows, colour correction, concealing birth marks and tattoos, painting prosthetic pieces to match the skin tone – all these and more provide a constant challenge to the make-up artist.

Guidelines in using colour

For more information on using colour see CHAPTER 3.

Do not be tempted to use too many bright colours in one make-up, as the result can be discordant. Using one or two pure colours can help to create a focal point in the face, more than that will be confusing. The eye will pass from one bright colour to the other and, because there is no contrast between brighter and more muted colours, the colours will fight for attention.

Not all cool colours are dull, and not all warm colours are bright; there are dull reds and yellows, and bright blues and greens. Whether cool or warm, subtle or intense, the mood can be determined by colour.

Do not worry about matching colours exactly. It is more important to get the tonal differences right – the degree of darkness or lightness of colours in relation to each other. (Consider a black and white photograph. Which are the light, medium and dark areas?)

Skincare

Make-up artists are expected to be up-to-date in their knowledge of products and skincare treatments. Leading actors are used to their skin being prepared properly before make-up, and having it removed with cleanser appropriate to their skin type. They often have a skincare routine which the make-up artist maintains when they are working together. By keeping the actor's skin looking healthy and clear, there will be less corrective make-up needed for the camera. A gentle facial massage can relieve stress when cleansing the face at the end of the working day.

Many beauty therapists progress into make-up, and make-up artists have made it their business to learn the techniques and skills of skincare. Being able to correct and prevent skin problems is part of the job; also applying face masks and removing the make-up with heated, damp face cloths.

Skin structure

The skin consists of three layers:

◆ **Subcutaneous** The deepest layer of skin (also known as the fatty layer).

◆ **Dermis** The middle skin layer (containing collagen and elastin).

◆ **Epidermis** The outer layer that we can see. This is the layer a make-up artist will work on.

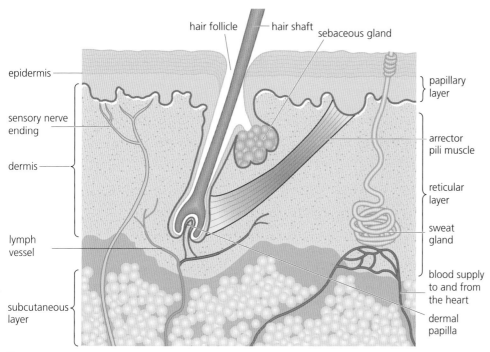

The skin

The subcutaneous layer

The subcutaneous layer protects the body and varies in thickness between one part of the body and another. It insulates against heat and cold and also determines the contours of the face and body.

The dermis

The dermis, which is the middle layer, connects the epidermis and subcutaneous layers with fibrous tissues of collagen and elastin, which is called connective tissue. The dermis contains the nerve endings and sweat glands, which regulate how we feel pain, pressure, temperature and touch. The dermis also contains the sebaceous glands which produce the natural oil known as sebum.

The epidermis

The epidermis, the skin layer we see on the outside, forms the body's first defence against infection. As the cells rise up through the layers of the epidermis, they die and form a hard surface on the outer skin. The epidermis also houses the cells that manufacture melanin, which produce a tan when the skin is exposed to the sun.

This layer makes the skin waterproof. If water touches the skin it will evaporate or run off the skin, but not penetrate. Using soap as a cleanser will wash away the natural moisture and sebum on the surface. The skin is soft and elastic when young and during puberty and may become oily, due to increased hormonal activity. If the sebaceous glands are producing too much sebum, it can cause the condition known as acne. The sun has damaging effects on the skin, especially fair or light-coloured skins.

The different skin types are normal, oily, dry and combination. Our skin types are determined by our genes and we inherit our skin type from our parents or grandparents.

Skin types

Normal

Normal skin is healthy, smooth and soft. Normal skin is often referred to as balanced, meaning the water and oil content is constant (neither too oily nor too dry).

Dry

Dry skin can be rough to the touch and dull in appearance. This skin type is lacking in sebum and therefore tends to also dehydrate more quickly as water can escape from the surface more easily. Premature ageing may be visible. A rich moisturiser is helpful for this skin type.

Oily

Oily skin may have large pores present and the skin may have a shine. The skin may feel greasy to touch and comedones and pustules may be present. Good cleansing is essential to keep this skin type clear and healthy.

Combination

This skin type can be a combination of any of the above types, but the most common is an oily t-zone with normal or dry cheeks.

Skin conditions

Sensitivity

Any skin type can become sensitive. This may be due to incorrect use of products, sun exposure, illness or medication.

Dehydration

This is where the skin is lacking in water. The skin may have a tight appearance. This can be in conjunction with the genetic skin type and can be temporary. The extent of dehydrated skin is dependent on the working environment, the weather and general well-being.

Skincare products

Cleansing

All skin types need cleansing to remove dirt, sebum and make-up, to keep the skin clear and healthy. Cleansing should be carried out using a product that suits the client's skin type. Soap is not a good cleanser, it is harsh with an alkaline pH that can unbalance and irritate the skin (which has a natural balance of pH5.5, being slightly acidic). After washing with normal soap and water the skin can feel tight, dry and uncomfortable.

The best way to clean the skin is to use a water-in-oil cream, without fragrance, with a warm, damp face cloth. Cleansing wipes and damp cotton wool are also used for quick cleans.

There is a wide range of products available on the market suitable for all different skin types. Make-up artists should research these products and stay updated with innovative products available.

Toning

Toners without alcohol (which is not good for the skin) should be used. They are used to remove traces of cleanser and to refine the pores. There are many types of products to choose from, according to the skin type.

Moisturising

Moisturisers correct the balance of moisture on the skin (either oil [sebum], or water to rehydrate) after toning. Depending on skin type, age and preference, there are ranges of different products available to all. Carefully consider the type of moisturiser to use prior to the make-up application. A product too rich may be detrimental to the make-up application and its durability to the longevity of the make-up.

Specialist products

Specialist products may also be required to help with a perfect make-up application. These may include eye gels, serums or pore minimisers.

Primers

Primers even out the skin texture prior to foundation and are a protective barrier for sensitive skins. There are various different brands on the market, including ones with skin illuminators.

> **TOP TIP**
>
> Look after your own skin and experiment with new products. Ask friends and family what they use. Regularly visiting department stores and checking magazines will help you keep up-to-date with the latest products available on the market.

Student kit box

It is always fascinating to see the contents of make-up artists' kit boxes, and which tools and products they favour.

There are certain items common to all, that everyone uses, whichever country they work in. Preference is usually given to a home-produced brand because it is usually less expensive than a foreign one. With globalisation most products are available through the Internet from anywhere in the world. Students will be influenced by cost; rightly so. In the beginning it is not necessary to spend too much money on designer brands.

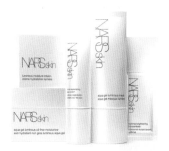

Skincare products

Recommended student kit

Tools & equipment

- A set of 20 assorted brushes:
  - angle eye blender brush
  - angle shader brush
  - blush brush
  - brow/lash brush – large
  - brow/lash brush – small
  - concealer brush
  - contour brush
  - crease brush
  - detail liner brush
  - eyebrow brush
  - eye detailer brush
  - eye shader brush – large
  - eye shader brush – small
  - finishing fan brush
  - flat eyeliner brush
  - foundation brush
  - lip brush
  - pointed liner brush
  - **powder brush**
  - smudger brush
- black gel eyeliner
- blusher palette
- Nars foundations (Barcelona, Sante Fe, Syracuse, Mont Blanc)

- neutrals eyeshadow palette
- oval sponges
- pencils (red, brown, black, nude)
- powder puffs
- *The Complete Make-Up Artist* textbook
- 1 black mascara
- 1 clear lip gloss
- 1 Denman brush
- 1 Dermacolour camouflage palette
- 1 headband
- 1 kit of assorted hair accessories, padding, one use mascara applicators and lip brush applicators etc.
- 1 Kryolan **aquacolour** palette
- 1 Kryolan lip rouge palette
- 1 Kryolan palette B supracolour
- 1 Kryolan stipple sponge, black
- 1 natural sponge
- 1 packet white wedge sponges
- 1 pair **false eyelashes**
- 1 set bag
- 1 Skin illustrator palette
- 1 stipple sponge orange
- 1 tail comb
- 1 translucent powder

Specialist cleaning products

It is important to know which product to use when cleaning off specialist materials from tools, equipment and the skin. Many of them are only suitable for tools and must not be used on the skin. It is vital to know the difference and understand their uses because the safety of actors' skin is in the hands of the make-up artist. This is a big responsibility and must be taken seriously.

Cleaning materials for use on the skin

- **Soap and water** To remove water-based products, such as face and body paints and artificial blood.

- **Cosmetic cleansing cream, liquid and oil** To remove all make-up products, such as foundations, eyeshadow, powder, lipstick and blusher.

◆ **Baby wipes or wet wipes** To remove casualty effects, or other heavy make-up quickly.

◆ **All Clear (Kryolan)** For removing spirit gum, latex, collodion, tuplast (scar plastic) from the skin.

◆ **Mild mastix remover (MME)** Made by Kryolan, suitable for sensitive skins to remove spirit gum from the face.

◆ **Proclens and proclean gel (or klene all)** Used in prosthetic work for removing Pros-Aide and latex from the skin.

◆ **Warm, wet flannel** Used with all products for cleaning the face.

◆ **Toners** Used to remove traces of grease from the skin.

CASE PROFILE: LOUISE McCARTHY, MAKE-UP DEPARTMENT HEAD

How long have you been working in the industry?

I have been working as a professional make-up artist for the last 14 years.

How did you get into the industry?

In 2000 I attended a three-month course. I worked for two years in London on television and then moved to New York. Knowing nobody in the industry, I had to start all over again to build up my contacts.

What has been your most significant project?

I moved to New York in 2002. To work in the industry here you have to be a union member. It took three years of independent work before I qualified for the membership. My first union job was a movie called *Across the Universe* as a make-up artist (doing background). On set, I met other make-up artists, who recommended me for work or I worked with them on their projects. Since then I've never looked back.

What do you enjoy most about the job?

I enjoy being part of a team, from the beginning of the movie when you read the script, to meeting with the director and actors, bringing the characters to life and seeing the movie at the end.

What do you enjoy least about the job?

Working outdoors, at night and in the cold ... it's never fun!

What advice would you give to a new make-up artist starting out?

◆ Always be on time.

◆ Be properly and thoroughly prepared.

◆ In the beginning, it's about establishing yourself, making contacts and building your CV. That means working for free or very little money but don't give up, all the hard work will pay off.

Lighting

How lucky for the new generation of make-up artists. With the advent of the digital age cameras are more sensitive and require less light. On the domestic market television screens have become larger, and high definition (HD) gives the audience a very sharp, clear picture. The cosmetic industry has developed a range of HD make-up and airbrush products and setting powders that are designed specially to work with the new technology.

As new digital cameras pick up so much detail, the television industry has had to raise its game in all departments, including make-up, where they do the hair as well.

In feature films the impact has not been so noticeable on the film crew. Make-up and hair have always been given the time and resources to produce detailed work. This has been possible for three reasons:

1 Films have traditionally divided make-up and hair into two departments.

2 Films usually have much bigger budgets and can afford to employ more specialists.

3 Most of all, because the make-up and hair artists have always worked towards close-ups on a 40-foot screen in cinemas, they are used to their work showing in detail.

If a make-up is too heavy, or badly applied, it will stand out in HD. Since technology is constantly evolving, the cameras will soon have even higher resolution than the standard HD. The make-up artists' mantra, 'Less is more' is very apt for students today. Less make-up, skilfully applied (only where it is necessary) is the accepted way of working, unless the production demands otherwise, e.g. horror, fantasy, drag make-up.

Principles of lighting

The principles of lighting have not changed. Lighting is the art of painting with light. Using light and shadows can make the subject look interesting, dramatic, beautiful, etc. Lighting can make or break a make-up artist's work.

Basics of lighting

1 A main light called the key light.

2 A secondary light, the full light, has less intensity, and can model or sculpt the subject.

3 A backlight, which separates the subject from the background.

It is not only the amount of light that is important, but also the direction from which it falls.

Cross-lighting is the illumination of the subject's face from two directions at equal distance but opposite angles. Cross-lighting will emphasise the character in an actor's face, including wrinkles, so is not good for beauty.

In film work the exterior work uses natural light; that is using the sun as the key light. The secondary or fill light is provided by reflectors (white boards) or arc lamps.

In theatre the stage lighting uses many filters and gels on the overhead lights to provide colour and drama on the actors and set.

Television lighting uses overhead fill lighting and side key lighting with floor fill lights to lessen the facial shadows.

On location, television lighting is the same as film, i.e. natural light plus reflectors and arc lamps at night.

Photographic lighting varies from using overhead lights with gels and filters for atmosphere and mood, to natural light and reflectors.

Lighting tests

There is always an opportunity for the make-up designer to see how the lighting affects the make-up.

Films There is a lighting test with costume, make-up, hair, set designer and all relevant personnel to make sure that the overall look meets the director's vision. Throughout the shoot there are monitors to view the action.

Television There is a technical run, which is a full rehearsal for cast and crew. There are also television monitors; in the studio the designers watch screens in the lighting gallery.

Theatre There is a full rehearsal for cast and crew. The wig mistress/master and make-up designer view the rehearsal from the middle of the audience seating area.

Photography The photographer is the director and lighting supervisor. He works closely with the make-up artist and clients. Photos are printed out between each set up for everyone to inspect and make adjustments.

Effects of good and poor lighting

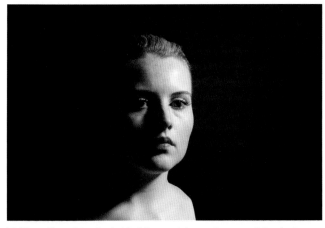

Light positioned too far behind the model, causing complete shadow on one side of the face

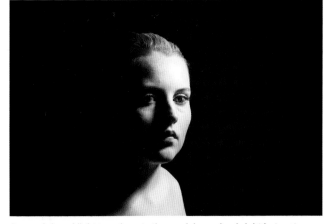

A non-defused light too close to the model causing bright hotspots and too much contrast

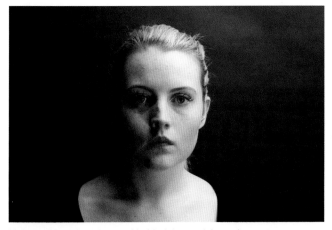

Light positioned too low and behind the model causing a strong unflattering uplight effect

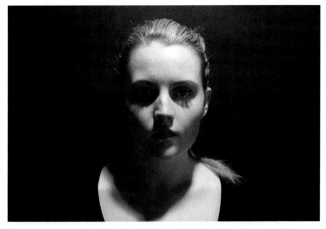

Light positioned directly above the model's head creating long deep shadows down the model's face

ACTIVITY

A simple lighting effect

Equipment required: 1 overhead light bulb, 1 table light, 1 chair, 1 model

For a basic light effect, seat your model under the overhead light.

Place a light on one side of your model.

Note the types of shadows cast on the face.

Move the light to the other side.

Place the light underneath the face.

By moving the table light around and switching the overhead light off, you can change the lighting dramatically.

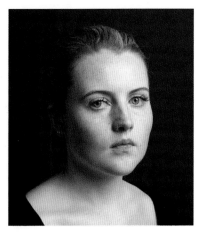

Good lighting

Fantasy make-up

Fantasy make-up satisfies the creative side of every make-up artist. The effect can be the simple painting of an animal face, a witch or a clown, or more complex designs of monsters and aliens using bald caps and prosthetics. Fantasy can be beautiful and charming (a fairy with pointed prosthetic ear tips), or dramatic and frightening (an evil stepmother in a fairy tale).

Any materials may be used to achieve the effect, but grease paints are best for stage make-up (as watercolours run when the actor sweats). For photographic, television and film work, water-based colours are good, with strong, clear colours. Ready-made prosthetic pieces such as latex noses and ears are ideal for creating fantasy characters such as animals. Some stiff hairs from a brush can be glued to the face for whiskers, as a finishing touch.

When making up dancers for light entertainment television shows, the brief given is often to produce a bold, striking effect. Shiny eyeshadows, glitter and shimmer that sparkles when the dancer moves are asked for, to complement the costumes and scenery. Burlesque and drag queen make-ups are also an opportunity to go for glamorous, exotic-looking make-up effects.

Of all the different areas of make-up, fantasy offers the make-up artist the greatest freedom of expression. Occasionally, when working in films, there will be a carnival scene with everyone in fancy dress costumes when fantasy make-up is required. Give your creativity and imagination free rein.

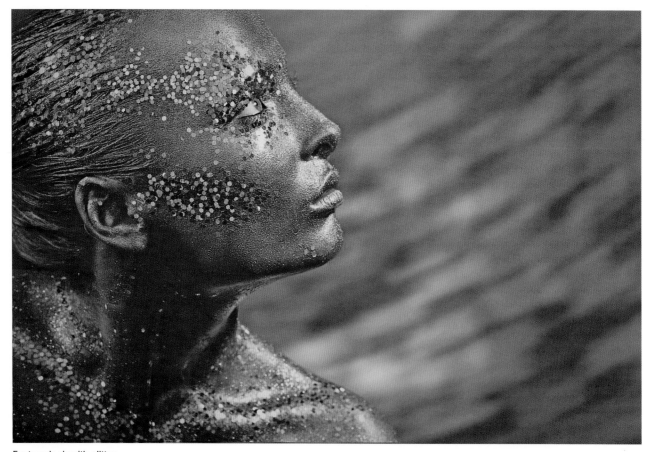

Fantasy look with glitter

CASE PROFILE: NAMRATA SONI, MAKE-UP ARTIST

Namrata has won the IIFA (International Indian Film Award) for the feature film 'Om Shanti Om' based in India, Cosmopolitan award for best make-up artist, Femina Woman of Worth awards and Vogue Beauty award.

How do you prepare each job?

Research is the key to every job done well. Every project that I work on I make mood boards for every presentation and do at least two to three look tests, before the look of the film is finalised, for every character. It is the most fun part prepping for a project. After every look is finalised I make a complete list of products that will be required and order them. I prepare for every kind of weather that will hit us, heat, cold and rain, so my focus is on ensuring that the foundations in the kit are suitable for any unpredictable weather changes.

What are your essential items in your kit box?

I love my kit and treasure every single product I have. I am a product junkie and buy every new thing that comes out to try and see how best I can accommodate it in my kit. My basics I cannot leave home without are:

- skin illuminating primer
- eye cream
- sunscreen
- eyelash curler
- concealers, foundations, powders
- tinted eye brighteners
- Tom Ford cream eyeshadows and palettes
- Estée Lauder gel liner pots
- Bobbi Brown bronzer
- Nars illuminating highlighters
- Charlotte Tilbury sculpt and highlight
- Chanel lipsticks
- YSL lipsticks
- Urban Decay kohl **pencils**
- Maybelline mascaras waterproof and normal
- individual eyelashes
- brush kit with all my favourite Kabuki brushes and Tom Ford brushes.

What different areas of make-up have you worked in?

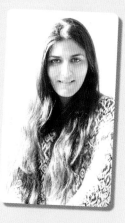

I have worked in fashion, beauty and film – yes, I am a skincare junkie! I do a lot of research on new products – what suits which skin type and what works with different foundations. It is important to understand skin so you can advise your clients and your make-up will always look flawless.

What advice would you give to a new make-up artist starting out?

It is important to keep working and practising. For my first two years I assisted a senior make-up artist and learnt all the behind the scenes tricks which a make-up artist will only get to experience on set. Being hands on is very important. Approach young fresh photographers, do **portfolios** and test shoots with them, build a portfolio and then start meeting all the industry professionals, magazine editors, art directors, fashion stylists, photographers, producers and production houses. The key is to be persistent, don't call once and let it go, call again and make sure you get a meeting set up.

Crowd scenes and dancers' make-up is the most fun and are where you can experiment with your work. You get loads of practice and you become faster. Always ask friends to join in and help, as you cannot do so many people alone.

What advice would you give to a new make-up artist on appropriate presentation and how to communicate with producers, directors, models, actors, etc.?

I am a big believer in what you see is what you get. Dressing smart and looking the part is important. I don't wear a stitch of make-up personally but I always ensure that my skin is flawless and I have a little bit of mascara and lip balm. Be polite and hear them out before anything. Be honest about your work and confident. Do not gossip, as the industry is very small and these things can damage your reputation.

Always be firm with your opinion but accommodating enough to listen to others' ideas like stylists, directors and models. People will call you back if you have a pleasant attitude, but don't be a pushover.

Sometimes you will meet people who are extremely opinionated, just be calm, hear them out and present your side to them.

I have had models sit on my chair telling me how to do my job and it can be frustrating. Hear them out, discuss with them what will suit them but do what you are best at doing.

What exercise could students do on one another to improve their awareness of techniques?

My favourite lesson to date was when my fashion make-up artist teacher asked us to do natural make-up with only brown shades of eyeshadow. I thought it would be so easy but it was a task.

I have realised over the years of working that liners have become very popular. Students should practice perfecting the winged liner. Every eye shape is different and it's not easy. It takes the longest to do and if you master that then it's one battle won. Students should also practice perfecting the red pout.

REVISION QUESTIONS

1 How often should your electrical equipment be PAT tested?

2 What would you do if your electrical equipment is faulty?

3 What is the difference between a contra-indication and a contra-action?

4 What are the primary colours?

5 Describe the main features of the three layers of the skin?

Notes

2 Basic beauty make-up

LEARNING OBJECTIVES

This chapter covers the following:

◆ Different products available.

◆ Step-by-step day and evening make-up procedures.

◆ Bridal make-up consultation and techniques.

◆ Camouflage application.

◆ Corrective make-up techniques.

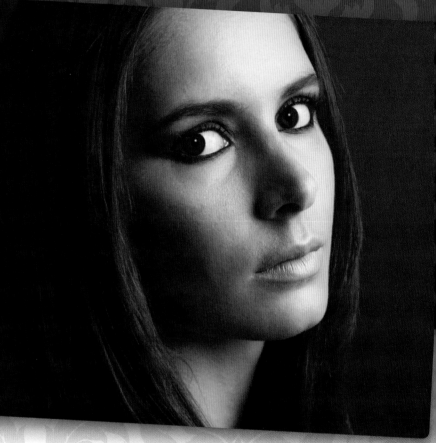

KEY TERMS

Blending

Camouflage make-up

Compressed powders

Stippling

Straight make-up

UNIT TITLE

◆ Make purchases for hair and/or make-up

◆ Acquire resources to meet design requirements

INTRODUCTION

Basic make-up application will be the foundation for all other specialist work. Knowing the correct techniques and procedures to apply a successful day, evening and bridal make-up will start you on your career as a successful make-up artist. In this chapter, you will explore the different products and textures needed to create the perfect results for your clients. The use and application of false eyelashes will also be discussed. The basic make-up application discussed in this chapter will cover everything a make-up artist needs to

know at Level 2. This chapter also explains the specialist application of camouflage make-up and highlighting and shading techniques to create the perfect face, which is covered at Level 3. These techniques are used extensively in the industry today; for instance, to help conceal an actor's tattoo or perfect a model's breakout on their skin. This chapter provides excellent preparation for advanced make-up techniques covered later in the book.

Products

See the student kit box in CHAPTER 1 for a list of basic tools and products.

Cosmetic stores are like sweet shops for anyone passionate about make-up artistry. All those alluring bottles and pots of paints, powders and creams promise so much magic. The very names on the bottles are chosen to attract and bewitch us into buying them all. We imagine the magical results we can achieve if we had them in our kit boxes.

But if you buy everything that is recommended by the retailers and manufacturers you will end up with more than you need – and broke. To start off you need some brushes, concealers, foundations, lip and eye colours, powder and a face to practise on.

Establish good habits when using products

A few good habits, established at the beginning of your career, will save you time and money in the future. Always squeeze tubes from the bottom. Shake bottles with the tops on before using. Always wipe the rims and necks of bottles, jars and tubes, and replace tops securely after use. The products will dry out if air gets to them and with tubes this happens very quickly.

Types of foundations

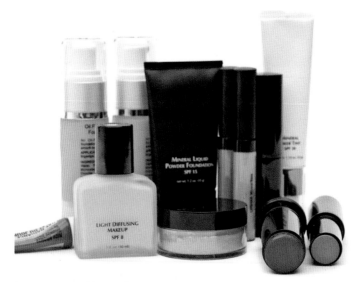

Different types of foundations

The most widely used foundations are liquids, cream-based, water-based, emollient-based, mineral-based and tinted moisturisers. Stick and cake foundations are used less frequently. All make-up artists carry a selection of these products, in various colours, in their kit. They are all applied with a sponge or foundation brush.

Liquid foundations

These are available in water, emollient and mineral-based formulas. Use a water-based liquid for oily or sensitive skin. An emollient (hydrating) liquid is good for dry and/or mature skin types. Liquid mineral-based foundation is excellent when used on sensitive, problematic skin types.

Mineral foundations

These are great for allergy prone skin types and are available in liquid or powder form. They have no parabens or talc in their ingredients, are water-resistant, contain UVA and

UVB protection and are not tested on animals. Mineral-based make-up gives good coverage, is long-lasting and is available in liquid or powder form. An increasing number of actors request this type of foundation.

Tinted moisturisers

Tinted moisturisers are useful on anyone with an unblemished skin. They are very sheer and look natural – often used on men and children, or on women for an 'un-made-up look'. They can be applied with a brush or sponge. No powder is used. Some clients may choose these for their daily coverage. Many also include a sun protection factor (SPF).

Cream foundations

Cream foundations come in compact and stick forms. They can be made very sheer when applied lightly with a damp sponge and blended with a brush. Good on dry skins, and need setting with powder. They are also good on mature skins.

Powder foundations

Powder foundations are applied with a brush or dry sponge. They are dry, so best used on oily skins. Good for quick touch-ups on set.

Types of make-up

Concealers

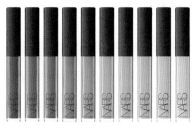

Concealers come in different skin tones, and are used for hiding shadows, spots, nose-to-mouth lines and any other blemishes that show through the foundation. They can be heavier in texture than foundations. Lightweight pen-style concealers are available for use in the eye area. These are formulated to brighten and illuminate the eye area. Apply first if you are using a powder-based foundation. For liquid and cream foundations you can use the concealer on top and before powdering.

Concealers of various colours

During application always start with minimal product and gradually build to achieve desired results.

Blushers

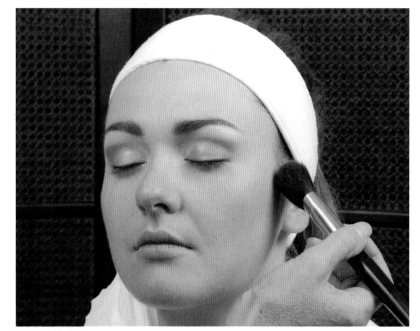

- ◆ **Cream blusher** Used sparingly, can look very natural when used on top of foundation, before powdering.

- ◆ **Pressed powder blusher** Used on top of the powdered foundation.

- ◆ **Tinted gel** Translucent, and comes in many colours. Does not rub off.

Blusher application

Eyeshadows

- ◆ **Cream** Comes in pots and tubes. Good on dry and mature skin.
- ◆ **Pressed powder** Comes in pots or palettes of colours. Stays in place well.
- ◆ **Loose powder** Strong colour pigments, used wet or dry.

Eyeliners

- ◆ **Pencils** Come in various colours, can be frosted and in kohl type. Can be waterproof and matt.
- ◆ **Liquid** Used with a brush for heavy, dramatic effect.
- ◆ **Gel** Used with a brush and is long-lasting. Usually packaged in jars or pots.
- ◆ **Cake** Applied with a damp, fine-pointed brush. Comes in pots and compacts.
- ◆ **Loose powder** Strong colour pigments, harder to apply than the other types.

Mascaras

- ◆ **Wands** Easy to apply with a built-in brush. Comes in different colours.
- ◆ **Cake** Applied with a damp mascara brush usually included in compact.
- ◆ **Fillers/extenders** Contain fibres to lengthen and thicken the eyelashes.
- ◆ **Waterproof** Dries quickly and is smudge proof.

Eyebrow products

- ◆ **Wax** Good for filling in, shaping and colouring the eyebrows. Used with a stiff eye brush.
- ◆ **Pencils** For drawing fine strokes to fill in and shape the eyebrows.
- ◆ **Gel** Used for holding the shape of the brows, in combination with pencil or wax.
- ◆ **Cake pressed and loose powder** Usually supplied in compact form with a brush.

Lipsticks

- ◆ **Cream** Comes in matte or shine in various colours. Creamy formula for moisturising the lips – most commonly used type in the industry.
- ◆ **Gloss** High gloss, shiny formula.
- ◆ **Frost** Frost and glitter formulas.
- ◆ **Matte** No shine, heavy consistency. Used in period productions, e.g. 1940s.
- ◆ **Lip liners** Pen or pencil form used to define or change the lip shape in conjunction with lipstick.
- ◆ **Lip balm** Used to soothe and smooth the lips. Good for dryness. Some have sun protection and moisturising ingredients.

Setting powder

Setting powder is loose, translucent, with no colour, used to set the make-up either with a soft powder brush or powder puff. It can be used without foundation to take away

---

TOP TIP

All cosmetic products will contain a little picture of a jar on the bottom. This indicates how long the product will last after opening. For example 12M will mean once opened use within 12 months.

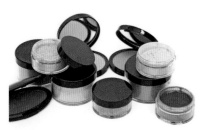

Various powder colours

shine on the skin. Powders are available in a variety of different shades. It is recommended to use a translucent or loose powder as this will not change the colour of the foundation. Loose powder is recommended to set the initial application of foundation and using a powder puff or powder brush. Compact powder (pressed powder) is used for quick touch-ups.

CASE PROFILE: JOANNE BYRNE, MAKE-UP ARTIST

How long have you been working in the industry?
Eighteen years.

How did you get into the industry?
I trained and then assisted the top make-up artists in the fashion industry.

Did you have a lucky break or a turning point?
Yes, my first job was a book cover with a photographer where the make-up artist had let him down. It was a worldwide bestseller and was in all shops, all train stations, etc. It was very exciting for my first job.

What has been your most significant project(s)?
Assisting on the fashion shows in Milan, London and Paris for the first time and getting to make up Kate Moss at a London show.

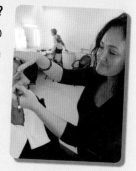

What do you enjoy most about the job?
Meeting exciting people and going to exciting places. Also doing what I love for a job.

How has the fashion industry changed during your career?
It has got a lot more competitive and you need to be your best at all times as there are people waiting to take your place – 'you are only as good as your last job' is my motto!

What advice would you give to a new make-up artist starting out?
Be punctual at all times. Be polite. Be tidy and work hard. And enjoy!

Day make-up

Tools & equipment

- blusher
- brushes
- cleanser
- concealer
- cotton buds
- disposable/one use applicators
- eyebrow pencil or powder
- eye liner
- eyeshadows
- foundation
- gown

- headband/section clips – if needed
- lip liner
- lipstick
- mascara
- moisturiser
- powder
- primer
- sponge or foundation brush
- tissues
- toner

Preparation

1 Place a gown around the client and a headband to secure hair off the face, if needed.

2 Discuss ideas, preferences and colours. Complete a consultation to ensure the products are suitable for the client. Check for allergies and contra-indications.

3 Cleanse, tone and apply moisturiser and/or primer if using.

4 Test for correct shade and choose the foundation. Using a sponge or foundation brush, take time to get a good even application of foundation. Start in the centre of the face and gently blend out to the hairline, sides of the face and jawline.

5 If required use a concealer to cover imperfections. Choose the correct tone and texture for the client.

6 If using cream-based products apply directly onto the foundation. This could be cream blusher or cream-based highlighting and shading products.

7 Cream-based products will need to be lightly set with powder. Always brush powders down on the face. This will help to lie fine, downy hairs flat.

8 Frame the face with eyebrow product application. Fill in any gaps and add colour or definition as required to achieve the desired results.

9 Eye make-up application. A soft natural application will be required for the day as this will be seen in natural daylight. Consider the client's eye colour, hair colour, outfit and personal preference. Start by applying a natural shade over the whole of the eye area. This will even out the colour and create a base for the other products to be applied, if needed.

10 Apply a coat of mascara on the upper and lower lashes, ensuring a good even coverage, helping to separate the lashes and create a natural finish.

11 Powder blusher may be needed to add warmth to the cheeks and add definition. Blend to add warmth to the cheekbones, if needed.

12 If powder highlighting products are being used they will need to be added at this stage.

13 Lip liner application. Using a sharpened pencil, gently line around the client's lip shape. Choose a colour to complement the eyeshadow and blusher. Corrective work may be needed on some clients. A strong mouth shape will not need lip liner application.

14 Using a lip brush, carefully paint the lips and then blot with a tissue.

15 Check the overall finish for balance and ensure the whole make-up application is even.

16 A setting spray may be used to add maximum durability to the make-up application, or blot the make-up slightly with a barely damp powder puff.

STEP-BY-STEP: DAY MAKE-UP APPLICATION

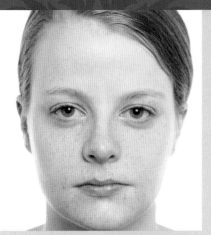

1 Cleanse, tone and moisturise. Choose the correct colour foundation by testing on the client's neck.

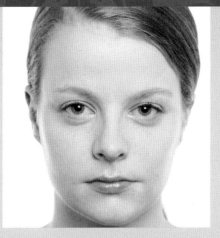

2 Apply with brush/hand and even out with sponge/buffing brush. Check you have even application of base and that it is not too heavy or visible, it is important to look like skin that is healthy but more even.

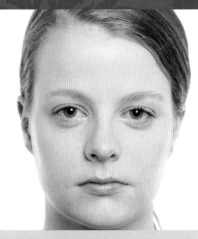

3 Conceal where needed using a creamy concealer that is the exact colour of the skin. Dust a little amount of translucent powder over the face to set it.

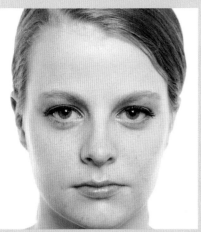

4 Comb eyebrows and fill in any obvious gaps with either pencil or shadow but keep it natural; you should not be able to obviously see it. Using a large, soft **blending** brush, sweep a natural soft colour all over the eye up to brow bone. Add a slightly stronger colour up to the socket blending all the time, no lines on show and no patchy mess. If needed apply some liquid liner thinly or gel liner/kohl to top of lash line.

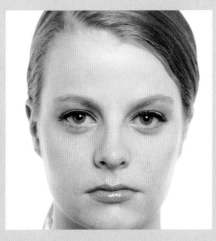

5 Curl lashes and add mascara. Sweep a little soft blush over cheekbones. Choose a lip colour or gloss that complements your model.

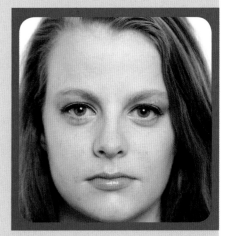

6 Groom hair and finish.

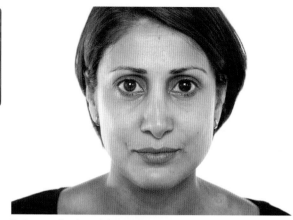

Before application of day make-up

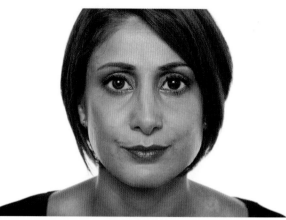

After application of day make-up

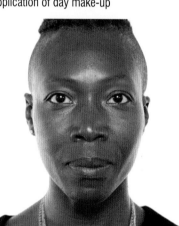

Before application of day make-up

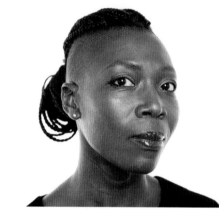

After application of day make-up

Evening make-up

Tools & equipment

- blusher
- bronzer
- brushes
- cleanser
- concealer
- cotton buds
- cream gel or liquid liner
- disposable/one use applicators
- eyebrow pencil or powder
- eyelash glue
- eyeshadows
- false lashes
- foundation

- gown
- headband/section clips – if needed
- lip gloss
- lip liner
- lipstick
- mascara
- moisturiser
- powder
- primer
- sponge or foundation brush
- tissues
- toner

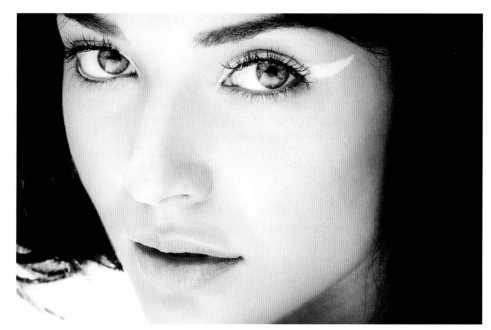

ELLE Magazine– India; Photographer: Suresh Natarajan; Make-up Artist: Namrata Soni; Model: Amy Jackson

Preparation

1 Place gown around the model, and a headband to secure hair off the face, if needed.

2 Discuss ideas, preferences, colours, complete a consultation to ensure the model is suitable for application. Checking for allergies and contra-indications.

3 Cleanse, tone and apply moisturiser and/or primer if using.

4 Test for correct shade and choose the foundation. Using a sponge, hands or a foundation brush, take time to get a good even application of foundation. Start in the centre of the face and gently blend out to the hairline, sides of face and jawline. (Some situations will require you to apply a tiny amount on the ears to blend the tones before photographic work.) An evening make-up look will not need a darker foundation but may need a heavier coverage.

5 If required use a concealer to cover imperfections. Choose the correct tone and texture for the client.

6 If using cream-based textured products apply directly onto foundation. This could be cream blusher or cream-based highlighting and shading products.

7 Cream-based products will need to be lightly set with powder. Always brush powders down on the face. This will help to lie fine, downy hairs flat.

8 Frame the face with eyebrow product application. Fill in any gaps, add colour or definition as required by the client for the desired results. Stronger brows may enhance an evening look.

9 Eye make-up application. A stronger eyeshadow application may be required by the client or needed for the look. A smoky eye make-up look may be created for a glamorous evening look. Consider the client's eye colour, hair colour, outfit and personal preference.

HEALTH & SAFETY

Always perform a patch test on the client before eyelash application, with the glue you will be using. This should be performed 24 hours prior to application.

TOP TIP

Always change your mascara regularly. They will hold bacteria and dry out quickly. Every three months is recommended.

TOP TIP

◆ Cream-based blushers need to be gently blended on the cheek-bones. These can be highly pigmented so apply gently to build up desired results.

◆ Highlighting and shading products will be applied to suit different face shapes, enhance features and hide imperfections.

See **CHAPTER 3** 'Step-by-step: Smokey eye application

◆ Start by applying a neutral shade over the whole of the eye area up to the brow bone. This will even out the colour and create a base for the other products to be applied.

◆ Choose one or two shades darker and apply over the socket area.

◆ To create a smoky eye, add a deeper shade, may be dark brown, grey, black or navy, to the outer corner. Using a fine brush sweep a soft line from the lower rim up to the socket line to help create the shape. Using a domed eyeshadow brush, blend and contour the darker shade in the socket line. Keep adding colour and blending until the desired depth and shape is achieved.

10 For a more glamorous evening look, liquid liner or gel may be applied. With a steady hand and using a fine brush follow the eye shape as close to the lash line as possible to add definition and interest. The thickness of the line needs to be considered by the client's eye shape and size. Client preference will help to define the style of finish, i.e. a strong cat flick or a soft joining of the top and bottom lines.

11 Apply a coat of mascara on the upper and lower lashes, ensuring a good even coverage, helping to separate the lashes, build the product to create a more defined look.

12 False eyelashes are an excellent additional media to use to turn the look into a sophisticated evening eye make-up. The eyelashes need to be sized up against the client's own and the lashes may need to be slightly trimmed to fit the client's eyes. A small amount of glue should be applied to the eyelash rim and allowed to go tacky for a few seconds. Using a pair of tweezers, gently sit the eyelashes above the client's own, in the rim. Ask the client to keep their eyes closed whilst the glue completely dries. It is wise to check the eyeliner application once the glue is completely dry. Blend the client's own lashes with mascara if required.

13 Powder blusher may be needed to add warmth to the cheeks and add definition.

14 Some clients may like a dusting of bronzing powder. This needs to be lightly swept across the forehead, down the nose and straight across the cheeks. This will create the illusion of a sun-kissed look.

15 If powder highlighting products are being used they will need to be added at this stage. Follow the client's face shape and any areas that need enhancing or concealing.

16 Lip liner application. Using a sharpened pencil gently line around the client's lip shape. Choose a colour to complement the eyeshadow and blusher. Corrective work may be needed on some clients. To help keep the lipstick in place a light colouring of pencil can be applied across the whole of the lips.

17 Using a lip brush carefully fill in the area shaped by the lip pencil. A lipstick with a stronger pigment may be chosen for an evening look or equally a nude lipstick may be used to create a contrast. If lip gloss is required, apply the lipstick over the lip gloss just in the centre area. This will help to minimise bleeding of the products.

18 Check the overall finish for balance and to ensure the whole make-up application is even.

19 A setting spray may be used to add maximum durability to the make-up application.

Bridal make-up

Tools & equipment

- assorted brushes
- blusher palette, natural colours – peach, pink, apricot
- cleanser, toner, moisturiser
- concealers
- cotton buds
- disposable/one use applicators
- eyebrow pencils, wax, powders
- eyeliners, pencils, gel, liquid, cake
- eyeshadow palette – neutral colours
- foundations

- lip pencils
- lipstick palette
- loose powder
- make-up chart
- make-up wrap and headband
- mascaras – brown and black
- powder puff
- skin primer
- tissues

A traditional bridal make-up is usually a classic natural beauty look for a ceremony that is performed during the day. The bride-to-be wants to look radiant and beautiful for the photographs that are taken that day and looked at many years later, in the family album. For this reason it is best not to have a stylised, high-fashion look that will date quickly. Of course much depends on the bride herself – if she normally favours a quirky type of make-up then she may decide to look the same on her big day. Different nationalities have their own customs, e.g. an Indian bride often has a high-profile ceremony with ornate clothes and a strong make-up with traditional henna designs on her hands and feet.

Whatever the look, there should always be a consultation and trial make-up and hair session a few weeks before the wedding day. Study her face shape, features, skin tone and skin texture. Discuss preferences, ideas and colours.

Trial make-up

1 Place a make-up wrap around the client's shoulders.

2 Cleanse, tone and moisturise her skin. If the skin is dry, allow time for the moisturiser to sink in. If oily, blot lightly with a tissue to remove excessive grease.

3 Apply primer, if using, to prepare the skin for the foundation.

4 Choose a suitable foundation that matches the skin tone. Test this on the jawline or forehead, as the light is good on these areas.

Applying the foundation

1 Use a barely damp sponge, natural or synthetic, or a foundation brush to apply a small amount of the chosen foundation, starting on the forehead, working down the face, lightly and evenly across the eyelids, avoiding the mouth, blending under the chin and onto the upper part of the neck.

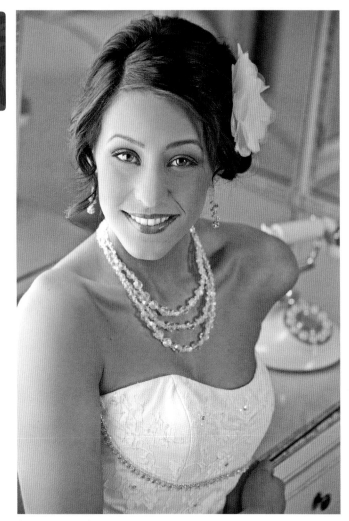

Complete bridal look

TOP TIP

You can use a powder brush to apply the powder instead of a powder puff, but the make-up will not last as long.

2 Use the clean side of the sponge or brush to blend the edges away at the hairline on the forehead, around the ears and onto the neck.

3 Use a clean brush to blend the foundation evenly around the sensitive eye areas, under the nose and around the nostrils.

Concealers or camouflage

Any shadows under the eyes, or blemishes that show through the foundation, can be lightly covered with a concealer of choice. Touche Éclat by Yves St Laurent is an industry favourite. For harder to hide blemishes, use camouflage cream.

1 Use concealer of choice for under eyeshadows, nose-to-mouth lines, and on any blemishes such as broken veins on cheeks or spots.

2 Blend away at the edges with a clean brush.

Setting the foundation

1 To apply loose powder, dip the powder puff into the powder. Shake off any excess, then tap the powder puff against the back of your hand to dislodge any excess powder. There should not be too much powder on the powder puff at one time.

2 Roll the powder puff over the face, pressing firmly but gently with a rocking motion until the entire face is covered. More powder is usually needed down the centre part of the face. Don't forget the eyelids, under the chin and onto the neck. Be very sparing in the eye areas, especially below the eyes.

3 Brush off excess powder with a soft powder brush for a smooth, even finish, using the tip of the brush to avoid streaking the make-up.

Cheeks

Only use blusher if it is necessary – not if the client has a high colour showing through the foundation.

To apply blusher, using a natural colour such as peach or pink:

Feel for the top of the cheekbones. Ask the client to smile and apply blusher to the apple of the cheeks, then brush upwards onto the top of the cheekbones. Use very little, simply to give the base colour some 'life'. More can be applied after working on the lips and eyes; by then you will be able to see the balance.

Eyeshadow

Use subtle colours for a natural look on pale skin tones:

1 Lighten the brow bone with pale peach or ivory eyeshadow.

2 Apply taupe, light brown (or client's choice of colour) on the eyelids up to the crease line. Blend gently at the edges.

Eyeliner

Use grey, brown or black. Keep this subtle. Use a fine eyeliner brush if using liquid or gel eyeliner, or use a soft eyeline pencil.

1   Pull the eyelid taut with your fingertip and paint a thin line as close to the roots of the lashes as possible. Begin at the start of the eyelash growth, but not too far into the inner corners of the eyes. If you want to blend the line, use a clean brush to do so. For a very natural look you can 'dot' the eyeline instead of using a continual line. Whether you use a flick at the outer corners is individual choice.

2   If you choose to use eyeliner along the bottom lashes, be careful not to draw the line further than the natural growth of lashes at the inside corner, or further than the outer end of the eyebrow. Hold a pencil or brush to check the distance (see image opposite).

Eyelashes

1   Apply mascara to the eyelashes in brown or black. Hold the eyelid stretched slightly upwards and, with the other hand, brush the mascara down through the lashes from the roots, then under the lashes brushing upwards from the roots. Repeat on other eye.

2   Brush through the lashes with a clean mascara brush or comb to separate the lashes and remove any blobs of mascara.

Eyebrows   If the client's eyebrows are normally waxed, threaded, plucked and/or tinted, this should be done well in advance.

1   Brush through the eyebrows with an eye brush or comb.

2   Fill in any gaps, or change the shape, as required. Use brush and powder, eyebrow wax, eyebrow pencil, or whatever is most suitable. Choose taupe, light brown, medium brown or dark brown according to the natural colour of the eyebrows.

Lips   Lips are often the hardest part of the make-up. The lips sometimes need balancing. Blotting, powdering or reapplying will make the lip colour last longer. To keep your hand steady, you can rest it on a powder puff on the face, or rest your little finger on the client's chin. To change the shape, the edges should be drawn in first and then filled in.

1   Discuss the shape and colour with the client.

2   Draw the shape with a lip pencil that matches the lip colour, then apply the lipstick with a brush, working from the corners of the mouth.

3   Lips can be evened out and enlarged. They can even be reduced if you apply a little foundation first. Work slowly but positively. Use the correct pressure; if you are too light it can tickle or irritate and it will be harder to create a line. If you press too hard you will move the lips. Once applied, blot the lipstick with a thin tissue and reapply.

4   At this point, define eye or cheek colour if needed. Discuss details with the client and if she is happy with the result, record all the colours used on a chart and take a photograph.

Hair   If a separate hairdresser is not being used, and the client is having an up-do, practise the shape and discuss arrangements for hair ornaments or a veil.

On the prearranged day and place, take your equipment, tools and products to the hotel or client's house and set up your workstation. Bathrooms are not suitable for doing make-up as the lighting is rarely good enough. The best place is a source of good light – daylight is best, close to a window.

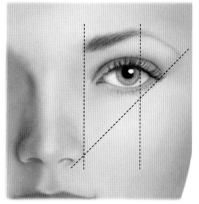
Measuring the perfect brow

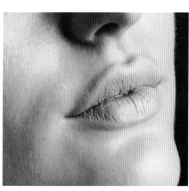
Lips

TOP TIP

When painting eyeliner, the lower down you hold the brush the more control you will have.

ACTIVITY

Using the same model, do a day, evening and bridal make-up. Take photos after each make-up. Also take a before photo without make-up to compare the results. Keep the photos in a file for future reference.

False eyelashes

From the natural look, using individual eyelashes, to the exotic, heavy lashed look for the stage, false eyelashes bring attention to the eyes. They come in different lengths, colours and types in beauty stores, chemists and online.

Preparation

Try the eyelashes without glue to see the fit. Place the strip at the base of the real eyelashes. If they need trimming cut them from the outside to suit the size and style. They should not extend beyond the natural lash growth. Lashes should be trimmed away from the client's face and eyes.

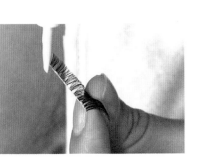

Adhesive applied to the false strip lash base

Tools & equipment

- choice of eyelashes
- cotton buds or q-tips
- duo eyelash adhesive – put a small amount on your palette
- eyelash tweezers
- mascara
- palette
- small scissors

TOP TIP

Ensure the client has been patch tested 24 hours prior to application.

Application of eyelashes

1 Use a cotton bud to place the adhesive under the strip in a thin line. Wait for 30–60 seconds before applying the lash to the skin. Allow the glue to go tacky to make the application easier and less messy.

2 Using tweezers or fingers, place the eyelash strip at the base of the real eyelashes close to the roots. With the client's eyes closed, press the strip gently into place with a damp cotton bud or q-tip. The cotton bud shouldn't be damp. The client can also just look down at the floor rather than closing eyes, to avoid glue seeping onto the lower lid and them sticking together.

3 For individual lashes dip the base of each one in the adhesive and place at intervals along the base of the real eyelashes. Use a selection of different sizes to create natural results.

4 You can use mascara before fitting the false eyelashes, or after, or both, according to the required look.

TOP TIP

Also available on the market are individual eyelash inserts. These are single-stranded hairs applied to each lash. The process can take an hour and a half but lasts for several weeks.

TOP TIP

For individual lashes your client may be advised to have their eyelashes tinted a few days before.

5 **To remove** – Place a finger on the client's closed eye. With the other hand pull the strip from the outside towards the inner eye. To help with safe and comfortable removal a small amount of oily eye make-up remover will help to dissolve the glue. Stretch/pull the eyelid gently from the outer corner to stretch the skin and make removal of the lash more comfortable.

HEALTH & SAFETY

It is extremely important that a patch test of the glue you will be using is performed at the bridal make-up trial. A small amount of the product should be applied behind the ear or in the crook of the arm. If the client experiences any itching, redness or sensitivity they are unsuitable for eyelash application.

Contouring (highlighting and shading)

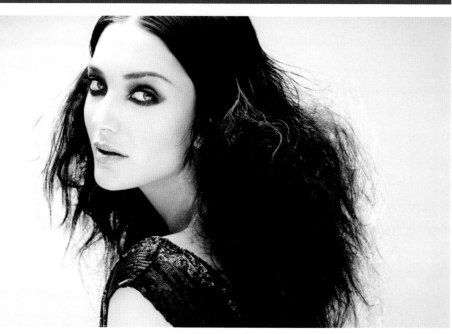

ELLE Magazine– India; Photographer: Suresh Natarajan; Make-up Artist: Namrata Soni; Model: Amy Jackson

In Chapter 1 we looked at how lighting is used to sculpt the subject with light and shadow. Make-up artists also use light and shade to contour and sculpt a feature with make-up.

Highlighting is the blending of a shade lighter than the foundation in order to project a feature forward, making it more obvious. Highlighting will enhance and bring out the best of a feature.

Shading is the blending of a shade darker than the foundation, in order to diminish a feature, pushing it back, making it less obvious.

The techniques of highlighting and shading can be used in corrective make-up, e.g. to correct a crooked nose or hide a double chin.

In beauty make-up, highlighting and shading is called contouring, and is often used to emphasise a good bone structure, or give the illusion of one. **Compressed powders** can be used to contour but the best way is to use cream-based colours from your basic palette and learn to blend with dark and light colours. Blending takes a lot of practice, but is used constantly in every area of media make-up and is a core skill.

Principles of light and shade

If you draw a round circle on a piece of paper it will appear flat. To make it look rounded you need to add some shadow and highlight. By placing some dark shading around the outer circle of the 'ball' and by blending this shadow to nothing, leaving a white highlight, you can make the circle look like a three-dimensional ball.

Read more about natural looks with contouring in CHAPTER 3.

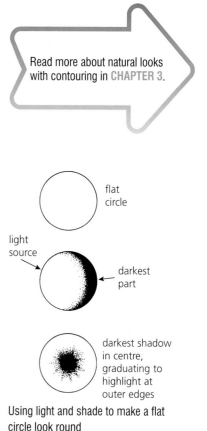

flat circle

light source

darkest part

darkest shadow in centre, graduating to highlight at outer edges

Using light and shade to make a flat circle look round

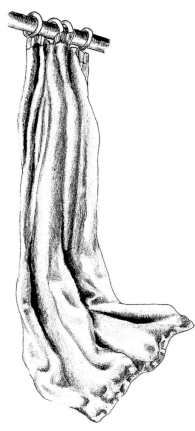

Lighting and shading

If you draw a similar circle and this time add a strong colour in the centre, blending this outwards to a highlight at the outer edges, the circle will again look like a rounded ball. This process is similar to the techniques used in blending cheek colour.

The object of this exercise is to improve your drawing skills, to develop your sense of observation, and to help you to become aware of the effect of light on any object.

ACTIVITY

Principles of light and shade

Equipment required: pencil and drawing paper

Throw a cloth over a chair near a light source, such as a window or side light. Draw the outline of the cloth first, then fill in the light and shade on the folds to make them look rounded. The parts nearest to the light source will be highlighted, and on the other side, furthest away from the light source, will have dark shadows.

The light from the window creates highlights on the folds of the cloth.

The darkest shadowed areas are furthest away from the source of the light.

The graduation of intensity in the shading makes the folds of cloth look rounded.

Applying these principles to make-up

Assessing what is needed

To begin the make-up, ask your model to tuck their chin down, and at the same time look up into the mirror without raising their head. Most people will have dark circles under their eyes. On younger faces the shadows will be slight, although even children may have dark circles from lack of sleep or by inheritance within the family.

On closer examination you will notice that there is a shadow running from the nose to the corners of the mouth. Apart from this, the face may have blemishes or patches of redness. After the foundation has been applied you can mix a skin tone somewhat lighter than the overall colour and use this to paint out the circles under the eyes covering any blemishes with a small brush. Blend the edges carefully. Redness can be toned down by adding more yellow to the concealing colour (concealing is not the same as highlighting, although both use a colour lighter than the base tone). The concealing colour should hide and tone in, whereas a highlighting colour is to draw attention to and emphasise a particular feature.

In certain contexts the performer is presumed already to be perfect for the part. The make-up is simply to make them as attractive as possible, but there are many people who appear on television who are not actors: people such as interviewers, weather fore-casters, politicians and people being interviewed. Slight adjustments can be made, such as darkening the eyebrows, covering a dark beardline, hiding blemishes, reducing bags under the eyes, or shading away a double chin.

Corrective colours

Basic make-up may not be sufficient to hide shadows under the eyes and minor skin blemishes.

◆ **Too much red in the skin tone.** Use a yellow-toned concealer after applying the foundation. Green can also be used to counteract red but should be used with caution – green can take away so much colour that it may look like illness (a very small amount must be used prior to foundation application).

◆ **Blue-black shadows under the eyes.** Orange works well on skin tones ranging from dark olive to black – apply a small amount to conceal the shadow and place the colour-matched skin tone on top.

◆ **Grey-blue shadows under the eyes.** Pink works well on pale skin tones, apply pink to hide the shadows – paint in the circles under the eyes only, and apply foundation on top.

Blending (contouring)

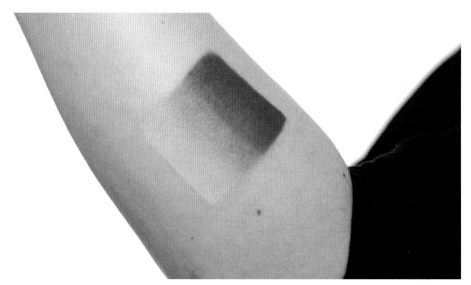

Blending

Blending means graduating the intensity of a colour. The technique of blending a colour from its strongest shade to its lightest, until it disappears into the natural skin tone is used constantly in every area of make-up.

ACTIVITY

Blending (contouring)

Equipment required: brush and colour

Practise blending by applying a line of make-up on the back of your hand. Use a brush to gradually reduce the amount of colour from the darkest point to the lightest, until the final edge fades into the skin.

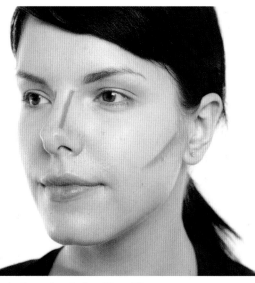

Apply shading colour to the sides of the nose and under the cheekbones

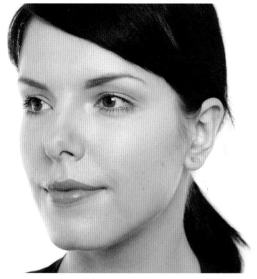

The strong lines are blended, resulting in a slimmer nose and more defined cheekbones

Correcting eye shapes

When we did a drawing of the face, dividing it into three areas, the eyes were used as a measuring technique to measure five areas from side-to-side on the face. They are:

◆ The eyes themselves.

◆ The space between the eyes.

◆ The two spaces between the outer corners of the eyes and hairline at the edge of the face.

Between the eye and the eyebrow there is an eye's depth of space. When the eye equals one length apart between the eyes, this is considered the perfect proportion. When there are variations from this category, there are ways of correcting the eye shape to conform to the ideal proportion.

1 For eyes that are deep set into the skull, and need 'bringing out' you can highlight the upper eyelids and lighten the crease line (or socket line).

2 For eyes that are too round, you can place eyeshadow on the lids putting the darkest shading at the outer corners, blending upwards. Eyeliner at the outer corners, blended upwards, will also help to elongate the eye shape.

3 Eyes that are too far apart can be corrected by using a dark eyeshadow on the upper eyelids, blending into the inner corners of the eyes. This technique is very attractive on Asian eyes. The eyeliner can also be taken further into the inner corners successfully.

4 Small eyes should be made up in the same way as deepset ones. Apply light coloured eyeshadow on the upper eyelids to highlight them and a light colour in the crease lines. Eyeliner should not be used as this would close the eyes even more.

5 Large eyes are generally considered attractive, but if they appear bulbous or protruding it may be necessary to tone them down. This can be done by using a dark coloured eyeshadow on the upper lids and crease line.

Remember dark colour will diminish a shape; light colour will bring it out.

Correcting lip shapes

Mouth shapes vary considerably, and so has the fashion in what size they should be. Small mouths were popular years ago when 'rosebud' lips were the vogue. Today the desired look is for full lips. When working on period productions it is often necessary to make the lips look smaller and neater, e.g. the 1920s or eighteenth century.

In general it is always considered desirable to have a fuller bottom lip than the top one. Fortunately, there is an inner and an outer lip line on everyone's mouth, so women have always been able to adapt their mouth size, and shape, to the prevailing fashion of the day.

1 Ensure the lips have been prepared well and concealer applied before corrective work begins.

2 For a thin bottom lip, find the outer line and apply a lip pencil liner on the outer line to make the bottom lip bigger. Apply lipstick to the rest of the mouth in the usual way – a light-coloured one will help it to look bigger.

3   To make a thin upper lip look bigger, use a lip liner pencil on the outside of the upper lip line and apply lipstick in the usual way to the rest of the mouth.

4   To make a large mouth look smaller, use a lip liner pencil inside the natural lip line, top and bottom, filling in with dark lipstick.

5   A mouth that is too small, with thin lips can be made to look fuller by placing a lip line on the outside line of the lips, top and bottom. Fill in with a light coloured lipstick.

Lip tips

◆   Use lip pencils in a colour close to the natural lip colour.

◆   Use dark reds to make the lips look smaller.

◆   Use light colours to make the lips look larger.

◆   Lip gloss, or any shine, placed along the middle of the bottom lip will make it look fuller. If too much lip gloss is applied it may bleed leaving unattractive results.

◆   The mouth can be turned upwards at the outer corners of the bottom lips for a 'smiley' look.

◆   Blotting, powdering and reapplying the lipstick will make the effect last longer.

Correcting the structure of the face

Earlier on, when you drew a face on paper, you learnt that the ideal face can be divided horizontally; from the hairline to the eyes; from the eyes to the bottom of the nose; and from the bottom of the nose to the tip of the chin. When the balance is not ideal, make-up can be used to improve it.

1   If the forehead is too high, darken the forehead around the hairline with a colour slightly darker than the base colour. The shading must be blended downwards until it gradually disappears into the foundation skin tone.

2   If the forehead is too low, follow the same principle, but this time apply a colour slightly lighter than the base colour. Paint it close to the hairline in an equal band of colour, then blend it downwards so there is no line of demarcation.

3   If the forehead is too wide, add shadow to the outer sides, above the temples. Be careful not to shade in the temple area, as you know from your previous skull drawing, the effect will be ageing.

4   If the forehead is too narrow, use highlighting at the outer corners above the temples, which will help to add width.

5   If the chin is too long, you can shade the lower part of it, blending away under the chin. If the chin is too short, highlight the lower part of the chin and blend under it.

6   If the face is too flat or round, shading under the cheekbones and highlighting the eyebrow bones is a classic way to create a more interesting shape.

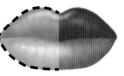

Thick lips

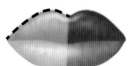

Thick upper lip

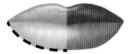

Thick lower lip

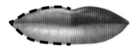

Thin lips

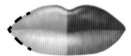

Small mouth

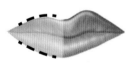

Uneven lips

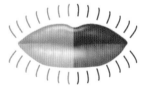

Lines around the mouth

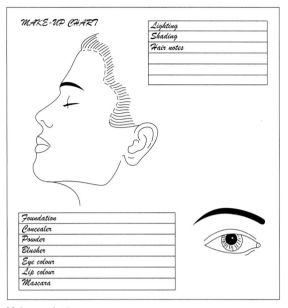

Make-up chart

ACTIVITY

Lighting and shading in make-up

Try some lighting and shading on one another, using brushes and make-up. Make the face look thinner or rounder with highlight and shadow. Try shortening a nose by shading underneath the tip or slimming it at the sides.

CASE PROFILE: LAUREN WHITWORTH, MAKE-UP ARTIST, BASED IN NEW YORK

Which area of the fashion industry do you work in?

Now I primarily work in advertising and celebrity work. But early on in my career I did a lot more editorial. I also do quite a bit of commercial video work nowadays as so much is online.

Did you have a lucky break or turning point?

Honestly, no. It was a gradual steady progression through hard work and perseverance. I was willing to work hard and for free. It paid off eventually. Gaining certain clients, though, would sometimes remind me I'd reached another level in my career and so, although they weren't 'turning points', they were 'points of no return'. Once you hit a certain level, there's no going down the ladder, so to speak.

What has been your most significant project?

That's a hard one to answer and I've been lucky enough to work with many talented and iconic people. And I also don't like to name-drop too much! As a make-up artist you learn discretion is key! However one of my long-time clients who I look after is Kathy Sledge from Sister Sledge. I've gained big iconic companies as clients such

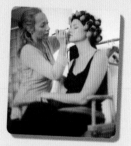

as Bloomingdales in New York. I've keyed the runway for Vera Wang. I've worked with A-list actors such as Kevin Bacon. Each project is so varied and rewarding in its own right. Being spokesperson for CoverGirl for me was a real accomplishment.

What do you enjoy most about the job?

Unleashing my creativity. Not being in an office all day. Every day is different. I meet so many talented and lovely people. I get to do something I love.

What do you enjoy least about the job?

Having such a heavy bag to lug around!

What advice would you give to a new make-up artist starting out?

Be prepared for hard work. And unpaid at that! Persevere as it's so worth it! And grab every opportunity you can, every job is another person who knows about you!

Camouflage make-up

Camouflage make-up should not be confused with concealer make-up. Camouflage creams are used in hospitals to cover burns, scars, severe acne, birth marks, skin grafts and all skin conditions where normal make-up is undesirable or insufficient cover. As a make-up artist you need to understand the use of camouflage creams, because many actors have birth marks, scars, tattoos and dark beardlines that need covering. It is the author's view that all professional make-up artists should be willing to use their skills to help people with skin problems. This is a challenging field of work, offering great satisfaction to the make-up artist in helping people with skin traumas. Some make-up artists specialise in this area, working alongside surgeons in plastic surgery clinics or hospital burns units. For make-up artists working in television and film, camouflage creams have their place in covering anything that cannot be hidden by foundations and concealers. Tattoos are hard to hide, and artists are frequently asked to do it. Camouflage creams are the answer, because they are dense, sun-resistant and waterproof. They are useful for hiding dark shadows under the eyes, cold sores, rashes, spots, freckles, shaving cuts and much more.

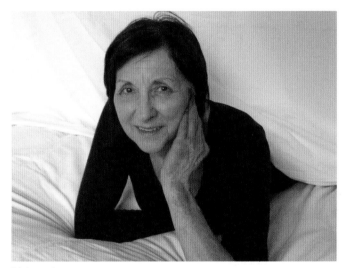

Birth mark on arm   Camouflage work to cover birth mark

Camouflage products

Veil Cover Creams by Thomas Blake & Co., UK

An excellent range of skin colours with good coverage, light in texture, good for light skin tones. The packaging is light and minimal in order to keep the costs down, so make-up artists usually transfer the colours into an empty palette or paintbox.

Dermacolor by Kryolan, Germany

The Derma range is well-known by make-up artists because Kryolan produces a wide range of professional make-up products and supplies worldwide. The Derma range has cover creams in strong metal boxes, and small plastic palettes that are easy for carrying in a kit box. Dermacolor light is now also available, this is an excellent product for clients to use at home.

Various skin illustrator palettes by Kenny Myers, US, including Flesh Tone, Dark Flesh Tone and Complexion.

Reel colour palette by Reel Creations are a popular range in the US, which includes Flesh Tone palettes for camouflage work.

Matching the skin tone

To begin with you need to find the underlying skin tone, ignoring colour produced by blood being close to the skin surface, such as red cheeks or freckles.

For pale, Celtic skin mix Veil medium with Veil tan. Veil medium has no pink and Veil tan has no yellow, so together they produce a very pale skin tone colour.

It is difficult to define particular skin colouring because every skin tone is a mixture of different ethnic mixes. Our skin tones are due to intermarriages, lifestyle and the climates of the countries we live in. The following guide is based on the country of origin and as a reference, because, as a student, it is necessary to start somewhere – although experience and practice are the best ways to learn.

The table lists skin tones from the palest to the darkest, with countries of origin and shades of camouflage creams that might be useful for mixing to find the exact skin match.

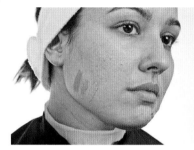

Perform a colour match test to select the appropriate foundation shade

Countries of origin	Camouflage creams
Norway, Sweden, Denmark, Finland, Canada, North America, Western Europe, New Zealand, Australia	Veil: natural, medium, natural medium tan, white peach Dermacolor: D0, D1, D2, D3, D6, D7
India, Pakistan, Bangladesh, East Europe	Veil: white, dark, natural tan, tan Dermacolor: D0, D3, D4, D5, D6, D7, D8
China, Japan, Middle East, Bangladesh, Pakistan, Northern India	Veil: white, dark, suntan, dark no. 2, dark no. 3 Dermacolor: D0, D4, D5, D8, D9, D10, D18, D19
Zimbabwe, Caribbean, Nigeria, Uganda, North American Indian, Southern India, Sri Lanka, Democratic Republic of Congo, Malawi	Veil: dark no. 2, dark no. 3, brown Dermacolor: D4, D5, D6, D8, D9, D10, D11, D13, D18, D19, D20
Uganda, Sudan, Zimbabwe, Tanzania, Zambia, Malawi, Democratic Republic of Congo, Mozambique	Dermacolor: D15, D16, D17, D40

TOP TIP

Ensure extremely small amounts of products are used as a little goes a very long way.

Orange

Dermacolor has a bright orange which is good for hiding dark shadows under the eyes on people from India and Pakistan, particularly elderly men. The orange will kill the blue-black colour without making it look grey.

When hiding tattoos, orange is also good for hiding the blue-black ink pigmentation.

Camouflage powders

Emphasis should be made about the importance of using a setting powder to ensure the product lasts on the skin without transferring. The client needs complete confidence that their area of concern will remain concealed.

All the companies that produce camouflage creams also make a loose powder for setting the colours. The powder is unperfumed and transparent so as not to change the colour. Baby talcum powder can also be used. Apply with an even application, allow to set well between each application and dust off the excess with a large brush.

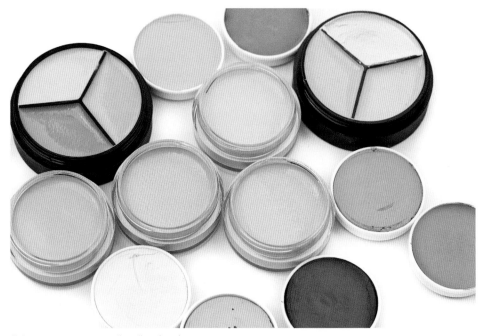

Colour correctors neutralise discoloration

Tools & equipment

The basic kit:

- brushes
- camouflage palettes
- cleansing cream, toner
- cotton buds

- cotton wool
- natural sponges
- orange sticks or spatulas
- stipple sponges – orange synthetic type
- translucent no-colour powder

Applying the camouflage creams

The skin must be clean and grease-free, so do not use moisturiser before applying. The cream should be applied very thinly so that the effect is natural and does not rub off. If one thin coat does not hide the blemish, powder lightly with cotton wool or powder puff, brush off excess with a soft brush and then blot the area gently with damp cotton wool to remove any powder left by the brush. Repeat the whole process on any area where the blemish is still visible.

Sometimes an additional cream needs to be added to match another skin area, e.g. **stippling** some pink on top of a cheek, to copy the flushed cheek colour on the other side of the face.

Tools for applying colours

For tiny areas, a small brush is best. Small, natural sea sponges are good for a stippled, natural look. The sponge should be made wet to soften it, then squeezed out until it is barely damp, but not wet. Place the chosen colour in the palm of your hand and press the sponge against the colour to load it.

Before testing on the person's skin, first press it on the back of your hand to test the strength of colour. The sea sponge method provides a good effect, which will tone down a blemish such as rosacea, while allowing some of the original colour to show through.

The sponges can be cut into pieces, and larger holes cut out if needed.

Stipple sponges, orange coloured synthetic ones, are also used for a denser coverage such as a tattoo. Natural sponges provide a looser, softer effect.

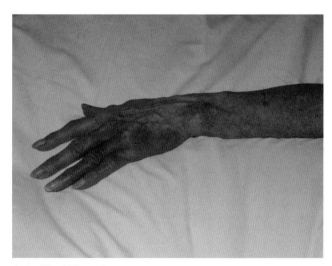

Arm with a birth mark

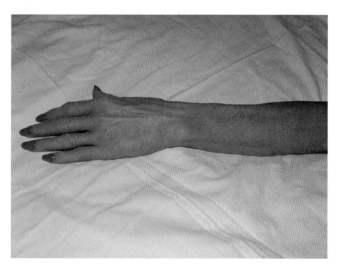

Arm covered in camouflage make-up

Covering a tattoo with camouflage creams

Everyone will be asked to cover a tattoo at some time. When the director says, 'Lose the tattoo' it can either be airbrushed away, or you can use Reel colour palettes or camouflage creams.

The easiest way is to start with a colour on the darkest part of the tattoo, which will be hardest to hide:

1 Apply Dermacolor D32, white, orange or Veil rose with a small brush; then powder as previously described.

2   Apply the next layer matching the skin tone.

3   Any bright red in the tattoo can be obliterated with Dermacolor 1742 or Veil olive.

For larger tattoos it is easier to use a sea or stipple sponge and to stipple on the natural skin colour at the end.

STEP-BY-STEP: COVERING A TATTOO

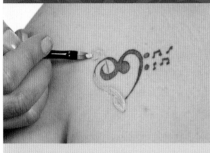

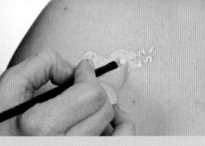

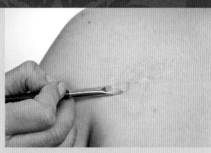

1 Apply corrector to discoloured areas with a small synthetic brush and then apply a light layer of translucent powder with a powder puff to set the make-up.

2 Cover the tattoo with a cream or paste that is closest to the client's skin tone.

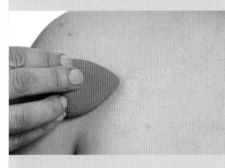

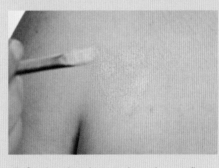

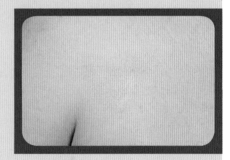

3 Blend by feathering out edges with a sponge and then apply a light layer of setting powder with a powder puff to set the make-up.

4 Continue layering powder and camouflage products until the tattoo is no longer visible.

The finished look.

Covering an indented scar

1   Cover the scar with a shade which matches the surrounding skin tone.

2   Use a colour one shade lighter than the skin tone and paint a thin line around the inside edge of the scar. Tap it with your fingertip to blend, and set with powder using a soft brush.

3   Using a colour one shade darker than the skin tone, paint a thin line around the outside of the scar. Blend it in by tapping lightly with your finger and set in the usual way with powder and a soft brush.

Covering a protruding scar

Use the opposite methods of lighting and shading. Paint a shaded line on the inside edge of the scar, and a lighter shade on the outside edge of the scar. Powder as above.

Filling in a beardline

To fill in bare skin patches on a man's beardline, simply stipple a greyish brown colour first, and then add a light stippling of whatever colour matches the natural beard colour. Use a stipple sponge to apply the colour.

Cross-infection

Orange sticks and spatulas should be used to transfer the creams to a clean plate or palette before mixing. It is the same for all make-up, but if you are covering a spot, cold sore or shaving cut you must use cotton wool to powder the area, and then throw the cotton wool away in a covered bin.

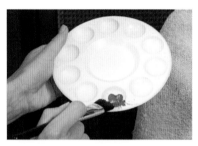

Hygienic placement of make-up product onto a make-up palette

Removing the creams

A simple, unfraganced cleansing cream will remove the camouflage make-up. Damp cotton wool or a clean, damp, muslin or towelling face cloth is good for wiping off the cream, followed by a mild toner and moisturiser to finish.

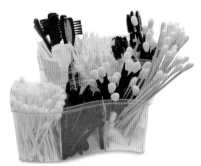

Make-up consumables, which are disposed of after use

Dot painting for an unmade-up look

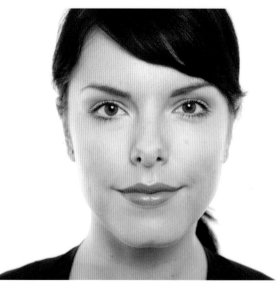

Natural make-up

This is a lovely way of making actors up to look as if they are not wearing any make-up at all – just naturally healthy and beautiful. No one will praise this make-up effort – because they won't see it. But that is the whole point of it.

Towards the end of the nineteenth century, the artist George Seurat developed a technique of painting that was later named pointillism. Using oil paints he worked with only pure colours (straight from the tube), to develop his method of producing pictures with only dots of colour. White, which he considered to be of no colour, was the only paint that he mixed. This was crucial to his work as he felt that it increased the reflected powers of the other colours and evoked a feeling of natural light.

Make-up artists are often asked for an unmade-up look and use the dot painting technique to apply dots of concealer, camouflage or even foundation base on the small areas that need covering, leaving the rest of the skin bare.

If the actor has a good skin tone, no foundation is needed and this type of dot painting is good on men, women and children.

Tools & equipment

- brushes
- derma colour palette
- palette knife or spatula
- palette or plate for mixing colours
- reel palette
- sea sponge and stipple sponge
- translucent 'no colour' powder
- veil palette

Application

1 Test on the jawline to find the exact colour match. Place a small amount on your palette.

2 Mix another small amount of the same colour, adding a tiny amount of white to make it slightly paler.

3 Prepare the skin: it should be clean but not greasy, so avoid heavy moisturiser.

4 With a small brush, apply the first matching skin tone to any spots or blemishes that need concealing. Blend the edges without going onto the surrounding skin. Work your way over the face, putting small dots of camouflage cream with the tip of your brush wherever needed. Sometimes you may need to add a spot of yellow to your palette mix. This depends on the person's skin tone and is the artist's choice.

5 Powder the dots lightly and brush away excess powder with a soft brush.

For a stronger colour correction you may have to apply another layer. But the layers should be thin because the look must be unmade-up to the eye. Blot the powdered areas to avoid an unnatural dry look. If it is obvious to the eye it is obvious on camera.

Dot eyeliners

Ideal for men's make-up as it is so natural. Use a tiny, pointed brush to put minute dots of grey or brown eyeliner between the eyelashes, leaving spaces between the dots. Cake eyeliner is suitable; liquids and gels look too strong.

Eyebrows

If the eyebrows are too pale and need definition, colour the hairs; not the skin. Again, stick to taupes and grey browns, but this depends on the actor's colouring. Use a mascara wand to apply to hair and not skin.

Brows can be set with brow-setting products, clear mascara or a small amount of hair gel on a clean mascara wand, but over time sealers can also start to flake so are not suitable on long shoots and big close-ups.

Eyelashes – mascara

Colourless if the eyelashes are good. If colour is needed, use a thin coat of brown, brushed through to avoid clumps.

Tinting On a long shoot the actor's eyelashes and/or eyebrows can be tinted every six weeks.

HEALTH & SAFETY

It is important to carry out a patch test on the client before beginning the tinting process.

ACTIVITY

Dot painting method

Practice the dot painting method on a fellow student or model. Take a photograph before and after. Try to perfect the natural look before moving onto beauty and fashion.

CASE PROFILE: SARAH JAGGER, MAKE-UP ARTIST

How did you get into the fashion industry?

After completing a three-month course I explored all areas of make-up. I won a place in the BBC's Vision competition, which gave me work experience in television. I assisted make-up artists in television, film as well as fashion, and basically went wherever make-up experience was offered. Fashion was my passion and the transition was organic – I kept saying 'yes' to fashion work and the television and film contacts dried up. Eventually all my contacts were in the fashion world.

Which area of the fashion industry do you work in?

I do a lot of close-up beauty work as well as editorial, commercial and high fashion. My work also crosses into celebrity and advertising.

What has been your most significant project?

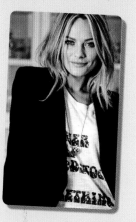

Vivienne Westwood is certainly one of the most significant; however, the greatest jobs are always the ones that give the most creative satisfaction – not necessarily the most money or prestige. I love working for *Elle* magazine because I get to do the kind of work I love – clean, natural, perfect complexions. I've become known as 'The skin girl' at my agency!

What do you enjoy most about the job?

Being able to use the face as a canvas because the skin is an amazing surface to work on. I love the creative collaborative process between stylists, photographers, models and everyone else involved that all bring something to the table to produce a work of art. To me a fashion shoot is like creating a painting – only you get to share the experience with other artists.

What advice would you give to a new make-up artist starting out?

Don't give up! There are only a lucky few who start out with the right contacts to get them work. The rest of us need to create them ... and that takes time. Contact all the make-up agencies and offer your assistance and regularly contact make-up artists to offer help (always attach a photo of yourself to your emails as make-up artists get so many emails from assistants, it's great to be able to put a face to a name). Take all the work you're offered and most importantly – be patient. Freelance work is gradual but it does grow quickly if you have a great attitude and work ethic.

REVISION QUESTIONS

1 List four differences between day and evening make-up.

2 Before using eyelash glue, what MUST always be done? Explain this process.

3 What corrective colour is used to neutralise redness and a high colour?

4 What is the 'dot painting technique' and what is it used for?

3 Working in beauty and fashion

Guest written by Jo Frost

LEARNING OBJECTIVES

This chapter covers the following:

◆ Different kinds of fashion work, including beauty, editorial, fashion shows and commercial.

◆ Researching the creative aspects of the design concept.

◆ Working as a make-up assistant.

◆ Working with an agent.

◆ Working on music promotions, working abroad and catalogue work.

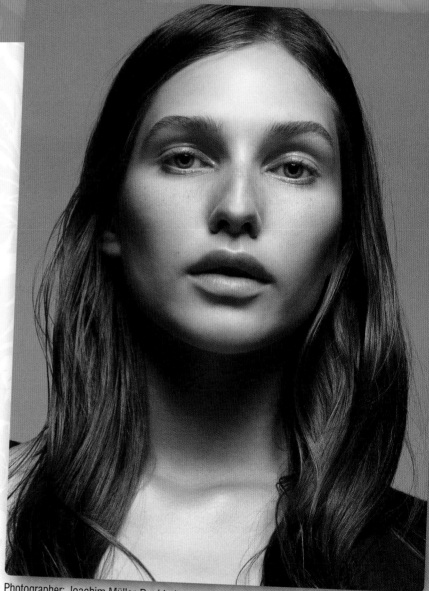

Photographer: Joachim Müller-Ruchholtz

KEY TERMS

Face powder
Look book

UNIT TITLE

◆ Research the creative aspects of the design concept

INTRODUCTION

Instead of dissecting beauty and fashion into dry theory, let us study the work of a leading fashion make-up artist. The looks she creates are influencing the current trends in beauty and fashion make-up today.

Jo Frost has been working in the industry since the end of 1998 and her case profile is in the second edition of *The Complete Make-up Artist* in which she said, 'It is the best job in the world'. Her passion and commitment to fashion is still strong all these years later. Here she talks about working in the different areas, with inside information on all that a student needs to know in this highly competitive field.

Working in beauty and fashion

The fashion industry is a complex melting pot of creatives, including: designers, photographers, stylists, make-up artists, hairstylists, nail technicians, models, art directors and casting directors. They influence each other and ideas are bounced around in teams, taking inspiration from street art to fine art, history, pop culture, art and socioeconomic influences.

Fashion by its very nature is obsessed with modernity and innovation: new ideas and aesthetics, which are constantly developed and mixed up with historical references, to create fresh looks as the old becomes dated. Even when an idea is revived it is never re-created in the same way; it is essential to remain current. Fashion experiments with sensory-emotional values. It is a reflection of art, culture and nature.

Make-up within the world of fashion experiments with semantics and semiotics: changing the way in which a look can be read, creating a narrative giving the models their character for the day.

How to succeed in the industry

With the exception of fashion editors, most jobs within the industry are freelance. To reach a supersonic level of career status, make-up artists need to work internationally and have their work shown in London, New York, Paris and Milan (also known as 'the circuit'). This includes editorial as well as shows and advertising.

Key players who can make or break careers are the agents who represent photographers, make-up artists, hairdressers, nail technicians, models, etc.

The fashion industry is inclusive of all sexualities, cultures, subcultures and races, and is where individuality is celebrated. Having a unique style at the right time will be recognised and rewarded.

It is of huge importance to have both a current and historical knowledge of fashion and beauty trends, as well as a deep understanding of their greater influences. As a fashion make-up artist you must develop your own individual style. This is a largely organic process which takes time, but is the basis on which you will be booked. Developing your style is a journey that depends on who you are as an individual, what has shaped your life and what has influenced your creativity. It may be challenging but should be enjoyed. Do not think about the destination because it is never what you expect.

Fashion is a really tough industry to break into, as the level of competition is extremely high but it is always the most fun, creative and innovative part of the market.

TOP TIP

Build up a reference library to work from.

TOP TIP

Absorb culture and the arts. Spend time observing and analysing other make-up artists' work. Break down what it is about the make-up that is beautiful and what makes it cool.

TOP TIP

"When you love what you do, you never work a day in your life.

Marilyn Monroe

- Have a deep understanding of reference material.
- Develop excellent technical ability.
- Be professional.
- Keep your kit immaculate.
- Dress practically for the location but appropriately for the industry and the client.

- Clean make-up.
- Make-up with an edge.
- Be friendly and positive; engage with the rest of the team while being aware of the hierarchy.
- Have current knowledge of all new make-up developments and products on the market.

White airbrush spattered portrait

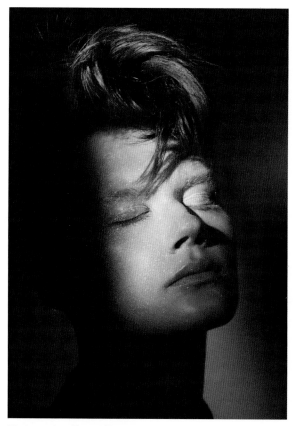

High concept beauty story conceived by Jo Frost entitled Japonica. Influenced by the Japanese marketing term meaning 'beautifully white'; a preference for pale skin free of blemishes. This look was achieved by extensive skincare, grooming brows and curling lashes then using an airbrush combined with hand splattering of white body paint.

Photographer: Rupert Tapper

Fashion make-up

Fashion make-up is a reflection of all aspects of fashion, such as trends within fashion, clothing, art movements, socioeconomic factors, politics, film and popular culture.

Fashion make-up pulls together the look, creating stories and trends. High fashion make-up conveys ideals and aesthetics and is usually not aimed at the commercial market. It needs to work harmoniously together with all the other looks and evokes a mood projecting who the person on the street is that day, often experimental, modern and chic. Make-up moves in cycles and trends and takes you on a journey and is about completing an illusion.

Typical trends

Fashion recycles old ideas but always in a new way, ongoing trends tend to be:

- graphic eyes
- natural look
- statement lip
- romantic
- new goth
- grunge
- starlet
- couture
- seventies glamour
- nineties
- masculine/androgenous.

Variations on eye graphics

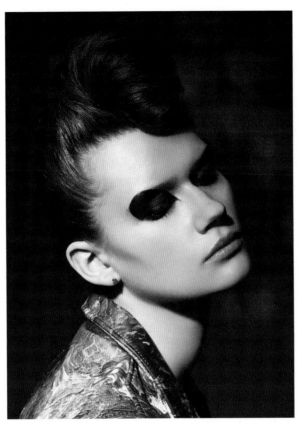

Photographer: Rupert Tapper

High concept beauty story conceived by Jo Frost. Entitled 'Japonica' this make-up look is influenced with the Japanese aesthetic for simplicity, clean lines and balance. This look was achieved by extensive soft contouring and highlighting. The graphic eye was first defined in black kohl pencil then set with a black paint-pot gel liner before a final coat of liquid liner was applied to achieve maximum colour intensity.

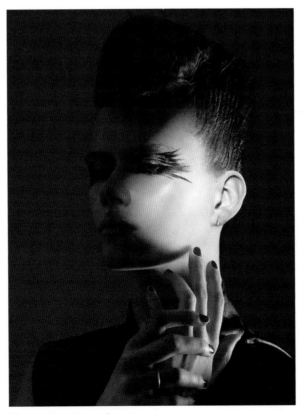

Photographer: Rupert Tapper

Another image from Jo Frost's 'Japonica' beauty story. This make-up look is influenced by the Japanese legend of Koi Carp – if a Koi succeeded in climbing the falls at a point called Dragon Gate on the Yellow River it would be transformed into a dragon. Through this legend Koi has become a symbol of worldly aspiration and advancement, perseverance in adversity and strength of purpose. This look was created by using textured brushes to paint on black liquid liner in bold, visible brush strokes. Gold body paint was then painted over the top of the lid (once the black has dried) and up to the brow in a rough freehand style. The gold was heightened with pigment powder and gold liner to intensify reflections.

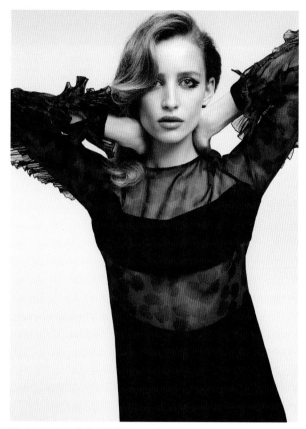

This was a 'new faces story' so Jo wanted to create a single look particular to each girl, to work with the styling and the photographer's lighting. Brows were softly defined and well groomed. Super-soft contouring was used to accentuate the model's bone structure. Finally the graphic eye shape was initially drawn on with black kohl pencil, once the shape was perfected it was set with black paint-pot gel liner, finishing the process with liquid liner to intensify depth.

Photographer: Oskar Gyllenswärd

Super-soft smokey eyes

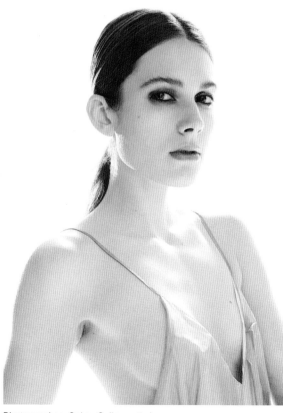

This super-soft smokey eye was created using kohl pencil and eye gloss. It was kept on the natural side to enhance the model's features for a 'new faces' story where the image is all about the girl. Skin was perfected and shine boosted for a fresh effect, and brows were filled and groomed to balance the look.

Photographer: Oskar Gyllenswärd

Fashion work

Types of fashion work

Beauty – Editorial

Fashion – Editorial

Portrait – Celebrity and art-based

Runway/fashion shows – New York, London, Milan and Paris

Advertising – Fashion and beauty

Commercial/catalogue/online

Editorial and advertising

Editorial work is when a fashion or beauty story is commissioned for a print or online magazine. This tends to be the most creative part of the industry but is the lowest paid. Generally speaking, the higher the level of kudos of the magazine/publication, the lower the rate. Many magazines have no rate available for make-up artists and often no budget for photographers. This means that the shoot will cost the photographer in terms of studio hire, retouching, flying in models, hotel for models, catering, etc. Stylists often have to pay for bikes and returns, plus courier costs of bringing the clothes in from overseas. More commercial magazines and glossies have a rate for the whole team.

Book (portfolio)

Within fashion, having a 'book' (portfolio) is of the utmost importance; it is on this basis, as well as your reputation, that you get future work. Your book illustrates your style and on this basis a team with a particular aesthetic can be put together. In the beginning you will be 'testing' to get images in your book. As your career progresses you will want to eliminate 'prints' from your book and replace them with magazine 'tears' of commissioned work. The industry standard 'book' is usually black, bound leather 28cm × 36 cm (11 inches × 14 inches), with your name embossed on the front. These come in different depths so you have a bigger book carrying more pages according to how long you have been working. A book that holds 20 sleeves (or 40 images/pages is perfect to start with). It is of fundamental importance how your book flows from one story to the next so that your style shines through. Clients may request a book drop or you may attend appointments with your book and have to talk through it, as well as talk about yourself and your work.

Times have changed recently and now books are often kept digitally, primarily on iPads, which is cheaper in the long-term, and it is easier to change the running order of the book according to the client. You should change your book frequently, so that it is appropriate to the job.

Websites

Websites are also of fundamental importance as they are often the first port of call for a client if you have been put forward for a job. Having your book online is a great way of promoting your work on the web in a professional capacity – Facebook and other social media has its place, but using them is not terribly professional. If a client or photographer likes your work, they may then 'option' you or request to see your book.

TOP TIP

Network in real life as well as social media. This business is about who you know not just what you know, or indeed talent.

Editorial and commercial work

The main difference between editorial and commercial work, aside from money, is the goal of the end-use of the images. Commercial work, like editorial, differs in levels from the lowest e-commerce (online) to high-end luxury advertising appearing in magazines and on billboards. There is a whole range in-between including advertorial and in-store (windows and point-of-sale). Rates vary according to usage and the client. Some clients want their advertising to look more editorial and less commercial, as this will lend the brand a cooler edge. They will sometimes give complete creative control to their team, but this is unusual. Generally speaking the brand will have a clear direction and brief for the team, which caters specifically to their target market. Anything that is too edgy will not have mass-market appeal; make no mistake we are in the business of selling a product.

A good understanding of the client, and what they want to achieve, is essential in creating an 'on-brand' look. Commercial make-up usually has mass appeal to the largest target market, although it will also be trend-driven and will reference show looks or editorial direction. Editorial tends to be more cutting edge and will explore concepts, be directional and experimental. This does depend on the magazine and its particular aesthetic. Some high-end magazines are more grungy or pared-down or art-based – these looks are not suited to mass-market, but may go on to be appropriated and absorbed into the mainstream. Luxury magazines have a similar editorial edge to the luxury advertising and reflect glossy, expensive and aspirational influences.

Credits

Having your name in print in the right publications is fundamental to a successful creative career, as it shows other people in the industry what you are doing and who you are working with. Everyone in fashion name-checks the credits to keep tabs on who is doing what. Credits are given by the photographer or stylist to the magazine and will include model details, hair, make-up and nail technicians' names. If it is a magazine title that a make-up company wish to sponsor or you are an artist who is endorsed by any specific brands, then in addition to your name and agency it will also state what brand you are crediting.

Some brands sell credits but only have a set budget per year, so a rate is given to the make-up artist instead of products. The amount of product given by a brand varies according to the magazine, the artist and if it is a cover, as well as the amount of pages. Covers carry extra prestige. Products are not usually given to publications unless it is a beauty story and the latest line of make-up from specific brands are going to be featured. Usually the beauty editor will call these in for the make-up artist to use on the day. There is an increasing trend for beauty shoots/stories to be sponsored by brands, as this raises the brand profile and is an excellent opportunity for them to showcase new collections. The brand public relations (PR) will usually contribute budget to the photographer or the magazine and pay the make-up artist a fee, but this is not an advertising rate and is not compulsory.

Contracts

Every make-up artist wants to secure a 'contract' when their career reaches a certain level. Contracts vary enormously and are generally secured by agencies who are best able to negotiate the legalities. Generally speaking a contract would give you the title of 'UK Ambassador', 'European Ambassador', 'Worldwide Ambassador' or 'Artistic Director'. By paying a retainer fee the brand will get a set amount of days per year with their chosen artist, who may be involved with press launches, advertising and advertorial shoots, social media (which is usually an ongoing concern) and the company may then want control of all editorial credits.

TOP TIP

Be industry educated. Research fashion designers, cosmetic houses, top make-up artists and hair stylists. Keep updated with catwalk models and how celebrities, television personalities and musicians wear their hair and make-up.

This means that the make-up artist will exclusively credit the brand with which they are under contract, both for editorial credits and quotes.

Ultimately, as the make-up artist you will be lending the brand credibility within the industry and raising its profile. The brand may also want to be involved in any catwalk shows that its artist is heading; this attracts particular attention from the beauty press. The artist will also have to be regularly available to give quotes and tips. Some brands will want the make-up artist to be involved in product development; famously Pat MacGrath for Giorgio Armani and Dolce and Gabanna, also Charlotte Tilbury for Tom Ford. Other make-up artists have launched their own brands such as Laura Mercier, Bobbi Brown and Charlotte Tilbury.

Some celebrities will request (through their agent) specific make-up artists for shoots and film if they have worked with them and trust them. This has to be agreed by the publication, photographer and/or director, as the magazine may want to completely change the way the artist looks and is therefore perceived. Celebrity work has become increasingly linked with fashion and many fashion periodicals often feature celebrities (actresses, models and singers) especially on the cover.

The working day

A standard working day will begin at 9 a.m. and finish at 6 p.m., although this does vary enormously. Often call-times are 8 a.m. or earlier if shooting on location and using daylight. Studios and locations do charge overtime so speed is essential.

> " Some photographers work late and I've shot on many occasions starting at 7 a.m. and finishing at 2 a.m. – so be prepared! The amount of shots required in a day can vary enormously; I've shot 36 commercial look-book images in one day and on other occassions just one simple portrait.
>
> *Jo Frost*

Morning planning/briefing meeting

It is always best to arrive 15 minutes early, allowing set-up time before the actual call-time. Usually there is a morning meeting with the whole team, when the look and concept are discussed and agreed. Make-up and hair usually take direction from the stylist/fashion editor and photographer. Sometimes you will receive a brief ahead of the shoot day or if you work in regular teams then the shoot may have already been discussed. Everyone works differently, but it is helpful to prepare references ahead of time, which will be in specific folders on an iPad or on mood boards. Sometimes it is appropriate to bring specific reference books. When shooting beauty always create mood boards in advance so you can email them ahead of the shoot date to the client and deliver them in the morning meeting. Mood boards also help you to remain focused throughout the day, especially when there are a multitude of make-up looks. Some of the ideas you deliver or create may be rejected by the photographer, stylist or client. Sometimes things simply do not work, so always have a back-up plan and be able to think on your feet. The look should be a collaborative effort involving all members of the team and has to be right for the clothes as well as adding narrative to the story. It also needs to work with the lighting and set or location.

Always stay on brief so that you are delivering what the client wants; if you firmly believe in another contrasting idea then deliver that idea in the morning meeting. If it gets rejected do not put it into practice as you will no longer be acting as a team member. Your idea may be right but allow the client to realise this; do not force them into it.

Research and references

It is essential to have a deep understanding of references and trends. You may not be shown any references but will be expected to know what the latest Prada/Chanel/Miu Miu look this season is. Often the look may not be specifically fashion but will borrow from popular culture, so a widespread knowledge of films, icons, cult classics, subcultures, art and literature will aid your creativity and ability to communicate ideas with the rest of the team.

The shoot

Generally within fashion there will be one or two make-up looks or a progression of looks. Sometimes there may be up to eight looks in a day, but this is more unusual. When shooting beauty, it is a minimum of four looks to a maximum of six looks in a day. Planning transition progression is key with this kind of work in order to create smooth and speedy changes.

The amount of time available for hair and make-up varies according to the look and the amount of shots needed that day. Some make-up looks will only take 15 minutes, whereas other more couture and extreme looks can take 1½ hours. Generally speaking hair takes longer than make-up, especially if extensions have to be glued in. It is often advisable to work with the hairdresser so that, as a team, you cut down on preparation time; giving more time to the photographer.

In high fashion there is nearly always separate hair and make-up. It is almost impossible to achieve outstanding brilliance in both areas as they are very different disciplines. In more commercial work such as catalogue and music videos one person will be expected to do both; this keeps costs down but quality is invariably compromised. Trips often require one person for hair and make-up, to keep both flight and hotel costs to a minimum.

Models

The key elements in fashion are the models – they can make or break the story. Models are usually cast by the photographer and fashion director, but sometimes there is a casting agent. Looks have to be tailored specifically to each model so they look amazing. Often it is all about the models. Some looks will not work on some models, generally speaking the better the model the more diverse looks she can carry.

> **TOP TIP**
>
> Discuss with the photographer how they want to light a story as this really affects how the make-up looks on camera and, essentially, as a make-up artist you are capturing light and playing with shadows.

> **TOP TIP**
>
> Look after yourself and be prepared. Long working days will mean tiredness. Take drinks and healthy snacks with you to help you through the day. Be prepared to eat and drink on the go – sometimes there is not time to break for lunch and there are never allocated tea/coffee breaks.

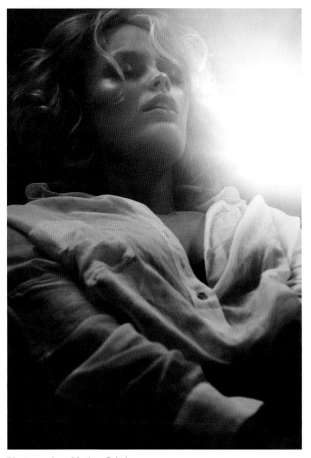

This story was based on Kim Basinger in the movie '9½ Weeks' and is a perfect example of great casting. The model already closely resembled the actress, so once hair and make-up had completed the transformation process the resemblance was incredibly powerful. This look was created but first tinting brows to match Kim Basinger (do not attempt this without extensive training as brows have to be dyed back to their original colour at the end of the day; if you can't do this you may be sued by the model agency). Skin was prepped and saturated with extensive skincare, moisturisers and oils to create a high sheen. The face was contoured and heavily highlighted. A soft smokey eye was achieved by layering up kohl pencil, metallic grease and eye gloss, followed by layers of mascara. Cheeks were flushed with cream blush and lips were stained to create a post-coital glow.

Photographer: Markus Pritzi

Fashion shows

There is such a buzz around doing the shows. It counteracts any of the stress and super early starts following late finishes as well as the logistics of getting from one show to the next. It's such an exciting experience it's hard to come back down to earth afterwards.

Jo Frost

'The shows'

Also known as 'runway', 'catwalk', 'prêt-à-porter' or simply 'the shows'. This is a bi-annual event in the four fashion capitals, running sequentially in New York, London, Milan and finishing in Paris. Each city has a 'Fashion Week' typically lasting four days (London) to a full seven days (Paris). Spring/summer collections are shown in September and October, and autumn/winter are shown in February and March. You are always working a season ahead. In addition there are two seasons of menswear shows, which also run around the world in January and June. The pinnacle and most exclusive of all the shows is haute couture, which is typically only in Paris and runs twice a year in January and July.

Hair and make-up test

When developing the look for the show both the hairdresser and the make-up artist meet with the designer. The designer will show them the collection (or what samples they have) together with fabric swatches and their inspiration boards, and discuss the concept for the show. The hairdresser and make-up artist will then do a hair and make-up test on a model for the show (also known as 1st looks). Once the look is confirmed then the make-up artist will take photos of the test model, all products used will be recorded so it can be re-created on show day. On show day the head make-up artist will demonstrate the look so the assistants can copy it. The idea is usually for all the models to look the same – like a fashion army on the catwalk. The look will have to be adjusted to work on each model. Photographs of the test are usually pinned up as a reference.

Call times

Call times in London are usually three hours before the show. All the models have to be made up and checked within this timeframe. The girls will also have to do fittings and rehearsals during this time, so it is essential to be fast. Often make-up and hair will have to work together in order for the show to run according to schedule. Usually make-up artists will have to pack a set-bag and work in the hair area, as that is where all the electrical hair equipment is. As soon as the hair is set the model can then travel to the make-up department with the make-up artist to have their look finished.

The more famous the model the more shows they will be 'walking' in and often models will arrive at the last moment still wearing the 'look' from the last show, which will have to be removed for the next look to work. If certain areas of the make-up can be saved and transferred to the current look to save time without compromising the look then that is preferable. Sometimes girls will arrive only 20 minutes before they have to open the show, so a whole team of three hairdressers, two make-up artists, nail technicians and dressers will descend on them to make the transition as fast as possible. You may have to work on your knees with the girl's chin on her chest while her hair is being done. In this situation, it is very high pressured and it is important to remain calm no matter how stressful or impossible the situation appears to be. The head make-up artist has to check each make-up and will probably want to correct and adjust it. Before the shows the models will be dressed and then stand in 'line-up', which is the order that they will be walking in. Final checks happen in line-up and the head make-up artist will be there, usually with their first and second assistants. The size of the make-up team is dependent on the number of models and also the complexity of the look. Often assistants are not confirmed until the day before the show when the model count is confirmed, once the collection selection is complete.

The look

There is usually a whole bank of photographers shooting the girls at the end of the runway. The images are sold on to the fashion press and in some cases the designers will employ a specific photographer to shoot a **look book** simultaneously. It is essential that the girls look flawless and the look is perfectly executed as the images will not be retouched and this is how the designers launch their latest collection. It costs the designer a lot of money to put on a show, so it has to be immaculate – there is no second chance. The make-up should not just stop at the face: hands, legs and any visible skin has to be moisturised and perfected so the legs are flawless and any imperfections are covered. Although it may be essential to use a light foundation on hands and legs it is of the utmost importance that no make-up transfers onto the clothes. Make-up artists can lose shows if the collection is marked.

Brands

Shows are often sponsored by cosmetic brands which provide key products, essential to the look. Some brands may also provide assistants or the money for the head make-up artist to pay their assistants. Increasingly, cosmetic and skincare brands pay the designer a fee for sponsoring the show. As an assistant, you may not always get paid, as it depends on the level of sponsorship that the artist is receiving. You will also need to bring your own 'show-kit', which is all your essential items – brushes, tools, skincare, foundation, concealer and basics such as contouring, highlighters, liners, mascara, neutral and black shadow. Most key make-up artists have favourite products which you will learn over time and it is advisable to buy those items and get them in your kit for future shows if you want to keep your place on the team.

Some exceptional make-up artists become synonymous with certain designers once they have a long-standing collaboration and have developed a look specific to the brand which is reinvented every season. The head make-up artist is often interviewed backstage regarding the look, concept and products. Sound-bites have become essential, as beauty editors love a snappy, catchy quote that sums up the look and paints a visual picture.

Creating the look

Show make-up can be cutting edge and experimental – an understanding of who the 'girl' is and the mood or concept that the designer wants to project is essential. Quite often the designer will want something brand new that has never been seen before. It is all about pushing boundaries and creating press interest to generate the most coverage possible for the designer.

Quite often this make-up is only suited to high fashion and is not aimed at mainstream appropriation. There are usually about six key trends running in show make-up. For every season, natural is a strong trend but there will always be a graphic eye and a strong lip coming through, colours change over time according to trends, technology and make-up collections. There are no rules within this area of work but the make-up must always work harmoniously with the collection and the hair. Any products can be used including tape, glitter, feathers, sequins, grease, powder and airbrushing.

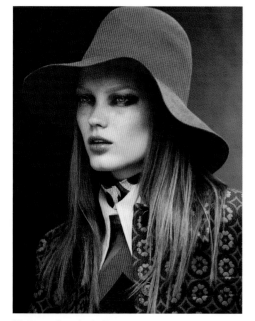

Photographer: Andy Eaton

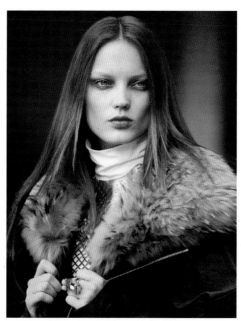

Photographer: Andy Eaton

This look was first created for a fashion editorial in *Black* magazine and was then used with great effect for the Antoni and Alison Spring Summer 2013 London Fashion Week Show. In the show three different colour-ways were used – extreme green, ultra-marine and intense violet. Each colour-way was predetermined for each model to work perfectly with their skin tone and eye colour. The clever variation on the smokey eye was created by first smoking out coloured pencil, then layering on greasepaint and setting with eyeshadow. A liquid liner also in the corresponding colour was applied at the root and smoked out. This layering of products gives real depth and intensity of colour.

HEALTH & SAFETY

Always be careful with your back when moving your kit from one venue to the next. Suitcases may be heavy. Consider 'manual handling'. Always bend your knees to lift something heavy. When possible, seat the model on a high stool and stand to work. If only low chairs are available then seat yourself at the same height as the model.

Essential qualities for a show make-up artist

- Being able to understand and communicate with a designer in the same language.
- Working fast.
- Remaining calm and grounded.
- Managing a team.
- Knowing who all the models are.
- Creativity with an edge.
- Technical brilliance.
- In-depth understanding of trends and references.
- Interview skills.
- Personal presentation.

TOP TIP

Have business cards when you are working. You never know when you may meet a new contact. But always remember the pecking order and never undermine the key artist.

Assisting

Assisting on shows is an amazing experience and the adrenaline rush is highly addictive. It is usually the best way to break into assisting fashion make-up artists. If a head make-up artist likes you and the way you work on a show, then you will probably be requested back next season or asked to assist on shoots and other projects. Being a team player is essential; be helpful and supportive to the rest of the team, never sit around doing nothing – keep busy as this will be remembered.

TOP TIP

Take every opportunity available to assist make-up artists as your learning curve continues for a long time after you have finished training.

What makes a good assistant?

Qualities:

- availability
- organisation
- speed
- awareness
- keeping calm
- punctuality
- positivity
- helpful
- loyalty
- discretion.

TOP TIP

Be prepared to work long hours for little or no money and never complain. Always be positive and diligent, inject fun where you can without compromising professionalism.

Actions:

- Do not ask too many questions.
- Understand etiquette and be able to read the situation.
- Anticipate the needs of the head make-up artist.
- Take responsibility for the make-up artist kit.
- Alleviate stress and do not contribute to it.
- It is not about YOU, do not show your work to other members of the team.
- Body make-up on the models.
- Take notes and process them quickly if asked.

TOP TIP

Keep busy and never be seen using your mobile phone or Facebook.

◆ Prepare a set-bag once the make-up is finished.

◆ Keep the station clean and organised.

◆ Stay in the background and do not dominate the shoot.

◆ Be prepared to work late and do not complain.

◆ Be able to communicate clearly and appropriately.

◆ Always look and act the part; as an assistant you are perceived as an extension of the make-up artist.

Types of assisting

First assistant

If you are first assisting but not on a full-time basis, then you will be booked when the key artist needs you. On editorial there is usually no fee but on commercial jobs there is usually a rate. You should know the kit inside out and keep it clean. You must be constantly available and be an effective part of the team, supporting and contributing positively to the lead make-up artist. This role may be shared with another first assistant or could be a single role.

Sometimes this can be a full-time position, according to the success of the person you are assisting. You will be expected to take ownership of the make-up artist kit and at times take it home with you. For top make-up artists there may be a wage or daily rate; although some jobs are not paid, especially editorial. It is usual for first assistants to be exclusive to that make-up artist.

Second assistant

Second assistants will always be on the show team and will assist on big production shoots.

Third assistant

Third assistants are a regular member of the larger team, key team, show team and larger-scale shoots.

Inspiration

Inspiration can literally be taken from any and every source: historical fashion and make-up, icons, nature, subcultures, music, art, films, women in the street, ethnic cultures and tribes. Often make-up trends will be strong for a few seasons before disappearing, only to be re-invented years later when the images are rediscovered and once again seem relevant and current. Fashion can either trickle-up or trickle-down, taking its roots from the street and real life or starting as a high-fashion concept before being gradually appropriated by the mass market. Typically, once the idea, such as false lashes or strong brows, has been adopted by the mainstream then the fashion industry will step away from it as it has lost its freshness. As soon as you see something everywhere it loses its novelty and is no longer 'cool'.

Certain elements will always be on trend because they are classic: a red lip, the natural look, glowing skin, eyeliner, a smokey eye. However, no matter how classic these elements are, there is constant reinvention regarding shape and texture every season to move the look on so it is current and chic.

Pop promos

Pop promos or music videos are vital in promoting a new release single or album. The director usually creates the concept for the shoot, which can be extremely diverse. The concept will then be approved and commissioned by the record company and the artist's management. The make-up artist and the rest of the team will receive a treatment consisting of story boards and a script, and will liaise with the director and the artist to create looks evoking the right mood. With a bigger cast the make-up artist will need a team. Often a band or singer will continue an ongoing working relationship with the make-up artist and use them for television appearances and concerts as well as photo shoots for the album, press releases and magazine features. When working with dancers, retouching the make-up regularly is of the utmost importance to keep it looking fresh after intense routines.

Catalogue

This is frequent and regular work. The daily rate is not great but often the shoots last for over a week so the block booking makes the work more lucrative. Shoots will either be in the studio or on location, where the light is good – generally in the tropics. South Africa, Miami and Spain are regularly used, as the light is warmer and the days are longer. Often the model will have to be ready between 6 a.m. and 7 a.m. so the photographer can start shooting at first light. The harsh midday light is usually avoided, so there is often a long lunch break and shooting commences later in the afternoon working through 'golden hour', which gives the best light, until levels are too low to continue work. Make-up is usually more commercial and classic, being easily accessible to the target market. The amount of shots per day can vary from 12 to about 36, depending on how tightly the budget is being squeezed. Often the make-up artist is also expected to do hair to keep costs down.

The agent

Most make-up artists want an agent, but it has to be the right agent. Some agents do not put the work in or simply do not have the contacts required to build a successful career. Many top agencies work like a management company and have a long-term plan for their artist: first focusing on the artist's editorial work and pairing them with particular photographers and clients. An agent gives the stamp of approval respected in the industry. Agencies have a much wider range of contacts available and will promote the artist verbally, on their website and manage the artist's book sending it out to prospective clients. They also influence the building of teams and set up meetings with clients, photographers, editors, cosmetic PRs and stylists. Many hair and make-up agencies are attached to photographic and styling agencies. They may also offer art directors and set builders on their roster.

As brilliantly used in an Uber agency of the same title, fashion is a mix of Art + Commerce. As make-up artists are usually creatives an agency will take care of the business side of things. Agencies are brilliant at negotiating rates, chasing payments and offering guidance. In return for their services, agencies take a cut of the artist's fee, which in London is 20 per cent from the artist, and another 20 per cent from the client – known as a booking fee. This rate varies according to country. Agencies also often charge a monthly fee for the web page that they manage for the artist, but this varies hugely according to the agent. There used to be a monthly charge for bike bills – sending out your book – but now as so much business is done over the web this has been massively reduced to a minimum.

Building your portfolio

Getting in with the right agent is extremely competitive as agencies will only take on the best make-up artists, generally those who have already done assisting work. To be taken on by an agent you usually have to have an amazing portfolio. Initially, build up your portfolio with test shoots which are non-commissioned and non-published shoots with a photographer working for no fee. It is through this kind of work that make-up artists build their skill set and develop a style. As your career progresses, work will be commissioned and published giving tear sheets for your book. An agent will not normally sign an artist until they have a book of a high standard and have built a reputation, having contacts who will travel with the artist to the agency. Agents will then spend six months to two years launching a make-up artist's career and making them bankable.

Professionalism

Presentation

Presentation is crucial for a make-up artist working in fashion. Always look cool, present-able and appropriate for the environment and client. Equipment must be scrupulously clean and well organised. Have fun but remember you are at work and keep it professional.

Planning or 'prepping' is vital to ensure you have all the correct products in your kit prior to the shoot day. Work out ideas in advance of the shoot and always have a back-up plan in case your first make-up or concept is rejected.

Before you start work, always lay out the basics: brushes and tools, skincare, foundation, concealer, mascara, eyeliner, contouring and bronzing, highlighters, essential lip colours, tissues, wet wipes and cotton wool, all arranged in a neat and organised manner so that products can be identified quickly.

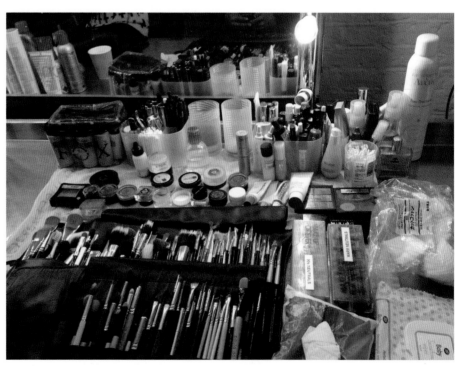

Workstation

ACTIVITY

Contouring

When shooting colour the photographer might want to take black and white shots simultaneously. It is important to understand the concept of contouring. Think of it as highlighting and shading. Look at a colour palette and imagine it in black and white. Which colours would show as shadows, mid tones and highlights comparative to the foundation you are working with? When contouring the face all contours must be beautifully blended into mid tones and highlights to create an illusion of natural shadows.

TOP TIP

Don't be seduced by gimmicky cosmetic collections.

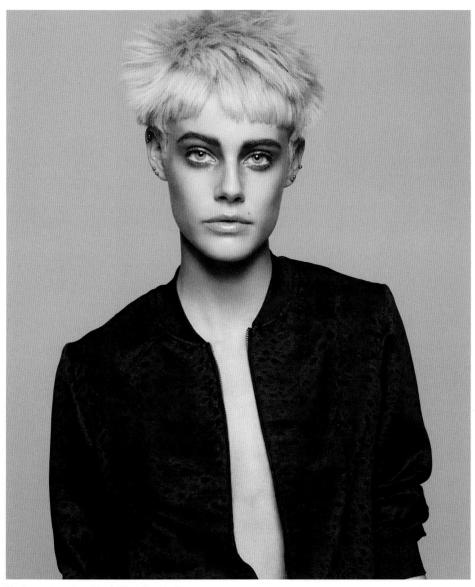

Photographer: Joachim Müller-Ruchholtz

This make-up combines detailed contouring with a strong brow. Skin was well prepped and very light foundation used. Eyes were contoured using taupe pencil with coffee closer to the lash-line, blending out before the next stage. Grease-paint was used over the pencil and perfectly blended, keeping the eye shape masculine. Highlighter and gloss were applied to reflect light. Brows were groomed and filled; redefined into a more masculine shape using a combination of neutral eyebrow pencils. Taupe greasepaint was used to contour the cheeks, temples, nose and jawline. Highlighter was used along the cheekbones, bridge of the nose and cupid's bow to enhance the contour effect and give the skin a luxurious finish. Lashes were curled but no mascara used. Lips were kept nude to preserve the balance of the look.

Core skills

All make-up is a combination of sharp lines and blending. These are your essential skills through which you can build and expand your make-up skills. You must be well-practised in playing with combinations.

Smoked red glossy lips

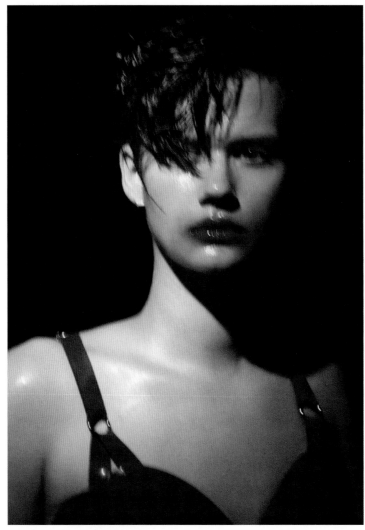

This image illustrates how well mixing techniques in an unusual way can work brilliantly in edgy fashion/beauty make-up. The smokey technique is usually used on eyes but here has been used on a glossy red lip.

Photographer: Rupert Tapper

Smokey eyes

The smokey eye has been in widespread use since the 1920s. The shape and strength of the eye changes according to time and fashions.

Smokey eye tips

◆ When using powders it is often best to do the eye first so any make-up spillage can be cleaned at the end.

◆ Always use pencils first and then gels or grease and set them with a corresponding powder.

◆ Apply product at the root of the lashes and blend out with each stage before commencing the next stage.

◆ Apply liquid eyeliner and mascara at the end (if you work quickly it is possible to blend out liquid eyeliner).

TOP TIP

To help create the perfect smokey eye, use a domed eyeshadow brush. This will help to contour the socket line. Remember BLENDING is the key.

HEALTH & SAFETY

Always make sure pencils are sharpened with a clean make-up pencil sharpener before and after use.

STEP-BY-STEP: SMOKEY EYES BY DELAMAR ACADEMY

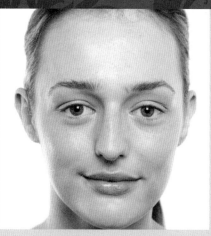

1 Apply clean natural foundation and powder to set.

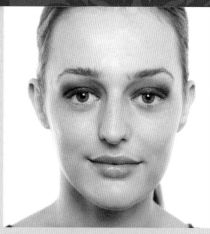

2 Start building up eyeshadow on top of the eyelid and blend into socket.

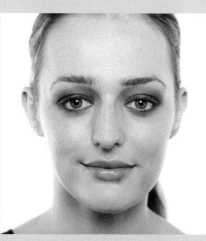

3 Apply eyeshadow under eye, blending and diffusing to join the upper eyeshadow.

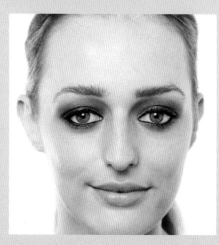

4 Apply kohl liner inside rim of eye for more dramatic intense look.

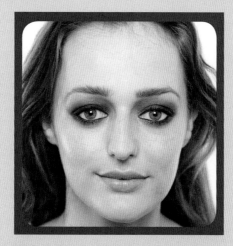

5 Strengthen the shadow, blending away the hard edges and groom hair for final look.

Natural make-up

To achieve this look it is important to remember the following tips:

◆ Have well prepped and moisturised skin.

◆ Colour match foundation to the collar bone (not the face or neck).

◆ Keep foundation light and only use where necessary.

◆ Conceal any blemishes and undereye circles gradually, building up concealer. It should never look thick or heavy.

◆ Groom the brow hairs through so they look lush and full. Keep brows light and natural and feather in any gaps with pencils or powder shadow. Eyebrows are normally ashy in colour tone, correspond your colour choice with the tones of the natural brow. You may also choose tones lighter than the actual brow to stop them looking heavy and strong.

◆ Softly contour the eyes, temple and cheekbone to echo and emphasise natural shadows.

◆ Well curled lashes are essential to any make-up; always curl at the root to achieve maximum lift.

◆ Highlight the inner corner of the eye and blend.

◆ You can open up the eye with a flesh tone liner inside the waterline. Avoid using white as this can look very 'made up'.

◆ Brown mascara looks more natural than black. Even on black skin use black/brown mascara.

◆ Always use neutral natural shades.

◆ Blush should sit on the apple of the cheek, blending into the contour seamlessly.

◆ Highlight on cheekbones using cream to give a fresh dewy, glowing, youthful effect.

◆ Lips can be left completely nude or a neutral toned lipstick or stain can be applied. Do not leave a crisp edge to the lip as this will look like make-up.

◆ Keep powder to a minimum to achieve a 'natural glow'.

TOP TIP

When applying mascara ask your client to look down, rather than directly at the wand. This will minimise the risk of watery eyes.

Natural looks

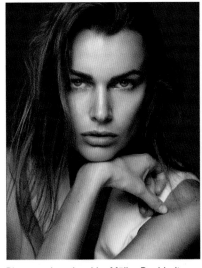

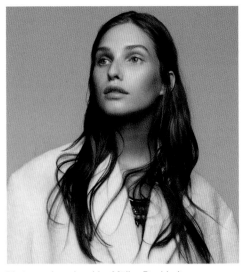

These images illustrate a modern fashion take on the natural look. Skin is well prepped and foundation minimised to look real and fresh. Soft contouring is used to enhance the models' features and work seamlessly with the lighting. A neutral palette is employed and reflections are boosted with highlights and glosses.

Photographer: Joachim Müller-Ruchholtz

Photographer: Joachim Müller-Ruchholtz

STEP-BY-STEP: COMMERCIAL LOOK BY DELAMAR ACADEMY

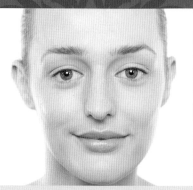 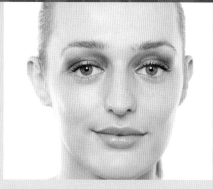 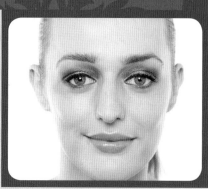

1 Apply light dewy foundation and powder to set.

2 Apply eyeshadow, blending well in a soft wash.

3 Apply thin liquid eyeliner to define lash line, and a cream blusher with natural lip gloss.

STEP-BY-STEP: EDITORIAL LOOK BY DELAMAR ACADEMY

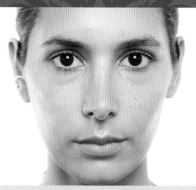 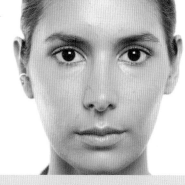 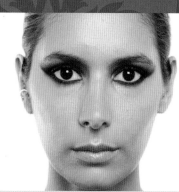

1 Prepare the skin with moisturiser.

2 Apply foundation and powder.

3 Do graphic outline of shadow underneath, building up layers of colour on top of the lid, and blend together.

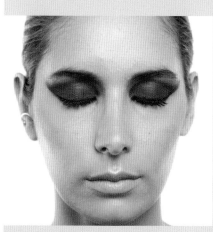 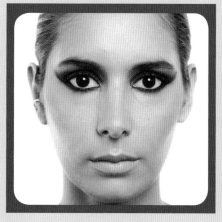 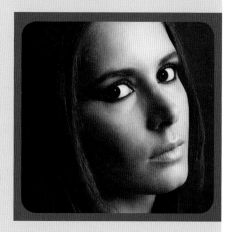

4 Apply kohl inside the eye rim.

5 Finished look.

CASE PROFILE: JO FROST, INTERNATIONAL MAKE-UP ARTIST

How long have you been working in the fashion industry?

Over 15 years. I am still intensely passionate about what I do and like to be heavily involved in the whole shoot, connected to the rest of the team and the work we do together.

What areas of fashion do you work in?

I cover wide areas of fashion including heading shows at London Fashion Week, editorial, designer and high street advertising campaigns and beauty – both campaigns and editorial. I sometimes work with celebrities and musicians too.

How did you get into the industry?

I was waitressing in Covent Garden when a hairdresser approached me to model in his final collection show (like a graduation show) for Vidal Sassoon. I got chatting to him and refused to model but offered to do the make-up. It went really well but I did make up 14 models in one day so it was a full-on first job. I bonded with the stylist and the hairdresser and we kept working together, and they put me up for jobs. Over time my circle expanded. I also knew a make-up artist before I trained so I assisted her straight away and we became good friends; she was my first mentor.

I chose to study at the Delamar Academy because I wanted to study all areas of make-up – not just fashion, although that was my chosen area. At the time Val Garland was collaborating with McQueen using bald caps with special effects so I wanted to learn everything.

Did you have a lucky break or turning point?

There was no single event that was life-changing. There is too much competition these days for that to be true. Key points were assisting certain make-up artists on big shows and shoots, getting my first story in *iD*, being made a Contributing Beauty Editor and signing to my agency.

Assisting was a big thing for me and I raised my game each time I assisted a different make-up artist on the shows. I started assisting Sam Bryant and Petros Petrohilos, then Alex Box, two years first assisting Miranda Joyce, spent three years on Val Garland's key team who then told me I had to leave her and assist Pat MacGrath. It took a long time to get onto Pat's team and in the interim period I was with Lucia Pieroni and on Charlotte Tilbury's international team for a few years.

What has been your most significant project?

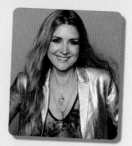

It's impossible to say. The very nature of fashion and its fast and fluid changes means that as soon as you finish one project you are straight onto the next and being continually seduced by the future. It's difficult for work to stand the test of time as fashion dates fast, but I do try and keep my work modern, chic and iconic to counteract this.

What do you enjoy most about the job?

I love being part of a creative team and developing ideas. It's like breathing life into dreams so they become real. It's important for me to flex my artistic and intellectual muscles and have a lot of fun while I'm doing it. I've made a lot of very close friends in this job, it's a very intense working environment especially on trips and you bond with people quite fast.

With the shows, I love collaborating with designers and creating a vision of who their girl is. I am driven by the adrenalin rush backstage and excel in working in high-pressured environments. Nothing beats the moment of a great finale when the girls walk in a union of grand vision, it's the stuff dreams are made of and the cutting edge of the industry.

What do you enjoy least about your job?

Super early mornings – I often have call times of 6 a.m.–8 a.m., which is fine if you haven't shot until 10 p.m. the night before, but when you are busy, you're mega-busy. I also work a lot of weekends and always have to be available, which plays havoc with your social life. It's also hard being broke for years – it takes a long time to make money in this industry.

How has the fashion industry changed during your career?

The Internet has changed everything, as has social media. Information systems are so much faster. It's a lot easier to carry out research with Google and websites rather than having to buy all the magazines, but it's good to mix it up as otherwise everyone has access to all the same images. I've kept and catalogued lots of my old magazines and won't allow other people to use them as they are specific and unique to me.

It's also much easier to contact people such as agencies and photographers than it used to be, which is great, but there are so many more people doing the same thing. I get bombarded by people wanting to assist me and it's just not possible to deal with all the enquiries while you are working and writing quotes, etc. on your days off. Everything is very last minute now so often you don't get confirmed on a job until the night before.

What advice would you give a new make-up artist starting out?

Get on a really good course where most of your time is doing practical work because make-up is a technical skill you have to develop through practice. The longer the course you can afford the better especially if you have no previous experience. Outside of college work, practice as much as you can on as many different faces as you can, this should never be underestimated. To develop what would be considered a genius level of ability takes about 10,000 hours of dedicated practice. This breaks down into 40 hours a week over five years. No one expects to be a concert pianist overnight: make-up is no different to any other creative, technical skill.

What do you see as the difference between the different parts of the fashion industry?

Fashion is a very small industry and most people tend to know each other but generally speaking there is a commercial side consisting of catalogue work, look books and beauty. The more creative side of the industry is generally the shows, editorial for high-end magazines-these are glossies or industry periodicals. The more creative side has less money behind it but is more artistically satisfying and off the back of a good editorial portfolio you can gain work on big ad campaigns which are seen as being aspirational.

What do you see as the difference between film and television and fashion shoots?

Film, fashion and television are worlds apart unless you are working with an extremely aesthetic director like Wes Anderson, Tim Burton, Baz Luhrmann, Ridley Scott, Tom Ford or Paul Michael Glaser. Often film work is less creative and does not offer up a fantastical visual treat. Most television and film make-up is kept in the palette of reality whereas fashion is about selling an ideal or dream and is more high concept based.

How do you think working in America differs from the UK or other countries?

America is a much bigger market and the fees are higher because of this. The top models tend to be New York based so most big high-end advertising campaigns and editorials are shot there. Los Angeles (LA) is where the film industry is located so there is a lot of celebrity based work out there; increasingly fashion shoots are happening in LA too. London doesn't have as much money but is often more creative.

What advice would you give to someone wanting to work in America?

You need a work visa and have to get sponsored by approximately 15 people in the industry as well as providing tear sheets and covers so that you can get an O-1 Visa for Individuals with Extraordinary Ability or Achievement. You have to be well-known and achieved a high level of status in the industry either nationally or internationally. This has to be backed up with evidence and you need a lawyer to submit and manage your application. It's a time-consuming and expensive process. I wanted to move to New York a few years back and had got a number of agencies who were keen to represent me but in the end I signed to a big London-based agency so I stayed.

You can follow Jo Frost's work on her agency website (www.clmus.com or at www.models.com). You can also find her on Instagram and Twitter as JoFrostMakeUp.

REVISION QUESTIONS

1 What is a mood board? And what would you use for inspiration?

2 What is a first assistant?

3 Why do make-up artists have an agent? And what can be the benefits?

4 List five key points that will help to create professionalism for a make-up artist.

4 Contemporary hair

LEARNING OBJECTIVES

This chapter covers the following:

◆ Contemporary hair tools and products.

◆ Hair types.

◆ Designing the hairstyle.

◆ Hairdressing, hair-up and styling techniques.

◆ Hair extensions.

KEY TERMS

Appliances
Synthetic hair

UNIT TITLE

◆ Apply techniques to performers' hair to create different appearances

◆ Apply and work with hair extensions

INTRODUCTION

This unit will introduce you to essential hairdressing techniques to help you succeed as a make-up artist. You will be introduced to products and tools that are essential knowledge for your success in this unit. You will explore different hair types that will help you with professional hair services. This unit covers how to design a hairstyle, different hair-up looks and a variety of key hairdressing techniques. All of this knowledge is essential for Level 2 hairdressing services; your knowledge will be advanced to Level 3 hairdressing by covering information on hair extensions. All hairdressing elements are important to help you complete a full service when working on an actor on a photo shoot or preparing a bride. This ensures that you are able to complete a total look.

Contemporary hairdressing

The hairstyle is as important as the make-up and, although they are very different skills, the make-up artist is responsible for both.

In television, theatre, fashion, commercials, music videos and increasingly more feature films, the make-up artist is in charge of the total look – hair and make-up. The techniques most often called for are styling and dressing the performers' hair, but not perming or colouring. Hairstyles have become softer and more natural looking, with an emphasis on healthy looking, shiny finishes.

Typical hairdressing equipment for styling and dressing hair

Tools & equipment

- assorted brushes – round and flat. A soft bristle brush for dressing hair up
- combs, assorted
- curling tongs
- diffuser

- handheld dryer
- heated rollers
- nozzle
- rollers and clips
- straighteners

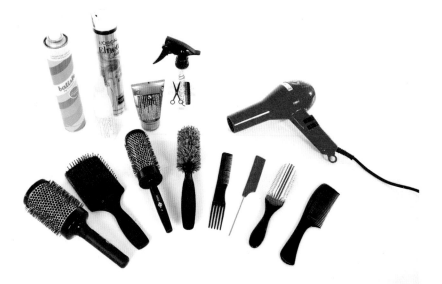

Hair tools and equipment

TOP TIP

When working on location, always make sure that lids are kept tightly on products when moving your kit. Take extra care when travelling abroad with aerosol products. Airlines may restrict the type and quantity of aerosol products you can take on a flight. Check with your airline and the rules for the country you are visiting before travelling with hairdressing products.

Products

- ◆ **Serums** Add smoothness and shine when setting or blow-drying.
- ◆ **Mousses** Add volume and texture.
- ◆ **Gels** Extra hold and sculpting the hair.
- ◆ **Waxes** Hold the hair in place, or smooth hair as a finishing product.
- ◆ **Creams** Smooth and control static hair as a finishing product.
- ◆ **Finishing sprays** Hold the hair in place as a finishing product.
- ◆ **Oils** Add shine to dry hair as a finishing product or when hair is damp.

It is important to refer to the manufacturer's instructions before using any hair products.

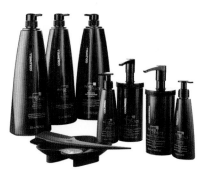

A range of products for hairdressing and styling

Hair types

Typical hair types are:

- ◆ dry
- ◆ greasy
- ◆ normal
- ◆ coarse
- ◆ thin
- ◆ soft
- ◆ thick.

> **TOP TIP**
>
> Always perform a consultation to determine the client's hair type; this will help determine how the hair will behave and the most suitable products to use to get the best results.

Designing the hairstyle

The hairstyle is designed according to the brief. In television, film and theatre it is a collaborative process, involving the director, costume designer, actor and needs of the script. For a fashion shoot the photographer, stylist, model and client will be involved in the decision-making.

Whatever medium, the make-up artist must take into account the type of hair, head shape, facial features, the haircut, and then work out what is possible. After liaising with the relevant people, a style is then designed, created, and shown to the director, photographer or client. A photograph is often taken for future reference, which can be added to the make-up chart.

> **TOP TIP**
>
> For continuity with hairstyling services make sure photographs are taken of the hairstyle from all angles. Front, back, both sides and top. The style can then be re-created for an exact match for television and film.

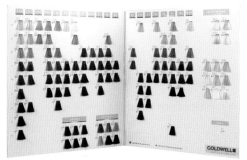

Hair colour chart

HEALTH & SAFETY

When working with electrical **appliances** always make sure that they have been PAT (portable appliance test) tested. Look after the plug and wires on your equipment.

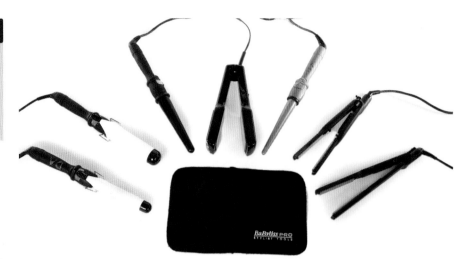

Electrical hairstyling tools and equipment

ACTIVITY

Hairstyle using hair additions

Working on a partner use wigs, hairpieces or crepe hair to achieve a look suitable for your given character.

◆ Research the look using different media such as library, Internet, magazines and art galleries.
◆ Design the look, taking into account face shape, hair type and length.
◆ Produce a mood board with a variety of styles.
◆ Evaluate the outcome.

TOP TIP

Always remember to consult with costume designers to determine what hairstyle will be achievable with the chosen hat or ornamentation that is being used.

CASE PROFILE: HAFDIS LARUSDOTTIR, MAKE-UP AND HAIR ARTIST

Which area of the industry do you work in?

I have been working in the industry since my graduation in 2013. I started by getting my degree in hair in Iceland. From there I wanted to do something more. I knew I wanted to go into the film and television industry more than fashion and beauty.

Did you have a lucky break or turning point?

My lucky break was only a few weeks after graduation. A make-up artist in Iceland was looking for an assistant for a feature film. She needed someone who could do hair as well, because the actors needed period haircuts and she didn't know how to cut hair. After this film she got me another job on another feature film. So six months after graduation I had already done two feature films!

What has been your most significant project?

My first project was on *Game of Thrones Season 4*. What an amazing first job for a make-up artist! Huge set, dozens of actors and long days. A perfect beginning for a career. Getting this job gave me the confidence to go after the projects I wanted.

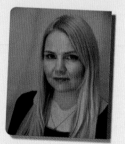

What do you enjoy most about the job?

It is so versatile and the bond between the crew members gets so strong after months of filming.

What do you enjoy least about the job?

It is very unstable, especially when you are just starting. It can be hard to get work, so luckily I have the hairdressing to get me through in-between jobs.

What advice would you give to a new make-up artist starting out?

Go for what you want! The worst thing that will happen is you won't get it and then you just move on to the next opportunity.

Styling techniques

Typical styling techniques that you will need to use and should be familiar with include:

- blow-drying
- straightening
- smoothing
- finger drying
- curling
- roller setting
- plaiting

- twisting
- applying hair extensions
- securing hair ornaments (on films and television productions the hair ornaments are supplied by the costume or wardrobe departments).

HEALTH & SAFETY

Always check that your client does not have any allergies. Some products may contain aromatherapy essential oils or ingredients that your clients are allergic to.

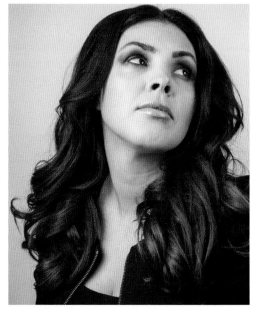

Curls created using a conical wand

STEP-BY-STEP: HEATED ROLLER SET

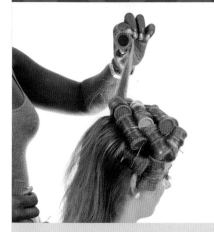

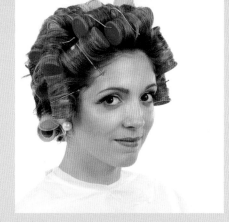

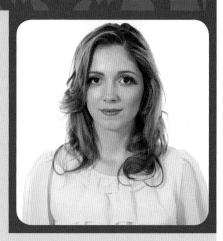

1 The heated roller is held on the outer edge to avoid burning the fingers. Be careful to not touch the client's ears with the heated rollers.

2 The finished heated roller set. Be careful that pins are not digging into client's scalp/skin.

3 Finished look. Tousled soft curls that have been finger combed and styled.

Hair-up styles

Typical hair-up styles that you will come across and should be familiar with include:

- knots
- twists
- braiding
- plaiting
- barrel curls

- chignons
- French pleats
- scalp pleats
- vertical/horizontal rolls.

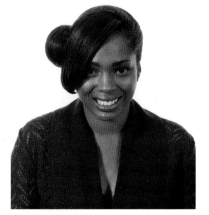

Horizontal roll

STEP-BY-STEP: BARREL CURLS

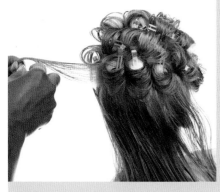

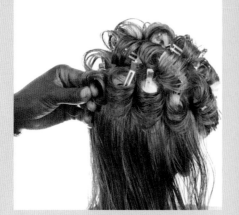

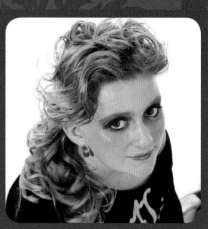

1 Rolling the newly formed barrel pin curl down towards the root area.

2 The finished barrel pin curl ready to be secured at the root with a Lady Jane clip.

3 The finished combed-out barrel pin curl set.

STEP-BY-STEP: FRENCH PLAITING

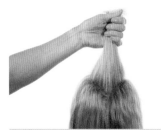

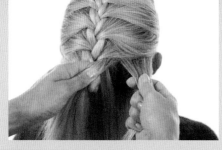

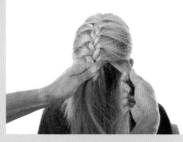

1 Section the hair at the front hairline into a triangle. Divide this section into three equal strands as if you were starting a basic plait.

2 Hold one of the strands in one hand and two of the strands in the other. Add a little extra hair from the front hairline into the outer strand.

3 Pass the outer strand and extra hair across and into the centre and into your other hand.

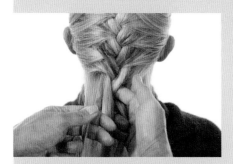

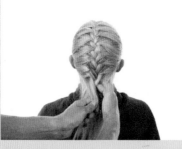

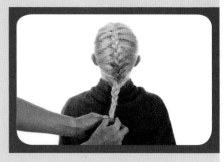

4 Do the same on the other side and repeat this technique all the way down the hair.

5 Continue steps 3 and 4 taking in a new section of hair from the hairline each time.

6 Your French plait will now start to form. Continue the plait in the same way until you finish.

STEP-BY-STEP: VERTICAL ROLL WITH ORNAMENTATION

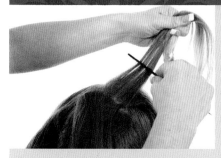

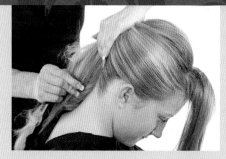

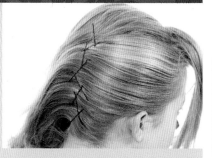

1 Taking each section and working throughout the head, backcomb the hair at the root area only.
All hair can be pulled back into this style, or some in the front area can be left out to be incorporated into the style later.

2 Smooth over the hair using a soft bristle dressing brush, gently sweeping the hair from one side back and slightly upwards.

3 Secure the hair in the centre from the nape to the crown with interlocking grips. The final grip should be placed just below the crown, facing downwards.

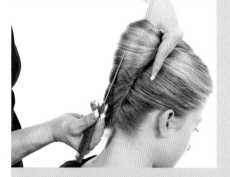

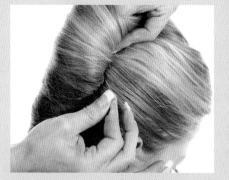

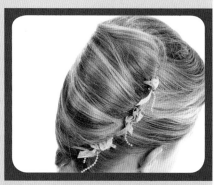

4 Fold the hair neatly over the grips, tucking hair under to form a roll. The end of a pin tail comb can be used to tuck in any stray hairs.

5 Secure the roll using pins, making sure that no grips or pins are visible. Use a dressing product and spray to smooth and hold the style.

6 The finished style is seen here with added ornamentation and finishing products applied.

STEP-BY-STEP: ASYMMETRIC CHIGNON

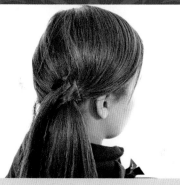

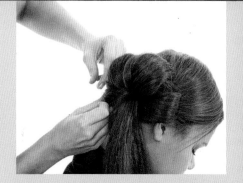

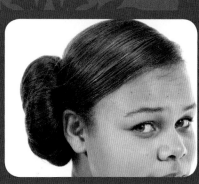

1 Comb the fringe section forwards and spray with hairspray then sweep back in a curve and pin around the base of the pony.

2 Divide the hair into five sections and lightly backcomb or brush to create a cushioned bed to place pins. Then smooth the sections and fold them in to secure the base.
A bun ring can be used if required.

3 The classic chignon is smart and stylish.

Hairdressing techniques

Typical hairdressing techniques that you will come across and should be familiar with include:

◆ backcombing

◆ backbrushing

◆ moulding

◆ shaping

◆ rolls

◆ knots

◆ twists

◆ plaits

◆ curls.

Hair extensions

Hair extensions, sometimes also called hair weaves, are lengths of real or **synthetic hair** that are closely attached to the scalp, adding length and/or thickness to the person's own natural hair. There are different ways of attaching hair extensions, some of which are longer lasting than others. When well-matched in colour and texture, and professionally applied, hair extensions are designed to mix in and move naturally with a person's own hair, making it difficult to tell the person is wearing them. They can provide volume, extend the hair length and add highlights or lowlights.

Types of extensions

Both human and synthetic hair extensions are available in a variety of lengths, colours and textures. Natural or human hair extensions are more expensive than synthetic ones, although usually much better quality. Synthetic hair is made from chemically processed fibres and, although more affordable, may not look as real and can be more difficult to work with.

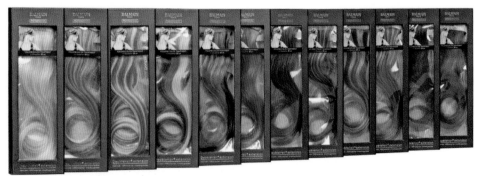

Hair extension packets

Application of extensions

Hair extensions can be applied using different methods:

◆ clipped-in

◆ glued with special adhesive

◆ sewn – attached to tight small plaits or cornrows of the person's own hair.

Gaining a qualification in hair extensions

To gain a qualification in hair extensions you will be required to:

◆ Establish suitable hair extensions for hair type.

◆ Describe the different consultation techniques used to identify service objectives.

◆ Recognise contra-indications of hair extensions.

◆ Recognise different hair and scalp disorders.

◆ Explain the factors that will influence hair extensions.

◆ Have a knowledge and understanding of client health and safety.

◆ Understand different attachment methods.

◆ Understand the client's hair length, texture and density.

◆ Understand the limitations of products on man-made fibres.

◆ Have a knowledge and understanding of differences between man-made and real hair.

◆ Apply hair extensions for a full head and partial head.

◆ Have a knowledge and understanding of product application.

◆ Have a knowledge and understanding of styling equipment that can be used for different types of hair.

◆ Understand how to maintain and style different types of hair extensions.

◆ Recognise the problems that can arise during a hair extension service and find a suitable solution.

◆ Have a knowledge and understanding of client aftercare.

Factors that you will take into account when applying hair extensions

◆ Client's lifestyle.

◆ Client's hairstyle, elasticity, texture, density, hair growth pattern and client's own hair length.

◆ Any evident damage that will affect application.

◆ The client's face shape and head shape.

◆ What attachment method will be required.

◆ Perfect colour matching.

◆ Possible contra-indications.

◆ A client's sensitivity and allergy test results. (e.g. an allergy to adhesive/glue)

STEP-BY-STEP: HAIR EXTENSIONS APPLICATION

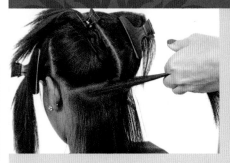

1 Part the hair horizontally in the nape area to create a base for your first track, make sure you leave up to one inch free around the hairline.

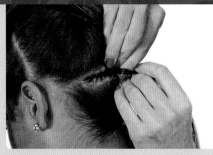

2 Create two cornrows starting from the outside and meeting in the middle; secure with a braiding band.

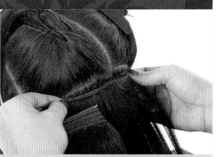

3 Measure the weft of weave to the exact length of your track and cut.

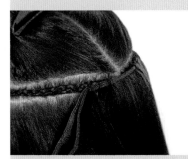

4 Using a weaving needle; sew the weft onto the track using a stocking stitch technique.

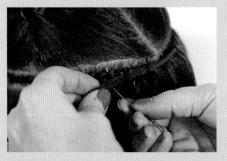

5 Repeat steps 2–5 creating and sewing another track just below the occipital bone and then again from temple to temple. Ensure the parted sections curve with the shape of the head.

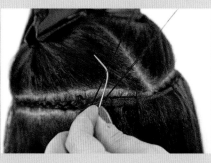

6 Parted sections.

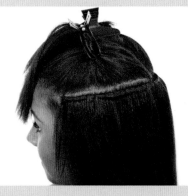

7 Cornrow.

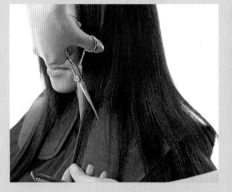

8 As with any hair extension technique the look is not complete unless the hair has been cut into shape. Use texturing techniques to blend the extensions with the client's natural hair.

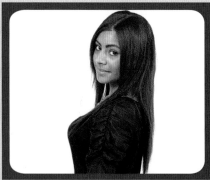

9 The finished extended look.

HEALTH & SAFETY

Always perform a tensile test to ensure a client's suitability for the service. This is where the strength of the hair is tested at the scalp in various different areas to ensure they have the strength to hold the weight of the hair extension.

TOP TIP

Recommend different hair extension techniques for clients to suit their requirements. For example, some clients may be allergic to the nickel in the clips of hair extensions, so another hair extension application method should be offered.

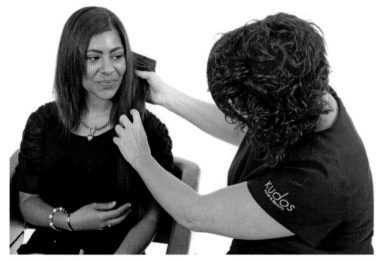
Consultation including suitability for type of hair extensions

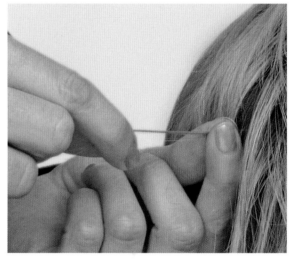
Tensile testing to check elasticity and strength of hair

Realistic expectations of what can be achieved with hair extensions

As a make-up artist, time will not be on your side. Generally you will use clip-in or glued extensions to create your desired results.

For a long-term performance/production, an actor may have permanent hair extensions applied by a professional. You may have to arrange for the actor to have the extensions rotated or removed by a professional.

Maintaining hair extensions

Always use recommended brushes and shampoos as defined by the manufacturer. Provide the client with after care advice and explain how to remove the extensions.

ACTIVITY

Research different brands of hair extensions currently available on the market.

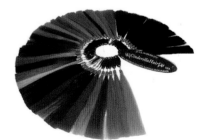
Colour match

Types of hair extensions

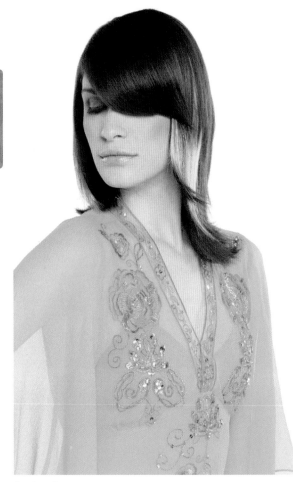

Pre-taped

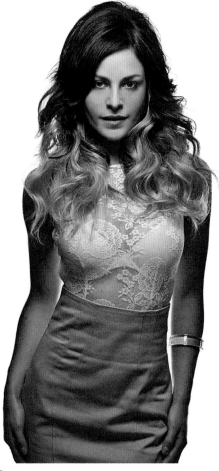

Sewn

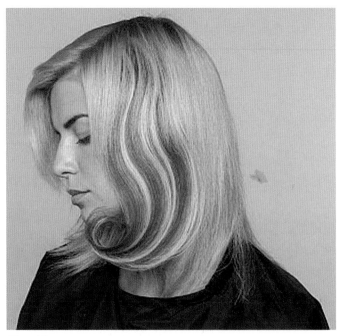

Clipped-in

CASE PROFILE: HOLLY EDWARDS, MAKE-UP ARTIST

How long have you been working in the industry?

I have been working in the industry for seven years.

How did you get into the industry?

After training on the one-year Course at Delamar Academy, I was very fortunate to be given an amazing work experience placement assisting a make-up designer on a feature film. I worked closely alongside her and was given my first glimpse of the industry. It was only then that I realised the extent of sheer dedication, hard work and skill that is required, a large proportion of which is behind the scenes. This gave me the opportunity to network within the industry. As a result of which I made some valuable contacts – some of whom I proceeded to work with over the next few years on films such as *Alice in Wonderland*, *Clash of the Titans* and *John Carter on Mars*. I am indebted to those people who enabled me to learn and grow with them.

What has been your most significant project?

Working in the hair department on *Game of Thrones* has been a big part of my life for the past four years. Having worked in the crowd department for the last three seasons, I am honoured to have joined the main team hair department. I am loving being a part of such an iconic show and it's been a pleasure to have worked on such a creative project with so many talented colleagues.

What do you enjoy most about the job?

The best part of the job has to be the buzz of seeing a production in the making behind the scenes and being privy to all the ins and outs – the blood, sweat and tears and all the excitement of creating something wonderful. Knowing you were a part of it makes you feel very privileged. Crew members become like family to you when working on long projects and I have had a great time building strong friendships and spending time with, and learning from, some extremely talented industry professionals.

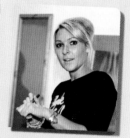

What do you enjoy least about the job?

The hours are usually long and it's perfectly normal to start work at 3 a.m. – sometimes for months at a time! But I'm used to it by now and I wouldn't change my job for anything.

What advice would you give to a new make-up artist starting out?

To a new make-up artist, the best advice I could give is perseverance. At times it's tough when starting out, trying to make ends meet and getting the experience you need – we've all been there! I think in reality, a make-up team just wants to have a trainee who is simply nice to be around – be helpful, be happy, be friendly and the rest will come. Be willing to put yourself out there and grab every opportunity which arises and always remember you never know who you're talking to and where your next job might come from. I once landed a great job through a woman I met on a bus who had a sister who was a producer!

REVISION QUESTIONS

1 What is a 'tensile test' and why would this be performed?

2 What product may a client be allergic to when applying hair extensions?

3 What hairdressing services are not usually part of a make-up artist's remit?

4 Describe four hair-up styles.

5 How will you determine a client's hair type?

5 Body art and airbrushing

LEARNING OBJECTIVES

This chapter covers the following:

◆ Body painting techniques, including brush and sponge and additional media.

◆ Freehand drawing and painting techniques used in body art.

◆ Planning and preparing the design for a body art application.

◆ Care of the model.

◆ Removing body paint.

◆ Airbrushing in body art: basic knowledge and make-up techniques.

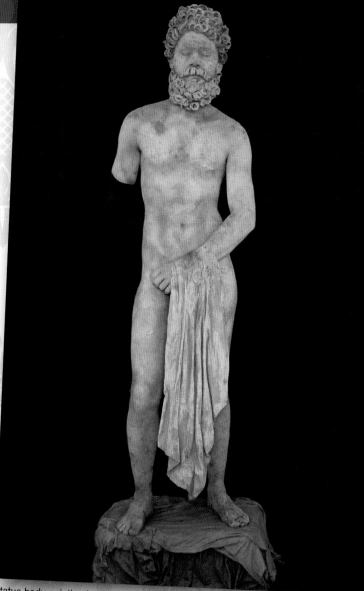

Statue body painting by Giorgio Galliero

KEY TERM

Chinese brushes

UNIT TITLE

◆ Research the creative aspects of the design concept

INTRODUCTION

This unit will introduce you to two different make-up elements required in the media industry. These are body art techniques and airbrushing. Body art techniques are covered in Level 2 and Level 3. Airbrushing techniques are covered in Level 3 only. You will look at different tools and products used in body art. For successful looks it is essential to plan and prepare the services beforehand, which will be discussed in this unit. Care of the model is very important for your results. Home care advice should be given after these services to ensure no contra-actions are produced after the treatments. This chapter covers all the processes required to use, clean and strip an airbrush. Basic make-up and exciting fantasy looks can be created with these techniques – the freedom is yours to create!

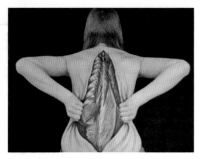

Painted body ripping

Body art

Body art is the technique of painting any effect, from a simple tattoo on the arm to a reproduction of a famous painting across an entire body, or even painting someone nude to look fully clothed.

To be successful in this highly creative niche, an arts background is desirable – or at least a familiarity with the skills of drawing and painting.

Areas of work include fashion, advertising, commercials, music videos, television, films, corporate events, competitions and high-end parties.

Since the process of body art is very time-consuming it is essential to plan the design on paper, and then try it on a model in advance. The materials used for body art are special watercolours, alcohol or silicone for the skin, available from professional make-up shops. These are supplied in liquids, creams and palettes of various colours. The tools used to apply the body paints are various sponges, brushes or any type of tool which gives the desired effect, including airbrushing. Stencils are useful for repeat patterns; masking tape is used to provide a clean edge effect; stipple sponges for textures; and feathers for marbling effects. For a statue look, a large natural sponge will stipple the effect of stone.

Chinese brushes are good for marbled effects, similar to using feathers. Specialist books on creating paint effects for furniture are a useful reference. So long as you use body art products instead of normal paint, you can employ the same techniques for gilding and tortoiseshell effects.

When painting clothes on the body, an idea that is used frequently in photography and advertising, you can use a combination of painting with artists' brushes, stipple and airbrushing techniques.

Body painting is truly an art, giving enormous potential for freedom of expression and imaginative use of different make-up techniques.

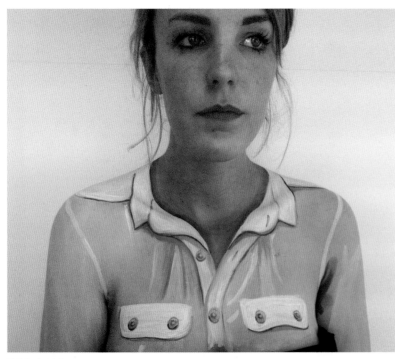

Painted shirt

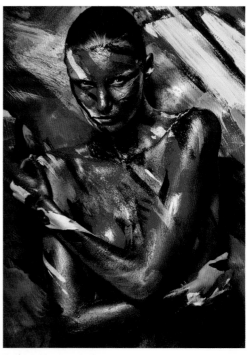

Colourful body painting

Body art techniques

The techniques used for face and body art are:

◆ freehand drawing and painting

◆ airbrushing

◆ a combination of freehand and airbrushing.

Freehand drawing and painting

Tools & equipment

◆ **brushes** all sizes, rounded, flat, pointed.

◆ **feathers** for delicate stone effects.

◆ **masking tape** for a clean edge.

◆ **specialist books** on creating interior design paint finishes on walls and furniture, for ideas on gilding, tortoiseshell effects, stencils, etc. substitute the industrial paint materials for body paints.

◆ **sponges** sea sponges, stipple sponges.

◆ **stencils** for repeat patterns.

It is important to remember that no other products should be used on the face or body other than those made for the purpose. Always read the manufacturer's instructions. This includes products for the hair, e.g. glitter and sparkle, as they will not be suitable to use on the skin.

Body art products

Water-based paints, made especially for use on the face and body, are available from professional make-up shops in various colours. The colour range includes glitter and sparkle. They are all used by diluting them with water, and come in different forms such as:

◆ **Liquid** In small bottles.

◆ **Cream** In small jars.

◆ **Palettes** In paintbox form; different colours in small compact form.

◆ **Lip and eye pencils** Used for drawing outlines of shapes before painting.

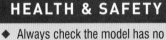

HEALTH & SAFETY

All body art products must comply with REACH (the European Registration, Evaluation, Authorisation and Restriction of Chemicals) to ensure they are safe and suitable for use.

HEALTH & SAFETY

◆ Always check the model has no allergies to face paints as some products can be highly pigmented. A patch test is advisable. Ensure all products are in-date, even water-based products can cause sensitivity on the skin when out of date.

◆ Ensure extra caution when applying paint/glitter around the eye area.

◆ Ensure your model is not wearing contact lenses as glitter can get caught behind the lens and cause great irritation.

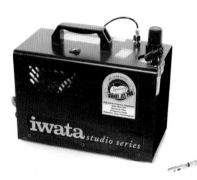

Airbrush and compressor

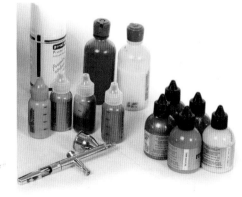

Products and equipment used for airbrushing

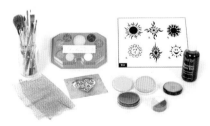

Body painting products

TOP TIP

Spattering techniques are also useful for camouflage. This will help to add different colour, texture and depth – especially good for freckles.

Spatter painting in body art

Spattering is when a shower of tiny dots of paint are flicked from a brush to cover an area with a spray of minute droplets of paint. The size of the spatter can be controlled by altering the distance between brush and support, and also by the choice of brush and the consistency of the paint. A toothbrush is a useful spattering tool. Hold the brush 7.5–10 cm away from the surface, load the brush with paint and then pull your thumb across the bristles. If you want to spatter a specific area, mask it off with newspaper.

A decorator's brush, loaded with diluted paint and simply flicked onto the surface will create a large-sized spatter. Either pull the thumb across the bristles, or bring down the handle of the brush onto your other hand so that the paint sprays forwards.

Spattering is a useful technique for body art, using body paints for the effects. It is also used for spattering blood in casualty effects, and artworking prosthetics for a very natural looking texture. Used by artists in watercolours for a softening effect, it has been taken by make-up artists and reworked into make-up design to good effect.

Tools & equipment

- ◆ **brushes** different shapes and sizes are available from art shops and professional make-up suppliers.
- ◆ **eyelash glue** for sticking sequins, or light body ornamentations onto the skin.
- ◆ **plastic stencils** made from plastic supplied by the roll, with adhesive backing, available from good stationery shops.
- ◆ **sponges** natural sea sponges, stippling sponges.

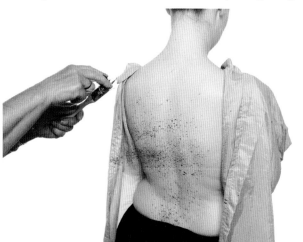

Spattering

Planning the design

- ◆ **Research** Look through magazines, television adverts and the Internet until you have an idea.
- ◆ **Plan the idea** Do sketches, make notes, work out how you will do it.
- ◆ **Trial session** Spend time trying out the idea on your model. When you are satisfied, take photos.

Preparing for body art

- ◆ Lay out your workstation with all the tools and materials needed for the design.
- ◆ Make sure you have everything ready.
- ◆ If the temperature is cool, have a heater nearby to keep your model warm.
- ◆ Supply your model with a dressing gown to stay warm when she has a break.
- ◆ Cover exposed windows/doors to maintain client modesty. Consider putting a note on the door to avoid unannounced entrances.
- ◆ Consider using folding screens/curtains to maintain modesty.

TOP TIP

Creating a mood board is an excellent tool for planning a body art service. This visual aid will help to pull all the ideas together.

HEALTH & SAFETY

When planning your design consider elements where your client can sit down and have a comfort break.

ACTIVITY

Additional media in a design

Use additional media such as feathers, lace, fishnet tights and much more to create different textures within a design.

Add glitters, sequins and gems to make a three-dimensional effect. Consider what effect the added media has on your design.

TOP TIP

When using additional media always ensure the adhesive has been patch tested on the client 24 hours prior to service.

STEP-BY-STEP: BODY PAINTING BACK STENCIL BY ALEXA RAVINA

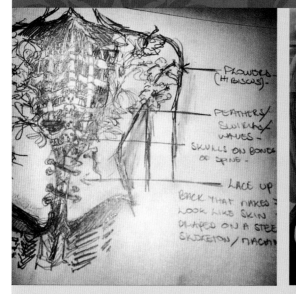

1 Sketch of design on paper.

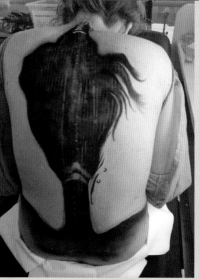

2 Paint and airbrush the outline on the body.

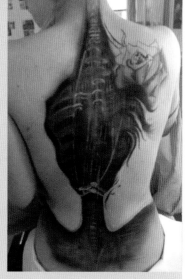

3 Start to fill in detail with colour.

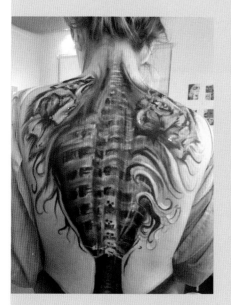

4 Build up the layers with lighting and shading.

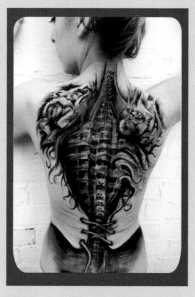

5 Final details to be added for finished result.

Body art projects

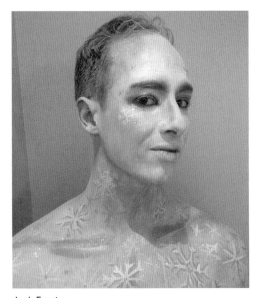

Jack Frost

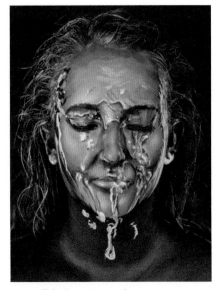

Dripping water on face

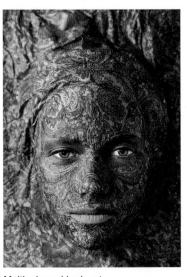

Multicoloured body art

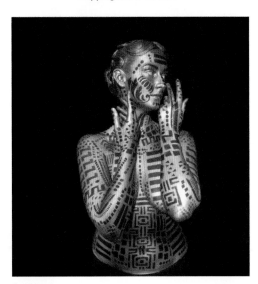

Gold body art

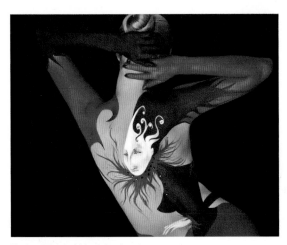

Red, white and black body art

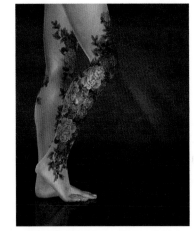

Rose tattoo body art

Airbrushing in body art

Airbrushing is perfect for body art effects. It gives fast coverage and delivers a finer film of colour than using the brush and sponge method. It is used not only for fantasy effects but also for contouring shadows on the human body.

It is also useful for a final finish to tie a look together on top of brushwork and sponged effects. It can give a fast, even-coloured background with hand-painted detail on top. Excellent for spraying hair instead of using aerosol can sprays, it can also produce perfect looking lines when sprayed against masked-off areas. Stencils can be used to create textures, shapes, patterns and fine detail within your design. Stencils will also help to speed up the body art service.

The airbrush

There are two types of airbrush:

◆ The airbrush that works with an electric compressor. This type is available in different shapes and sizes with silencers, fans and extra fittings. The airbrushes have different storage facilities for the make-up. Some have a small well on top of the brush for smaller areas. Some have small jars that attach to the bottom of the airbrush to contain the make-up; these are good for covering larger areas. Some have both attachments. This type of airbrush is more commonly used in industry. Ensure you are set up within reachable distance of electric plug sockets.

◆ Also available are the smaller, more portable kits in which the airbrush propellant comes in the form of a gas can. These are less expensive in outlay, but the cost of the gas cans adds up if used regularly.

Both types are good, but the compressor set-up can achieve a more detailed effect – although it is more expensive and less portable.

The ventilation should be efficient when airbrushing, to prevent inhaling airborne paint vapour.

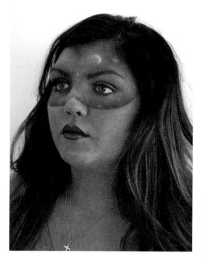
Fantasy airbrushing

Care of the model during body art

1 Allow regular breaks for your model.

2 Provide drinks at frequent intervals: water, tea, coffee, whatever is appropriate.

3 Make sure the temperature is comfortable – not too cold or too hot.

4 For the model's comfort, any areas on the face that need painting around (the eyes, nose or mouth) should be done last.

5 Provide a mask, if necessary, to avoid your model inhaling airborne paint vapour.

6 Make sure the ventilation is sufficient.

7 At the end of the session let your model walk around to stretch their legs while you set up an area for taking your photographs.

When you have finished, take photographs of the final effect. Choose the background carefully, taking into account the colours used and type of design.

HEALTH & SAFETY

When using an airbrush always follow the requirements set out in the Electricity at Work Act. Ensure there are no trailing wires, equipment is stored safely, training is given and all airbrushes are PAT tested in line with current legislation.

TOP TIP

Airbrushing a full body can take hours to complete. Models often become cold during the process as they are sitting or standing still for long periods of time. Keep checking your model is comfortable and make suitable adjustments to make them comfortable.

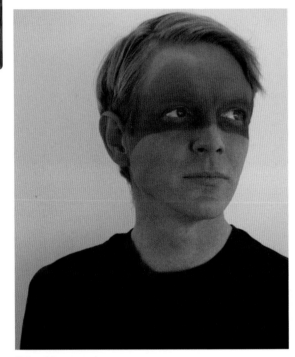

Airbrushing a mask

Removing the body make-up

Normally a shower is the only way to remove the make-up, but soap, sponges or a flannel with a large bowl of warm water will also do the job. Depending on the type of product that has been used in the body art application, you will need to consider the following options for removal:

◆ **Water-based body make-up** Removed in a shower with soap-based products or make-up wipes.

◆ **Silicone-based body make-up** Removed in a shower with soap-based products or make-up wipes.

◆ **Alcohol-based body make-up** Removed in the shower with oil-based removers or shower gels with a high percentage of alcohol.

◆ **Exfoliation** An effective technique for removing body art.

Ensure the shower is rinsed and any excess paint or water is removed from the shower tray. Make sure the shower area is completely clean after use – especially if it is in shared facilities or facilities that are not your own. Have towels ready for your model after showering.

CASE PROFILE: RAPHAELLE FIELDHOUSE, MAKE-UP ARTIST

How long have you been working in the industry?

I had already been face and body painting for seven years before I set up Body Canvas (www.bodycanvas.co.uk) back in 1999.

How did you get into the industry?

Looking back, make-up is something I was always interested in – I had my first kit around the age of nine. I was inspired to teach myself brush and sponge techniques after having my own face painted several years later. I started with face painting but never saw a reason to stop at the jawline or to restrict the artform to children's events.

Did you have a lucky break or turning point?

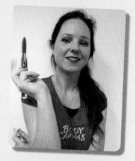

In 2004 I started competitive body art with my husband. We went on to win or be placed highly in every event we went to. This gave us international recognition of our level of skill and I have been on the jury panel for many body art competitions since. Having a good reputation has led to work passing those skills on through teaching classes all over the world.

What has been your most significant project(s)?

My competitive projects have always been significant both in satisfaction with the creative process and the worldwide acclaim that comes from winning. More recently the projects that give me complete artistic freedom and enough time to prepare have been the ones that I have really enjoyed and have produced good images.

What do you enjoy most about the job?

Stepping back from a finished piece of work and feeling pleased with it, seeing people's reactions to it. Plus the difference between what I do and a piece of canvas art or a sculpture is that once I am finished it really does come alive. The model's movements change the shape of what is painted and give added meaning or style to the design. Collaboration with dancers and performance artists are the most rewarding.

What do you enjoy least about the job?

Lack of time. Quite often the make-up artist is given an hour to do hair and make-up but they expect me to do the entire body in just two hours!

How has the industry changed during your career?

My work has mainly been in the entertainment and marketing industries, providing live artwork for varied events. Over the years I have noticed that new bookings are coming in more and more last minute, as clients wait until their budgets are finalised before even enquiring – though established customers book a year in advance for fear of me missing their event.

What advice would you give to a new make-up artist starting out?

Always carry your business cards with you – and remember to give them out! I have had work from a card given out years before, passed from one person to the next until it reached the relevant person. Work hard and always aim to be professional in everything you do.

Airbrushing

We are fortunate to have Raphaelle Fieldhouse, our expert on airbrushing who teaches at Delamar Academy, as a guest writer. Here she explains in detail the theory and key make-up techniques used for airbrushing.

The airbrush is a great tool for applying make-up, giving a wide range of effects from sheer and natural to more dramatic looks. It has a very fine application making it particularly suitable for HD (high definition) cameras. With practice it is possible to achieve beautifully subtle blending and shading both on the face and body. With good cleanliness, it is also a very hygienic application system as the tool never comes in direct contact with the skin.

Types of airbrush make-up

There are three main types of airbrush make-up. They all have different bases/mediums and it is very important to know what base your product has in order to use the correct solvent for cleaning. Never mix different mediums together in the brush as they separate (like salad dressing) and will clog the airbrush. However it is possible to layer different mediums on the skin as long as the brush is cleaned well in-between.

Water-based airbrush make-up

Easy to use and clean. It washes off with water, making it less durable than other mediums.

Silicone-based airbrush make-up

The most popular base for airbrush foundations. It is more durable than water-based products, making it great for long-wearing shoots and bridal make-up. Silicone-based cleanser must be used to clean the airbrush. Make-up remover is needed for washing the skin.

Alcohol-based airbrush make-up

The most durable make-up product as it is both waterproof and wear resistant. It is great for humid conditions and underwater work. Alcohol-based products should not be used on the face, delicate body parts or on laser resurfaced skin. Be particularly careful to ensure good ventilation to avoid inhaling vapours or getting alcohol in the eyes. Isopropyl alcohol (IPA) must be used to clean the airbrush and the skin.

HEALTH & SAFETY

- ◆ Never airbrush into the eyes, ears, mouth or nose – if this happens by accident seek medical attention.
- ◆ Eyes should always be closed during application.
- ◆ Ensure all airbrush products are clearly labelled and are suitable for use on the skin (no acrylics such as Createx or graphics inks).
- ◆ Make sure that the airbrush is cleaned well and flushed through with IPA when changing between mediums, i.e. alcohol, silicone and water-based products.
- ◆ Never use the airbrush without a nozzle cap in place – the needle can seriously damage someone.
- ◆ Always make sure there is suitable ventilation in the make-up room.
- ◆ Always use a suitable pot for colour change and cleaning in order to minimise excess airborne product.
- ◆ Always ensure the compressor is on a stable flat surface.
- ◆ Be aware of trailing cables and air hoses. Try and keep all products easily to hand to avoid getting tangled in the air hose!

Make-up techniques

Colour mixing

Most products can be mixed if they have the same base, for best results use the same brand product. Add several drops of the different colours to the cup and back-bubble to mix. Test as usual on the jawline for colour match.

Preparation

Prepare the skin as you would normally, paying particular attention to removing all traces of mascara as this prevents the make-up from getting to the under-eye area. Special moisturiser can be applied through the airbrush. If using normal moisturiser ensure it is oil-free.

Conceal blemishes with a small amount of airbrush foundation using a conventional brush, blending the edges well and making sure to only cover the blemish. With practice it is possible to use the airbrush.

Foundation

Once you are happy with the colour match, keep the airbrush in your eyeline and spray downwards on the face, this will make the fine downy facial hair lie flatter and feels more comfortable for the model. Ten drops is usually sufficient product for face and neck foundation. Hold the airbrush around 10–15 cm from the skin with the psi no more than 7–10. Always start with just air so that the face relaxes, before pulling the trigger back to apply the product. If the model is tense or screws up their face, the make-up creates a very wrinkled and crêpey look around the eyes. Smooth out straight away with a blending brush as airbrush foundation dries very quickly and is impossible to touch up once it has dried. For best results airbrush slowly, evenly, smoothly and continuously across the face. Work methodically so that all areas of skin are covered. Build up the product slowly, stepping back frequently to see the overall effect. Make sure that the face is well lit and check in the mirror to see the effect.

Contouring

Once the foundation is finished, contour the face with highlights and shadows applied in drastically lighter and darker shades of foundation. It is better to use a sheer cover of a very dark colour than building up a thick coverage. Shimmer products can be used to highlight and bronze, but be careful not to give an all-over shiny or sweaty look. Blusher can also be applied with the airbrush. Practice ensures that the product ends up where it is meant to be. Always make sure that the airbrush is pointing directly at the area to be covered – a slight change in angle could mean a red nose rather than a healthy blush!

Eyes

Lower the psi to around 2–5 for eyeshadow application, products may need to be diluted slightly to avoid spattering. Hold the airbrush much closer to the skin to get the maximum detail and accuracy. With the face relaxed and eyes shut, gently pull up the model's eyebrow to tighten the skin. Again, concentrate on the angle of spray to avoid getting colour above the eyebrow and leaving a void where your thumb is. Make sure the eyes are kept shut until the product is dried to avoid creasing. For dramatic effects, eyebrow shape can be stencilled, otherwise shape and darken freehand.

Finishing

Eyeliner, mascara and lip colour should all be applied with conventional tools. Gently wipe any product over-spray off the hair and mens' facial hair. For a matte look, a touch of translucent powder can be used to set the make-up. For a dewy look, Jojoba oil can be sprayed through the airbrush. For a wet or sweaty look, spray glycerine through the airbrush for a fine mist or use a pump spray bottle for larger droplets.

STEP-BY-STEP: AIRBRUSH MAKE-UP APPLICATION

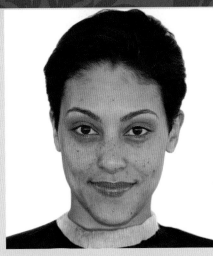

1 Before airbrush make-up application

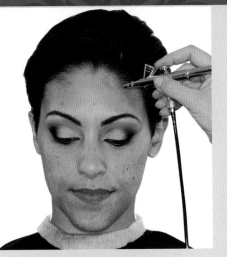

2 Airbrush foundation application

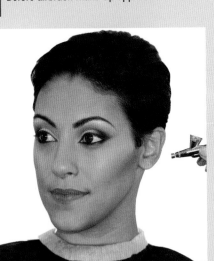

3 Airbrush contouring application

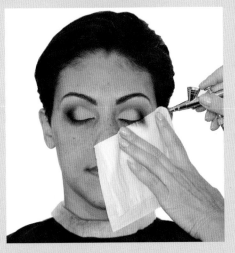

4 Airbrush eye make-up application

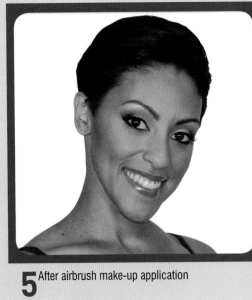

5 After airbrush make-up application

Airbrush basics

Different types of airbrush

The airbrush is the small metal tool through which the product is applied. It must be connected to a compressor or tank of compressed air via an air hose.

Single-action airbrush

When the button is pressed, both air and product are released simultaneously, similar to a can of spray paint. It is difficult to vary the brush strokes with this type of brush so it is best for areas of similar coverage, i.e. spray tan.

Dual-action airbrush

Press the trigger down to release air and pull back to release product. The distance that the trigger is pulled governs the amount of product that comes out. This gives the most control for all the required effects.

Gravity feed/top feed

The product is dispensed from a cup in the top of the airbrush. Cups come in different sizes and are easily accessed for topping up/changing colours. This is the best type for make-up as only small amounts of each colour are needed.

Bottom feed

The product is dispensed from a bottle attached to the bottom of the airbrush. This is best when a lot of product is needed. Bottles can be swapped to change colours.

Side feed

The product dispenser is attached via a side connector enabling either a cup or bottle to be used. This is very versatile but slightly harder to clean.

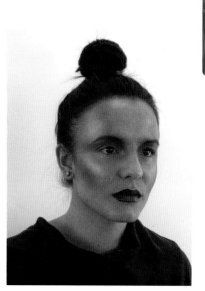

Beauty make-up by airbrush

Compressor

The compressor compresses air to a given pressure in order to blow particles of product out of the airbrush. Electricity is needed to power the compressor. Larger compressors have a tank which keeps the pressure until it is all used up, then the motor kicks back in to top it up. This means that it can be used continuously on larger projects or multiple models without the motor overheating. Smaller compressors are much lighter and more portable but the motor needs to run continuously to give air pressure, these are better suited to

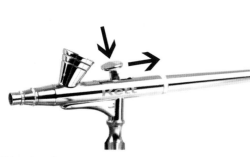

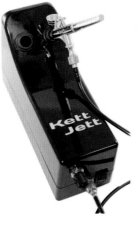

Airbrush and compressor

fewer make-ups or on-set work, they also tend to give lower pressure. Where there is no access to electricity it is possible to use small canisters or tanks of compressed air though these are not as reliable and are harder to control.

Pressure gauge

Most compressors have a pressure gauge that shows the psi of the air coming out of the hose. This is very helpful to see whether the correct pressure is being used or not. It is only a guide so it is always sensible to check the pressure on yourself before airbrushing your client/model. Smaller compressors do not have a gauge but the pressure can still be varied via a small dial.

Moisture trap

Larger compressors can also have a moisture trap that is useful when working in a moist or humid environment. This is less important when working with water-based products but very handy for not contaminating silicone or other hydrophobic products.

Basic airbrush principles and techniques

There are a lot of variables with an airbrush that do not need to be considered with a conventional brush. This gives an enormous amount of control and means that a lot of different effects can be achieved, although it takes a while to master. The following description is for dual-action models of airbrush. Hold the airbrush balanced on your middle finger and supported by your thumb. Your index finger is then free to operate the trigger. It is important not to grip too tightly in order to ensure a good flowing movement.

Narrow spray pattern

Small dot, narrow dash spray pattern

Large dot, wide dash spray pattern

Finger position

Press the air button down to release the air, then at the same time pull it back to release the product. The further it is pulled back the more product is released.

Airbrush position

The distance that the brush is held from the surface governs how wide the spray pattern is. To get a very fine line, hold the brush very close to the surface and hardly pull back the trigger at all. To get wide even coverage, hold the brush quite far from the surface and pull the trigger as far back as possible.

Bearing this in mind it is possible to create 'dagger strokes' that start and end with a point by moving the airbrush closer, further away and then closer whilst also pulling the trigger back a little, a bit more and then back again.

Speed of movement

The speed with which you move the airbrush affects the amount of product that settles on the surface. Therefore, if you linger in one spot while spraying a line, that area will be darker or if you speed up, that area will be lighter.

Wrist position

The angle that you hold your wrist affects where the airbrush is pointed, the slightest change in your wrist makes a big difference to where the product goes and how even the coverage is. For even coverage make sure that the airbrush is pointing straight at the surface. Where the surface is curved (e.g. an arm or forehead) remember to change angle as you are spraying. If the airbrush is held at an angle there will be more product at the nearest side and it will blend away on the furthest side.

Air pressure

Air pressure has an impact not only on the visual effect of make-up but on its safety. For the purposes of body art the air pressure should never exceed 20 psi, for face make-up no more than 12 psi and for eye make-up no more than 2–5 psi. The correct consistency of product will come out smoothly at the correct pressure; if the pressure is reduced a splattery or freckled effect can be achieved. When working at lower pressures it is sometimes necessary to dilute the product to avoid a speckled texture if it isn't wanted.

Back-bubbling/colour mixing

To mix two different colours or to dilute a product, put both products in the cup/bottle. Put your finger or a paper tissue tightly over the end of the nozzle to prevent the air coming out then press down and slowly pull your trigger finger back. This will force the air back up into the product cup creating bubbles and mixing the contents together. This technique is used to mix different colours, dilute a product with its solvent and to rinse the brush between colours.

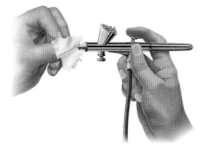

The back-bubble method is used to clean the airbrush after use

Cleaning

It is possible to simply spray though the remaining colour, rinse with solvent then add in the next colour. But it is important to thoroughly clean the airbrush between contrasting colours, or after pearl/metallic colours, to prevent contamination and even more essential to clean thoroughly when you have finished using the airbrush. Due to the very precise mechanics of an airbrush, the needle perfectly fits the tube that it sits in. When the needle is pulled back a tiny gap is created for the product to flow past it and spray out. If the smallest amount of dried product or a particle of glitter gets stuck it will block the airbrush and stop it from working properly. To start, rinse the airbrush by back-bubbling with the relevant solvent and tipping the waste product back out of the cup. Continue doing this and spraying into a cleaning pot until the spray is clear. Then dismantle the airbrush and clean each part individually. Reassemble the back-bubble with solvent, spray onto a clean paper towel, then take out the needle and wipe it on the paper. It should not leave any marks or hints of colour; if it does repeat the process until clean.

The sections about airbrushing on pages 109-113 were written by Raphaelle Fieldhouse.

ACTIVITY

Airbrushing technique

To help learn technique and control perform the following exercises on white paper.

◆ Make a pencil grid on paper, the aim is to perfectly get a dot in the centre of the crosses.
◆ Using the airbrush make five different shapes on the paper.
◆ Using the airbrush practise writing your name to get an even flow of make-up.

REVISION QUESTIONS

1 Research the terms 'PSI' and 'BAR'.

2 List five considerations for your model during body art services.

3 What are the limitations to using the airbrush?

4 What is the most suitable environment for airbrushing?

5 Research the PPE required for airbrushing.

6 Working in theatre

LEARNING OBJECTIVES

This chapter covers the following:

◆ Hair and make-up skills for theatre.

◆ Products required and preparation needed.

◆ Establishing a design and maintaining continuity.

◆ Maintaining the make-up.

◆ The effects of lighting.

◆ Live-to-cinema relays.

◆ Working conditions and auditorium sizes.

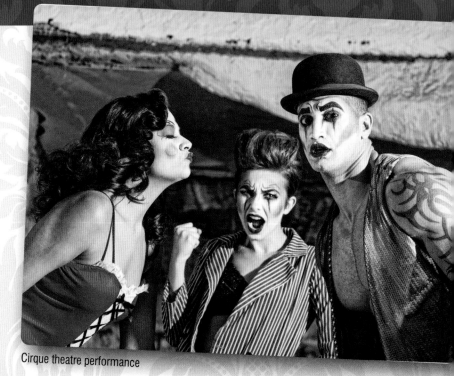
Cirque theatre performance

KEY TERMS

Gelatine

Modelling tools

Mortician's wax

Sealer

Witch hazel

UNIT TITLE

◆ Prepare to change the performer's appearance

◆ Assist with the continuity of the performer's appearance

◆ Apply make-up to change the performer's appearance

INTRODUCTION

In this unit you will cover all the requirements for working in the theatre. You will look at the different hair and make-up skills required and understand the importance of preparation and continuity. You will learn to establish design plans and understand how working with others, such as costume designers, actors and lighting technicians, will help you with your work.

There are many technical aspects to working in the theatre, including the effects of lighting, which are covered in this chapter. You will learn how to enhance the performer's or model's features with the use of modelling wax and casualty effects that may be required when working in theatre. You will also explore the elements of live-to-cinema relays. This chapter covers Level 3 media units and preparing to work in this disciplined area of the industry.

Working in theatre

The history of theatre dates back to ancient times as the earliest form of entertainment from Shakespeare, music hall and burlesque, to the spectacular, sophisticated form of stagecraft today. Despite television, film and computer effects, there is no substitute for the experience of watching actors, singers and dancers perform live on stage. Each performance is unique and the excitement generated by an appreciative audience creates a buzz which is only experienced in this area of entertainment.

The importance of hair skills

To work in theatre, the make-up artist must have hair skills in modern hairstyling and period wigs. The make-up and hair designer is known as the wig master or wig mistress.

The make-up

Stage make-up needs to be clearly defined and broader strokes are needed to provide definition, especially in opera where the performers are cast for their voices and not how they look. Contouring is used to good effect, and placement of colour is used to emphasise facial features.

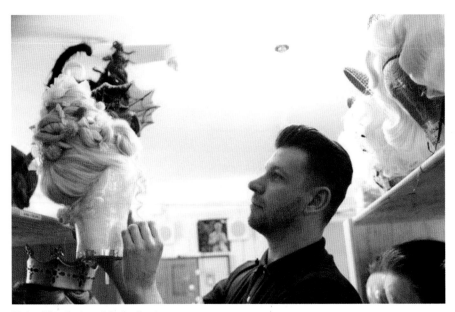

Stefan Musch at work in the theatre

Products

The products used are the same as for television, with many of the actors working across the media having their own preferences for make-up, hair and skin products.

Preparation

The wig master/mistress refers to the production designer who decides on the 'look' of the sets, costumes, lighting, hair and make-up. The overall design having been set, it is up to the various department heads to design and work out how to apply and maintain the required image. The wig master/mistress takes into account the practical needs of the production, such as quick changes, how many assistants are needed and ordering stock, wigs and facial hair.

Establishing the design

During rehearsals – both dress and technical – the lighting, costume, hair and make-up designs are adjusted as the show is watched from the audience point-of-view. Collaboration with the director, actors, lighting and costume designers ensure that the details are perfected. The show is viewed from the audience seating, usually the middle of the house.

Maintaining the design continuity

Once the style and method of working have been established, the routine is rigidly upheld. With two performances a day the show has to run like a well-oiled machine. If it goes on tour to different venues in other countries, the formula must remain the same. When local make-up artists are employed on tour they are taught exactly how the wigs are set, make-ups applied and every detail of the quick changes. Sometimes there are only two or three minutes to change an actor's costume, hair and make-up backstage. Quite often in productions there will be a quick-change area that is set very close to the side of the stage. Here the make-up and costumes will be ready, saving actors time as they will not need to go to their dressing room. The make-up artist must stand in the same place at precisely the same time for each performance, and change the hair and make-up in exactly the same way every time. The performer depends on this strict continuity. Wherever the show is performing it must be identical down to the last hairpin.

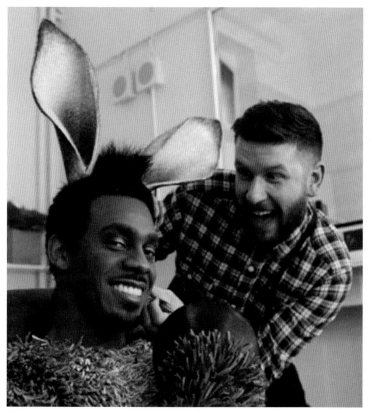

Stefan Musch working on *Shrek the Musical*

Maintaining the make-up

Another important aspect of the make-up is that it has to last without touch-ups throughout the entire scene. Whether dancing, singing or fight scenes, the wigs must not fall off and the make-up must not run. This is often a challenge for the make-up department. For example, if the dancers have to change from one look to another, it might be easier to remove water-based make-up quicker than oil-based creams. But watercolours are tricky because they run when dancers sweat. Powder make-up would be better, but powder can cause dancers to slip if it gets on the floor or on their feet. Pressed powders are recommended for safety and quickness. The safety of the cast is a priority. The wig master/mistress has to make many decisions before the final rehearsal.

Work prospects

For anyone wishing to work in theatre, it is best to contact the wig master/mistress at a local theatre in order to gain some work experience. Many make-up artists with hair skills begin their careers in this way. To learn from an experienced wig master/mistress is the best possible training. It is easy to cross from theatre to television and film by doing crowd work. Film make-up designers often hire theatre assistants for big crowd scenes because of their ability to work swiftly under pressure. Throughout the media, theatre is recognised as the most disciplined craft of all, employing dedicated, creative people.

TOP TIP

Set all make-ups with a fixing spray.

HEALTH & SAFETY

All make-up artists working in theatre must have public liability insurance to safe guard themselves and the actors.

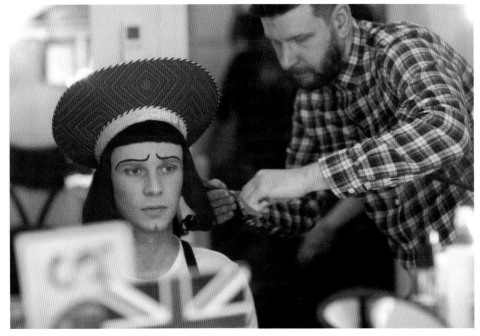

Stefan Musch working on *Shrek the Musical*

Live-to-cinema relays

Many theatre productions are shown live in cinemas. HD cameras are used to film stage performances, which are then shown in the cinema in real time. This involves a film crew moving into the theatre and collaborating with the theatre technicians. The desired effect is not a film but an authentic theatre production. Adjustments are needed to tone down an over-theatrical make-up or obvious hair laces on wigs that do not look good in close-ups. This is a highly skilful co-operation between film and theatre and the process is best described by Robin Lough, our guest writer.

CASE PROFILE: ROBIN LOUGH , MUSIC DIRECTOR AND PRODUCER

Robin Lough is an award-winning director who has worked in all areas of television arts and entertainment. His documentary work includes films about André Previn, David Putnam and Joan Miro, and he was a producer/director on the seminal BBC Arts series, *The Shock of the New* written and presented by Robert Hughes.

Currently he is specialising in live-to-cinema relays and was responsible for the first transmissions from the National Theatre (*Phedre* starring Helen Mirren), the Royal Opera House (*Don Giovanni* with Simon Keenlyside in the title role), and most recently the Royal Shakespeare Company (*Richard II* starring David Tennant).

What are live-to-cinema relays?

'What you're doing isn't cinema and neither is it theatre. So what is it?'

The question came during a question and answer session following a screening of *Richard II* at the Barbican Cinema in London. It was the Royal Shakespeare Company's first venture into live-to-cinema relays of live theatre events and followed in the footsteps of the Metropolitan Opera in New York and the Royal Opera House and the National Theatre in London.

Live-to-cinema relays from the world's opera houses and theatres are now almost commonplace. Around the world, from New Zealand to Finland, there are audiences who book months in advance to sit in a cinema and watch David Tennant performing *Richard II* 'live' from the Stratford stage, or Helen Mirren reprising her role as the queen in *The Audience* from London's West End. So why has the relatively recent phenomenon been so successful, and how did it happen?

The techniques for filming opera and theatre have been around since the days of black-and-white television and generally involve five or six cameras. The camera operations work to a carefully detailed camera script, devised by the director. They are guided through several hundred shots by a script supervisor (who calls the shots) and a vision mixer (who switches the camera outputs). However, there are many crucial differences between those pioneering days of monochrome television and the sophisticated relays of 50 years later. Advances in lighting, sound and lens technology allow for far greater flexibility in the way events are filmed. Just look at an early colour presentation of a football match and compare it with the detailed coverage today. But now we use HD technology, first introduced in the 1990s, which allows electronic images to be transmitted to giant cinema screens with picture quality that is comparable to film.

The introduction of HD pictures was a qualitative breakthrough but it led to concerns in some quarters.

In the theatre, for example, actors were rightly concerned that a performance, developed and honed for the theatre auditorium would look mannered and exaggerated if it were transferred to a giant cinema screen.

Adjustments required when cameras were present

The National Theatre transmitted *Phedre* starring Helen Mirren, in 2009. It was the first live-to-cinema relay from the stage and was directed by Nicholas Hytner who is not only the National's artistic director, but also the man whose idea it was to bring live theatre to the big screen. Just before that first pioneering relay, he assembled his cast on the stage of the National's Lyttelton Theatre. 'We're not making a movie tonight,' he said, 'we're filming a stage production.'

For the actors it was a crucial definition. The cameras were there to convey the stage experience to an audience in the cinema. The actors were free to do what they did on that stage every other night of the week. But not all aspects of a theatre relay can be so easily accommodated.

Costume and make-up

Here the context of a stage production was not enough to excuse tired costumes, theatrical make-up or noticeable wig lines; all of which are, to a greater or lesser degree, acceptable to a theatre audience if only by virtue of physical distance. So a closer alliance developed between the stage and screen director, the costume and make-up departments, and the camera and sound supervisors. In preparation for a live-to-cinema relay, the stage performance is recorded once, generally without an audience in attendance, so that every department can see what works on screen, what doesn't and what needs attention.

Theatre make-up artists are frequently joined by film and television specialists during this process to work out what can be done to accommodate the demands of the HD images – this is the area where the demands of film/camera have to be met, there is no halfway house.

Shot sizes are discussed with the camera director, the position of radio microphones (frequently placed in the actor's wig) agreed with the sound department, and the general credibility of an actor's make-up considered in terms of cinema presentation. And, given the amount of time required to fine-tune an actor's make-up on a film set, it is a huge testament to the talents of film and theatre make-up artists that they can do a comparable job for a live-to-cinema relay in considerably less time.

Compromise between cinema and theatre

So do these live events require compromise from those taking part? I don't think so. Live-to-cinema relays are now as popular as mainstream cinema, partly because they are 'one-off' screenings (although repeat screenings also attract large audiences), and partly because they bring the added excitement of the live event.

No, it's not cinema, and it certainly isn't theatre. Peter Gelb at the Metropolitan Opera in New York described these relays as a new genre and perhaps he is right. Our techniques have been fashioned from both film and television but at the end of the day Nicholas Hytner is absolutely correct: with all the techniques and advanced technology at our disposal we're still filming a stage production.

The section on pages 121 and 122 was written by Robin Lough.

TOP TIP

Good time keeping, planning and preparation are vital to ensure the success of the production. The cast must be out on stage in perfect time with perfect changes of costume, hair and make-up.

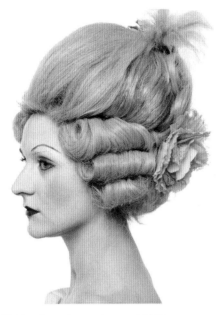

Eighteenth-century make-up and hair for theatre

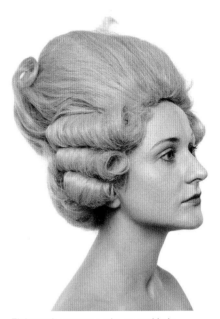

Eighteenth-century make-up and hair for television and film

CASE PROFILE: CAROLINE O'CONNOR, OPERA WIG AND MAKE-UP TEAM LEADER

How long have you been working in the industry?

I have worked in the theatrical industry since 2000. At the age of 30 I realised that it was time for a career change, from a sales and marketing executive. I had always been involved in amateur dramatics societies and loved the excitement and atmosphere that a live performance provided. Along with a life long interest in hair and make-up, I knew that the only option for me was to pursue a career incorporating both. I studied at Delamar Academy and was fortunate to be offered my first position with Pam Orange working on Matthew Bourne's *Swan Lake* and shortly afterwards I was offered my first permanent post with *The Lion King* as a junior make-up artist. I stayed within musical theatre until 2003 when I heard of a casual position at the Royal Opera House. On my first day, I realised that this was where I wanted to be and I am fortunate to say that 11 years on I am still there and enjoying every minute.

How did you get into the industry?

I am now a permanent member of the team and have been privileged to have worked with some of the world's leading opera singers, including Dame Kiri TeKanawa, Alfie Boe and Sir John Tomlinson. My work at the Royal Opera House is extremely varied as each production will have its own unique design. We currently put on about 18 productions a year so this offers much variety and scope for using our complete skill set.

What do you enjoy most about the job?

The most rewarding part of my role is to deliver a designer's vision. Sometimes the designs can be complicated and challenging and to see a designer really happy with my work is a wonderful feeling. It can however, be quite tricky if your performer has their own fixed ideas and they may not necessarily agree with the designer. My role is always to find a happy compromise.

What do you enjoy least about the job?

The one downside to working in theatre are the hours that are required. I work many evenings and am quite often not at home until midnight. Some weeks can be in excess of 60 hours, so socially it can be a bit difficult. I have had to miss out on many an event over the years, but I still wouldn't change what I do.

What advice would you give to a new make-up artist starting out?

It has taken me a few years to be completely confident in my abilities. Don't put yourself under too much pressure. Our art form is constantly evolving. Over the first few years absorb as much as you can. Observe other colleagues that you work with and be open to new ideas and different techniques. Finally, leave your troubles at home. A happy manner is infectious and when people like having you in their team, they tend to find a way of keeping you.

Basic principles of theatre make-up

The main considerations when applying make-up for the theatre are the distances involved and the colours normally used in theatrical lighting. Usually these are cold colours in the blue and green range. To deal with the distance between the actors and the audience, the make-up artists apply the make-up strongly and cleanly using the basic corrective techniques; strongly because both the strength of light and the distance will reduce the impact of the make-up; cleanly because otherwise the facial definition will fail to register at a distance.

To cope with the cool lighting the faces are made up with warmer tones of red and orange. The make-up should not be heavy or overdone. The foundation can be as lightly applied as for television and film. What matters is that the right colours are applied in the correct places to give definition to the face.

In general, the eye make-up should be stronger than would be normal for television or film, plus darker or brighter lipstick and stronger colour on the cheeks. The placing must be exact, and the blending subtle. Corrective lighting and shading or contouring can be used effectively because there are no close-ups in theatre.

Effects of theatre lighting on the make-up

The lighting is usually set at a 45-degree angle to the stage to counteract any shadows. Overhead lighting is also used. These lights are operated and changed during the performance. Colour gels such as 'mid sapphire blue' are used over the lights. These bleach the make-up, draining colour from the faces, which is why more red and other warm colours such as orange and pink are used to put vibrancy back into the skin tones. Lighting changes the make-up colours:

- ◆ white make-up looks blue – so use cream
- ◆ blue make-up looks black – so use brown
- ◆ yellow make-up looks washed-out white – so use pink, orange or red.

Make-up for small and large auditoriums

In intimate theatre there is often no need for the actors to have strong make-up, especially if set in the modern day. Stylistic effects will look wrong when the audience is seated close to the performers, unless this is required, such as in burlesque or drag queen effects. Normal beauty make-up can be applied, according to the needs of the script and characterisation.

In a large auditorium such as the Royal Opera House in London, only a small proportion of people will be able to distinguish the make-up. As you cannot meet the needs of everyone, it is best to apply make-up that will look good to the front and middle sections of the house. The back rows will simply view it as part of the overall picture of the performance, costume, lighting, wigs and make-up.

Working conditions

The hours of work in theatre are long: matinees in the afternoons and evening performances. But the hours are regular: the curtain goes up at a certain time, and down when the performance has finished. So the work schedule is fixed: the same every day. When a show goes on tour the crew stays in digs, which generates a close relationship where

TOP TIP

Set bags should be prepared beforehand so that you have everything you need on hand for make-up changes and are prepared for unforeseen events that could occur during the performance. For example, spirit gum to re-attach a beard.

TOP TIP

False eyelashes work well to enhance the eyes and make them look bigger.

TOP TIP

Detailed make-up changes will help to define the character.

everyone bonds. Key qualities for working in theatre are social skills, self-discipline, passion for the work and good time keeping.

A typical day working at the Royal Opera House

Wendy Topping, Wig Supervisor, describes a typical day working at the Royal Opera House, with two performances.

The Royal Opera House normally has several operas and ballets running concurrently so I may be working on three different productions at once. This makes things really interesting as it is so creative and the work can be so varied. For example, I might be doing an elaborate make-up on a character like the 'Queen of the night' on the *Magic Flute*, then applying a bald cap on another production or working on a production like *Tosca* where the leading lady can have three wigs so there's a lot of wig dressing.

A typical day on the principal floor at the Royal Opera House would involve a fairly early start. Sometimes it can be as early as 8 a.m. if it is a rehearsal and the finished 'look' hasn't been decided with the designer. Usually it will be 9 a.m. if I am working on two productions and I have a matinee or evening performance.

After I collect my kit from our make-up room I can start my preparation for the first show. I might have one wig or even a few and these need to be set and dressed in time for the matinee performance. Depending on the design of the style, this will determine how much prep I need to do. It may involve cleaning, brushing out, re-setting and a short time in the wig oven, so as with most theatre work I need to work fairly quickly.

When my wigs are in the oven, I will 'set up' in my artist's room and lay out all the make-up and hair equipment that I will need. The ladies' principals are made up in their dressing rooms, so it is essential that everything is in the room before I start.

Sometimes I will have time for a short break before I start but again this will depend on the production, the design and how time consuming the make-up is. Singers may want to be made up early as they may want to do a singing warm up.

The matinee performance normally starts around 2 p.m. and I will start the make-up an hour before. Once I have finished the hair and make-up I will check my show notes, which are notes that have timings and quick changes for all the information I need for my show plot. Each person who works on the show has their own show plot which is unique to them and it is basically a list of things you need to do during the performance. Each musical or opera or ballet is different, so requires a different set of plot notes. You may be really busy during a performance with several wig and make-up changes, some changes can be very quick or you may have little more to do than wait stage-side for your artist to make sure the wig is secure and maybe powder them a little. At the end of the performance, the wig comes off and then you can tidy up, clean your brushes and get ready for the evening performance.

Sometimes I have time to prepare for the second show throughout the day and may have had time to set my wig if I have one. It is important on a busy day that you think ahead and are organised, as time management is very important in theatre.

Once I have set up for the evening performance, I can then take a break. Luckily the Royal Opera House has a café and coffee bar so if I am short of time I will go there.

The evening performance usually starts at 7.30 p.m. so, again, I would start an hour before and as with the previous performance I will check my plot notes and work accordingly.

I would normally leave the Royal Opera House quite late, after I have taken off my wigs and tidied up all equipment. Sometimes I don't leave until after 11 p.m. so it can be a very long day. However, it is usually interesting, creative and fun!

HEALTH & SAFETY

As a make-up artist you must wear the correct footwear to ensure you can work safely around lighting and cables. The health and safety manager will give you a briefing to outline any special effects you must be aware of, such as dry ice or smoke machines.

CASE PROFILE: WENDY TOPPING

How long have you been working in the industry?

I have been working in the theatre for 23 years. Prior to that I studied hairdressing and make-up for film, theatre and television.

How did you get into the industry?

I was a student at the London College of Fashion and just about to finish my course when a position of 'swing' came up at the Old Vic theatre on the musical *Carmen Jones*. A 'swing' is someone who covers other members of the department when they are not available. Luckily I was offered the job.

Did you have a lucky break or turning point?

I was lucky in the people I met and worked with over the first few years in the business. They were successful and well respected in the industry and they taught me so much and gave me work as a wig assistant on the new productions they were working on in the West End. After three years working as a wig assistant, I was offered the post of wig-mistress at the Cameron Mackintosh production of *Oliver* opening at the London Palladium. This then led to wig mistress positions on several top West End shows such as *Chicago, Oklahoma* and *The Witches of Eastwick*.

What has been your most significant project?

I have been fortunate enough to have worked in the West End for many years and also at the Royal Opera House where I have been a freelance wig and make-up technician for 11 years. The Royal Opera House is a very interesting and creative place to work. Having a freelance position gives me an opportunity to work on other projects, such as the London 2012 Olympics, where I did the hair for the headline talent for the opening and closing ceremonies.

I have managed to retain my link with musical theatre and I was assistant wig supervisor on the UK tour of *Oliver* and *The Phantom of the Opera* and wig and make-up supervisor on the recent Japanese production of *Les Miserables* in Tokyo.

What do you enjoy most about the job?

I absolutely love my job but the unsociable hours can be difficult. Sometimes a show may not come down till late and therefore you may not get home until midnight. I normally work weekends and bank holidays, so my family time can be compromised, but the good parts of the job outweigh the bad.

How has the theatre industry changed?

Theatre has changed in many ways in the last 20 years. From the products used to the increasing demand for live cinema relays, and the ase with a which theatre hairdressers can switch from working in theatre to working in film.

What advice would you give to a new make-up artist starting out?

You never stop learning. Be open to new techniques and ideas. Work hard. Have a good attitude and be nice!

Theatrical make-up

See **CHAPTER 13** Character make-up for more information on ageing.

ACTIVITY

How to enhance the ageing effect

The use of wigs, hair mascaras and reel palettes will help to enhance the overall ageing effect.

◆ Age three of your peers using different ageing techniques. Take photographs and compare the results.

◆ Research three hairstyles that will complement a character through the different stages of ageing.

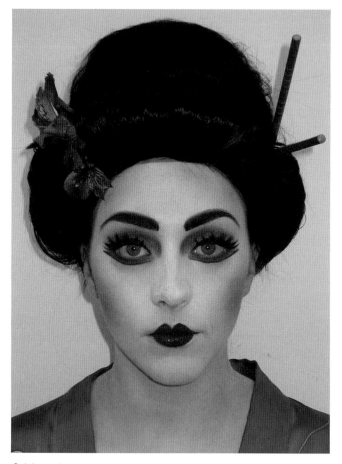

Geisha make-up

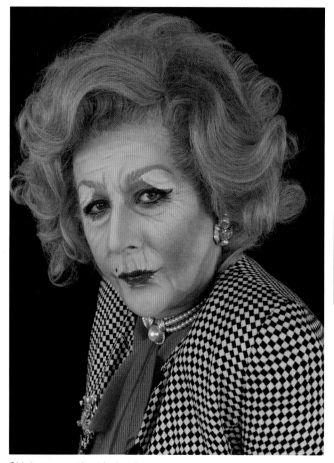

Old drag queen theatrical make-up

Modelling with wax

Sometimes lighting and shading (contouring) are not dramatic enough and a three-dimensional effect is needed without making or commissioning prosthetics. In such circumstances putty or wax can be used to reshape a feature or create a casualty effect. **Mortician's wax** is often used by make-up artists and there are different brands to choose from. The wax is covered with a **sealer** and allowed to dry. Make-up is applied on top of the sealer to blend with the natural skin tone.

See **CHAPTER 12** Prosthetics, for information on modelling, casting and how to produce a false nose.

HEALTH & SAFETY

Patch testing is required 24 hours before application, to identify any allergies to the products. Be aware that the actors may build up a sensitivity to products that are being used excessively night after night; therefore it may be necessary to modify the type and quality of products used over time.

HEALTH & SAFETY

Always store your products as per the manufacturer's guidelines. Always use a spatula to decant products from containers to avoid cross-infection. Ensure equipment and products are stored correctly.

Most theatres commission prosthetics from specialist suppliers. They are usually made from foam latex, which is easy to apply and light for the actor's comfort. On a low budget production directly applied wax or moulds filled with gelatine are sometimes used, or a less expensive alternative.

Tools & equipment

- bowl of water – cold
- foundations
- isopropyl alcohol – to clean the brush when using sealer
- **modelling tools** – wooden and metal
- moisturiser
- make-up brushes – assorted
- make-up palette – camouflage colours or illustrator palette
- Make-up wrap

- powder – translucent
- rough textured towel
- sealer
- segment of orange or grapefruit peel skin
- stipple sponge
- student or model
- toner
- wax – Mortician's wax or Kryolan wax

Wax nose

Although wax may be placed anywhere on the face, it is most successful in changing a nose shape. A small amount can produce a striking change in appearance, and does not affect the actor's ability to speak. If used too far up, between the eyes, the wax will lift and look unnatural when an actor smiles or frowns. It is best to use it on the middle section of the bridge of the nose for it to sit securely on the bone. Wax takes practice to use; the hands should be kept cool and dry otherwise the wax becomes very sticky.

Research and design

Plan the proposed nose shape on paper.

Preparation of model

Put a make-up wrap around the model and make sure the skin is grease-free, using toner if necessary.

Applying the nose

1 Apply a thin coat of wax to the area of the nose you are working on, as a base.

2 Soften a small ball of wax with your fingers.

3 Mould a rough shape and apply it to the nose. Work cleanly – keep your hands cool to prevent your fingers from becoming too sticky. Dip fingers into the bowl of cold water from time to time.

4 Use a modelling tool to sculpt the shape and blend the edges.

5 Work up and out from the natural bone and nose shape. Build width, keeping a contoured shape, without ridges. View your work in the mirror in profile.

6 With a modelling tool blend the wax into the natural shadows and folds of the real nose. Work quickly and positively. For the best result, use the minimum wax.

7 When you are satisfied with the result, viewed from all angles, smooth a little moisturiser onto the surface to smooth the wax and remove tackiness. Use the tip of your finger to smooth away any imperfections.

8 Apply texture, if needed, using a rough towel, segment of orange peel skin or a stipple sponge. This will give an open-pored look if needed.

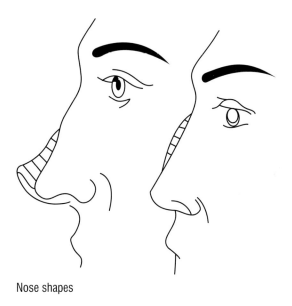

Nose shapes

9   Paint a thin coat of sealer all over the wax with a brush. Allow to dry. Apply a second coat, and allow to dry.

10 Add a third coat, and tap a little translucent powder onto the surface whilst it is still tacky. This will prevent any shine from the sealer and wax showing through the make-up. Use a soft powder brush loaded with powder; tap the stem of the brush for the powder to drop onto the sealer making it matte.

STEP-BY-STEP: MAKING A GELATINE PROSTHETIC NOSE

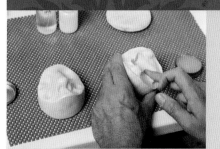

1 Warm moulds with an oven or hairdryer. Apply Vaseline to the mould.

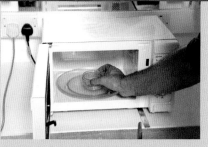

2 Place the **gelatine** in the microwave.

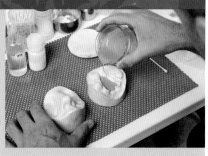

3 Pour liquid gelatine into the mould and allow to cool until it is safe to handle.

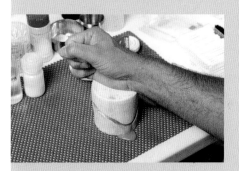

4 Close the mould (wait 5–10 minutes).

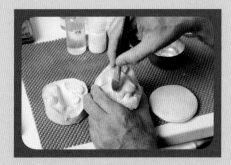

5 Release the mould, powdering the gelatine to remove any grease.

STEP-BY-STEP: APPLYING A PROSTHETIC NOSE

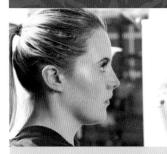

1 Before in profile.

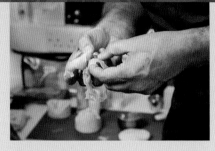

2 Removing flashing from around the edge of the gelatine mould.

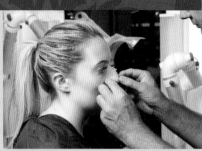

3 Position the nose. Powder the edge of the nose so when the mould is removed from the face the powder will show the outline for positioning the nose.

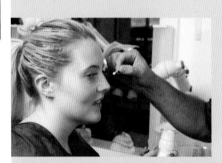

4 Apply betabond adhesive or Pros-Aide to the area of the nose inside the powder.

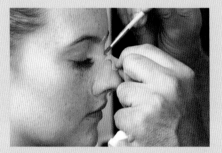

5 Apply the nose onto the glue using a brush.

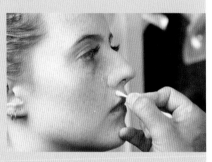

6 Use a cotton bud dipped in **witch hazel** to blend the edges of the gelatine around the nose.

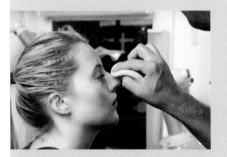

7 Powder the nose.

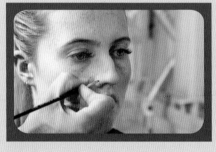

8 Apply sealer over the nose ready for applying make-up.

For modelling and making a cast see **CHAPTER 12** Prosthetics.

Making up the nose

When the top coat of sealer is dry and powdered, the nose can be coloured.

1 Study the colours and tones of the surrounding skin on the model's face.

2 Check out pigmentation marks – freckles etc.

3 Use a sponge or brush to apply make-up to the nose. Start with rose pink or pale pink under the lights. Powder and add skin tone colours on top. Finish with foundation on the nose and rest of face.

4 Powder and finish the make-up according to the design.

Safe removal of wax

After the performance the wax must be removed safely using adhesive removers. As the actors may have adhesive removers applied night after night, special home care products may be recommended to help desensitise the skin and keep it in optimum condition.

Using spirit gum

If the actor has to move a lot during the performance there is a way to make the nose stronger and stay in position, by applying spirit gum to the natural nose before the wax is put on. Whilst the spirit gum is still tacky use a small amount of cotton wool to bond the surface. Place the wax on top and model in the usual way, applying sealer and make-up to match the rest of the face.

Casualty effects in theatre

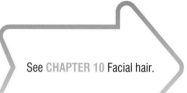

See **CHAPTER 8** Wigs and hairpieces.

Theatre productions often commission prosthetics if the budget is good, but some productions have a low budget in which case theatre make-up artists make their own effects in the same way as for low-budget television and film. *(See Chapter 11 Casualty Effects.)*

Period hair work is the same in theatre as television and film except the wigs are made with thicker hair lace.

Facial hair is also the same as for television and film, except that it is knotted on thicker hair lace.

See **CHAPTER 10** Facial hair.

Recipes for blood effects that are cost-effective

1 Flour, water, red food colouring – vary the proportions to make the 'blood' thicker or thinner.

2 Red and yellow food colouring, karo clear syrup, methyl paraben (preservative) and photoflo (from photographic dark room suppliers).

Recipe for wound filler

Use black treacle, red food dye and something to bind it – for example, fine bread-crumbs, crushed cereals or talcum powder.

CASE PROFILE: STEFAN MUSCH, WIG SUPERVISOR

How long have you been working in theatre?

I have been working in professional theatre since 2000.

How did you get into theatre?

From a young age I was a fan of theatre and live entertainment, and it was always clear to me that I would work towards a career in theatre.

Did you have a lucky break or turning point?

Back in Germany it is incredibly hard getting a foot into the theatre industry. One morning I decided to drive to the neighbouring city, where a big musical was playing at the time. I didn't know anyone in this theatre, but was hoping that I might have the chance to talk to the head of wigs and could ask for advice on how to get into the industry. I was very lucky that the HOD [head of department] had a spare ten minutes and she gave me a few tips. We exchanged numbers and she asked me to keep her in the loop about my future. When I arrived at home I had a message from her on my answering machine, offering me a full-time position in her department.

My turning point was in London. I had a great career in Germany already and moving to London wasn't on my list. In December 2006 I came to London for a week to look over the shoulder of the wig team on *Wicked*. It was a great experience, because it was very different to how theatre is back home. I had the chance to do a bit of wig work that week. Back home in Germany the make-up supervisor on *Wicked* asked me if I wanted to go for an interview for a new production that was coming up in 2007. I went back to London for the interview and I got the job offer straight away. I just thought, why not give it a go? I had three months to pack up my life in Germany in boxes and find a flatshare in London. So I finished my job on *The Phantom of the Opera* in Germany, took my bags and five days later I started my first ever West End job as deputy wig master for *The Lord of the Rings*.

What has been your most significant project?

Every project I am working on teaches me something, either for my career or for life. Therefore every project is significant to me, it doesn't matter how big or small the project is.

What do you enjoy most about the job?

I always learn new techniques and challenge myself. There are always new situations coming up. I meet incredible people, with great talents. My job takes me around the world and I have made great friends, some of them are for life.

What do you enjoy least about the job?

The non-existing gratitude that wig, hair and make-up artists can sometimes receive. I have crossed a few individuals in the theatre industry who have no awareness of how much skill, knowledge and effort it takes to create what we create eight times a week.

How has the theatre industry changed during your career?

Many productions these days are stage versions of films. People come to see the show and expect the characters will look exactly like the film. It makes it hard for designers because creativity is limited. On the other side it is a great skill to be able to convert from film to stage, but I wish more original ideas would get produced.

What advice would you give to a new make-up artist/ hair dresser starting out?

Be yourself. Observe what is going on around you. Push yourself out of your comfort zone from time to time. Never think you know it all. And remember, if you are working on the worst production with the worst boss and you think you aren't learning anything- you actually are learning! You have learned to be a better boss for your team on the worst production day in the future.

www.stefanmusch.com

Make-up for the ballet

Ballet make-up is traditionally a pale skin-toned look, whitened shoulders and arms, and strong eye make-up. The hair is drawn back neatly into an elegant bun.

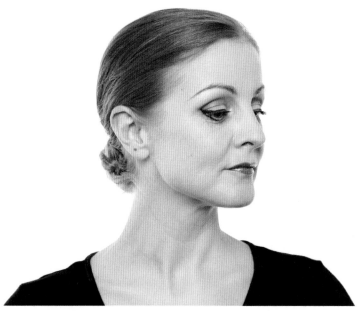

Traditional ballet make-up

REVISION QUESTIONS

1 What are the principles of live-to-cinema relays?

2 What other professionals do you expect to be working with when working at the theatre?

3 How will you alter your make-up techniques for a small auditorium as opposed to a large?

4 How will the effects of theatre lighting affect a performer's make-up?

5 Why is the continuity important when working in a theatre and how will you maintain this?

7 Working in television and cinematography

LEARNING OBJECTIVES

This chapter covers the following:

◆ A career in television and film make-up.

◆ Make-up design for television and film.

◆ Pre-production planning.

◆ Production filming.

◆ Who does what on a film.

◆ Working on set.

◆ Working as a daily.

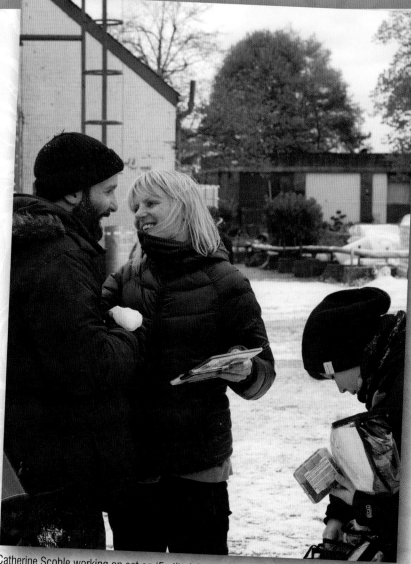

Catherine Scoble working on set on 'Fortitude'

KEY TERMS

Breaking down the
script

Chamois leather

Contact lenses

Standing by

Test shots
(cinematography)

UNIT TITLE

◆ Prepare to change the performer's
appearance

◆ Assist with the continuity of the
performer's appearance

◆ Apply make-up to change the performer's
appearance

INTRODUCTION

In this chapter you will gain invaluable
understanding of a make-up designer's role in
television and film. You will cover what is required
for pre-production planning including: meetings,
research, ideas, scripts, costs and the actors. The
chapter will discuss what is involved in production
filming including call sheets and continuity. You
will also learn how to conduct yourself on a film
set and understand who does what on a film.

This unit will assist with various elements of your
training. This chapter will encourage you to apply
your knowledge and understanding of basic
Level 2 make-up, airbrushing, camouflage, creative
hair and wigs to help you work effectively in the
television and film industry.

Working in television and film

Digital technology has brought television and film industries closer together. The clarity of high definition (HD) picture reception and larger television screens has resulted in domestic viewing more similar to the cinema experience, plus a raising of standards throughout the industry with more focus on design detail than ever before.

Whether a television drama series, or blockbuster film for cinema, the ability to tell a story is what matters. This is made possible through the collaboration between writers, producers, directors, cast and crew. It starts with a script and budget, followed by casting of the actors and hiring the crew to work together in order to serve the story.

A professional crew, working well together, is a good thing to see. Not every team gels, but, when it does, the combination of technical expertise and professional grace can look like a choreographed dance. To be part of something like that, when it happens, is a unique experience.

A career in television make-up

The make-up artists working in television are responsible for both the hair and make-up.

On news, documentaries, weather, sports, and quiz and chat shows only one make-up artist may be required. On dramas, films for television, series and light entertainment shows, the make-up department might include a designer, senior make-up artist and several assistants, depending on the number of actors and the size of production budget. On costume dramas more staff may be needed for the wigs and facial hair. For special effects, such as prosthetics, the designer hires out the work if the budget allows. If not, the make-up artists make the piece, and it is up to the designer to decide which is the best option. On busy crowd scenes extra make-up artists are called in on a daily basis. Television make-up artists are expected to have skills in all areas of make-up and hair, but in most cases where hair bleaching and colouring are called for, the designers take the actors to specialists and brief them on the required looks. Nail technology is not part of the make-up artist's brief, except for special effects such as witches' nails; neither is shaving an actor's face. However, the make-up artist's kit should include manicure and shaving equipment for the actors' use.

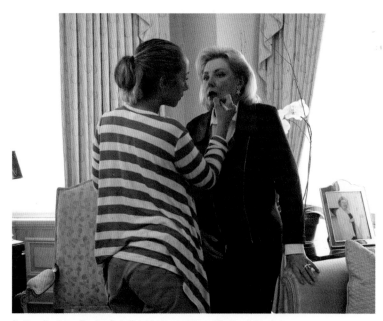

Author Barbara Taylor Bradford being made up for an interview

A career in film make-up

On major feature films the make-up artists are not responsible for the hair, which is a separate department, but are responsible for all facial hair - beards, moustaches, sideburns, eyebrows – because they relate to the face. Prosthetics is also a separate department, employed by the film if there are numerous effects, e.g. *Harry Potter*. When there are only one or two pieces they will be made by an outside workshop, and often applied by the make-up artist responsible for the actor's make-up. The hair department's work consists of managing all the hair requirements, such as cutting, colouring, hair extensions, wigs and hairpieces.

Sometimes there will be another team in charge of making up animals if they are featured in the film. Non-toxic colours are used to colour in patches when several animals have to stand in for one another, for example, in the filming of Spielberg's *Warhorse*.

Many leading actors have their own personal make-up and hair artists: people whom they know and trust.

The make-up designer in television and film

Advances in technology have had an impact on the art of make-up design. Yet, at the same time the role of the designer has remained the same: conducting research, visualising the characters and contributing to the director's brief in helping to tell the story.

CASE PROFILE: CATHERINE SCOBLE, MAKE-UP DESIGNER

How long have you been working in the industry?
Almost 20 years.

How did you get into the industry?
I got into the industry after meeting a family friend who was a make-up designer. I was doing my A levels at the time and considering career options. After meeting her I studied hairdressing for three years, then completed a course in make-up for film and television. I then worked on student and low-budget films until I built up experience and contacts.

Did you have a lucky break or a turning point?
Relatively early in my career I worked as make-up designer on *Lock, Stock and Two Smoking Barrels* which was a very successful film. This was a turning point in my career.

What has been the most significant project(s) you have worked on?
This Is England would have to be the most significant project that I have worked on. I designed both the film and then the two television series. They were so important to me because I had admired the work of the director, Shane Meadows, for a long time. To get to work with him was a massive honour. The scripts were so brilliant and all set in the 1980s which was such a rich time for hair and make-up. My team and I worked extremely hard on capturing the

look and feel of the period and so it was fantastic to go on and win a Bafta for our work on the first television series, *This Is England '86*.

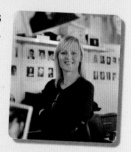

What do you enjoy most about the job?
I enjoy the fact that I never stop learning. I love that I never know what the next script will contain and I find it very rewarding to work as part of a team.

How has the television and film industry changed during your career?
Right now, it's a very exciting time in television. There are so many high-quality television series being made, especially in the USA. This means that the audience here too are demanding better and better television. Scripts are getting better. The ante has been upped.

During my career there have been changes in the way we, as make-up artists, work. Ever evolving technology means we have to keep adapting and moving forwards with our make-up techniques. For example, we have to know how to work with high definition cameras and monitors, and how to work alongside CGI (computer-generated imagery) technicians. Very exciting times!

Pre-production planning

First meeting

Having read the script, the make-up designer attends a meeting with the producer, director, art director, costume designer, hair designer, director of photography, script supervisor and all relevant people to discuss the script and style of the production.

HEALTH & SAFETY

The actors will be contacted to ensure they do not have allergies to any products to allow time for alternatives to be obtained if necessary.

Research

After further meetings with the costume and production designers about the colours to be used, and the characters in the story, the make-up and hair designers proceed to research and interpret the needs of the actors according to the script. Inspiration can come from vintage photographs, art books, old films, fashion, street characters, libraries, art galleries or the Internet. Drawings and sketches are made, contributing to the ideas.

ACTIVITY

Television make-up budget

Plan a make-up for a television character and cost the budget. The budget should cover all aspects of the hair and make-up design.

Presentation of the ideas

Whether using photographs, magazine cut-outs or sketches, they should be presented neatly in a file or portfolio to show people who will accept or reject the ideas. A drawing can save time, and may eventually be passed on to the various specialists to show how the wig, facial hair or prosthetics should look. Once the design is on paper, it can be looked at by everyone involved, particularly the actor – although the director has the final word.

Design concepts can be shown on a model, and talked through verbally. In practice, many make-ups are designed directly onto the actor's face and presented to the director for further discussion. The design element in make-up is present throughout the make-up artist's work, but communication at the beginning is important: drawing the idea on paper can save hours of talking.

The sketches should be covered with a layer of paper to protect the artwork from getting dirty. Notes, instructions and comments should be included to help those involved to achieve the concept. The designs can be simple charts or photos of the actor. Many make-up artists use Photoshop (image editing software) to work out their designs; using them for discussions and following up with testing on a model to become familiar with the products before trying out on the actor.

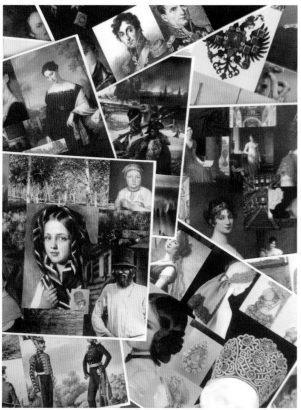

Moodboard

Make-up design for an accident victim

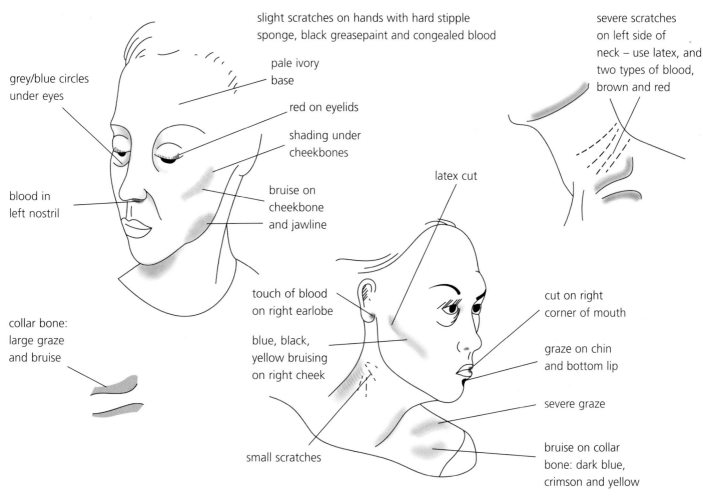

slight scratches on hands with hard stipple
sponge, black greasepaint and congealed blood

severe scratches
on left side of
neck – use latex, and
two types of blood,
brown and red

grey/blue circles
under eyes

pale ivory
base

red on eyelids

shading under
cheekbones

blood in
left nostril

bruise on
cheekbone
and jawline

latex cut

collar bone:
large graze
and bruise

touch of blood
on right earlobe

blue, black,
yellow bruising
on right cheek

cut on right
corner of mouth

graze on chin
and bottom lip

severe graze

small scratches

bruise on collar
bone: dark blue,
crimson and yellow

Collaborating with actors

Actors will often discover their look during costume, make-up and hair tests. They will transform themselves into the person they are seeking to become. The change in make-up and hairstyles, together with the clothes, enables the actor to shape his role and create a new look. His posture, facial expressions and entire physicality will often change before your eyes in the make-up chair.

Script breakdown

The designer breaks down the script, listing the number of characters and crowd artists involved in the scenes.

Cost breakdown

A cost breakdown is worked out for the producer, which is then discussed and a budget agreed. The costing includes the number of staff to be employed, make-up materials, equipment, special effects (if not a separate department), facial hair and wigs, hair products and tools (if not a separate department).

Contacting the actors

The make-up and/or hair designer proceeds to contact the actors through the assistant director (AD) or production office, to meet and discuss their make-up and hair.

More script breakdown

A more detailed breakdown of the script takes place to take into account any changes. Continuity involved for scenes being shot out of sequence is discussed. Notes are made of make-up changes, e.g. crying or injuries in fight scenes. All the other department heads do the same, so that everyone is working to a common end.

ACTIVITY

Theme: victim of a car accident

Either write a small script or download a script from the Internet. Break down the script and plan the make-up products required for this theme. Your plan should include:

- a budget
- description/details of how to create the look
- visuals
- an evaluation.

Employing staff

The designers now contact their choice of people to work with them on the film. Normally this will be an experienced senior make-up artist, sometimes called a supervisor, who will assist with wig and facial hair fittings or any other pre-production planning, plus several make-up artists as assistants, and often a trainee or work experience graduate, to work on the shoot.

Dental work and contact lenses

Appointments are made with dental technicians and opticians for actors requiring dental veneers, or optical effects, such as **contact lenses**. A make-up artist is usually given the task of looking after the dentures or lenses, sterilising them after use and storing them safely.

Lighting tests

Before filming begins the director of photography (DOP) arranges a lighting test for the principal actors to be filmed in costume, make-up and hair, or particular special effects. This enables the director to discuss any changes to be made.

Organising the make-up room

The designer organises the make-up rooms at the studio base, and location facilities with the location manager: such as make-up trailers, and marquees for extras, with portable mirrors and lights.

HEALTH & SAFETY

Ensure all electrical equipment is PAT tested. A risk assessment should be carried out to determine how often PAT testing is required. Visit the HSE website for further guidance (www.hse.gov.uk)

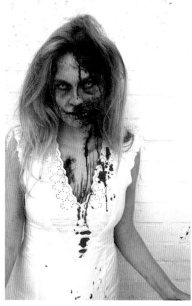

Zombie with specialised contact lenses

HEALTH & SAFETY

Always check manufacturer's instructions. Check use by dates on sterilising products.

TOP TIP

You may need to arrange extra electrical points for electrical equipment such as airbrushes, tongs, hairdryers, rollers and hot sticks.

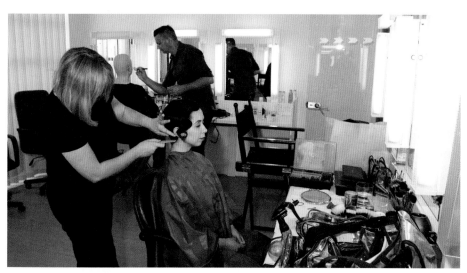

Working in a make-up room

Final fittings

Final fittings are done on actors for wigs, prosthetics and facial hair. Wigs may be custom-made because on a long shoot it might be less expensive than weekly hire. Facial hair cannot be hired, for hygiene reasons, so must be bought.

Arranging the transport of equipment and materials

Before going on location the equipment is loaded and checked by the designer before it is taken to the arranged place.

Pre-production planning is now finished.

HEALTH & SAFETY

When helping with transportation and equipment always remember to consider 'manual handling' best practice. Think of your back and posture when lifting boxes and heavy items.

CASE PROFILE: CATE HALL, MAKE-UP DESIGNER

How long have you been working in the industry?

Ten years.

How did you get into the industry?

I started off by answering adverts that required make-up artists for short films on websites like Mandy.com and Talentcircle.org. I also assisted a make-up artist I had met when at university and this led to further paid work.

Did you have a lucky break or turning point?

I worked unpaid on a short film in London with an actress called Sophia Myles. We got on well and she liked my work and mentioned me to her agent. They happened to know an experienced theatre/television director who was making his first feature film so recommended me. We met, and whilst I had never designed a production before, he decided to give me a chance. It was my first opportunity to hire a paid team and manage a make-up budget. Since then designing has been the main focus of my career.

What has been your most significant project?

In late 2013 I was offered the job designing the sequel *Woman in Black: Angel of Death*. Not only was it the largest budget film I had worked on, it was also my first studio picture with a guaranteed international distribution. The design demanded 1941-period hair and make-up as well as significant character and special effects make-ups. It's rare that a job comes along combining so many different looks, so it was a real treat to research and set up.

What do you enjoy most about the job?

I love that every day is different. Because I head a team, I have the pleasure of hiring and working with some of my best friends which is a real privilege. I love the moment a character's look is signed off on set or at a camera test, after a long research period and some nerve-wracking fittings and make-up tests.

What do you enjoy least about the job?

Having to sort and repack my kit for different jobs.

How has the television and film industry changed during your career?

The amount of make-up artists seems to have increased but so has the amount of work available. It feels like more productions are coming to the UK, but that may be only because I now know about them. The industry itself feels pretty similar, though my experience of it is very different since my frequency of work has stabilised.

Is research important?

The knowledge or understanding of specific periods and cultures is partly what you are hired for and the more specific you can be in your references, the more believable your character will be as a result. Even if you decide to disregard certain rules or trends from a different period or culture, it's important to know them initially and allow them in their absence to inform, shape or inspire the final image. Before I interview for a job I spend days saving images that I think might be relevant. I probably only end up using 20 per cent of those images in the moodboards I take to interview. But distilling so many images down to a relative few really focuses the tone of the board and gives it its distinct mood or theme. If I then go on to design a job, I find already having completed this process takes the pressure off the research stage, since I already have an idea of what I'm looking for.

What advice would you give to a new make-up artist starting out?

Make yourself as desirable as possible in your skill set. Remember your career might be 45 years long or more, so taking your time to become specialised is a long-term investment. Personally speaking I don't cut hair, so I'm reliant on hiring hairdressers on my team. Equally, someone who is really good at prosthetics and SFX [special effects] as well as straight hair and make-up is valuable. And don't give up – it's a really wonderful career once your amount of work becomes consistent.

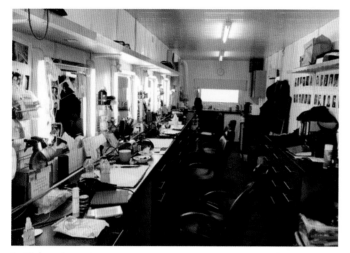

Inside a make-up bus

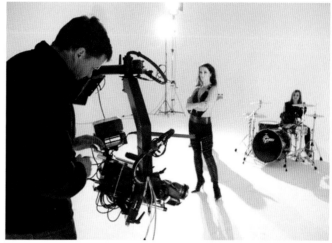

On set

Production filming

Continuity

Continuity Breakdown						
Character:				Artist:		
Sc	Time	Day	Location	Special Make-up/Hair	Details of Scene	F

A continuity breakdown

> **TOP TIP**
>
> Prior to leaving the house before filming on location always check the weather reports to ensure you are wearing the correct clothing and footwear. The weather will also dictate the durability of the hair and make-up. See example of call sheet on page 145.

In television and film the scenes are shot out of sequence for various reasons, e.g. availability of the locations and actors. Scenes may be re-shot long after filming has officially finished if the producer and director decide to change the scene. If the crew members are working elsewhere new people may have to film the pick-up shots on a re-shoot.

The script supervisor deals with the general continuity of the filming, type of film stock, and marking the film unit's daily progress in shooting the action dictated by the script. When the script is changed they issue the changes to all the crew to insert in their copy of the script. It is still up to the individual make-up artists to work out their own continuity – taking photographs of all the main actors' front, back and profile views – plus notes on products and techniques used. All changes of hairstyles, costume and make-up are logged with the scene number and day number of the film sequence and kept in the department's continuity files.

MAKE-UP CHART

TITLE OF PRODUCTION: ....

ACTOR'S NAME: ....

CHARACTER NAME: ....

Foundation: ....

Concealer: ....

Shading: ....

Highlight: ....

Eyes: ....

Cheeks: ....

Eye make-up

Lips: ....

Eyebrows: ....

Body make-up: ....

Hair notes: ....

A make-up record chart

The call sheet

	CALL SHEET 12
	THURSDAY 4TH FEBRUARY 2016
	UNIT CALL: 1000 ON SET
	Breakfast @base from: 0900
	Lunch from approx.: 1500
	Estimated wrap: 2100

SPLIT DAY 1000-2200	
Crew cars: RUSKIN HOUSE, OFF STAFFORD RD, WA4 1GR	John Hughes (2nd AD)
Unit base: UNDERGROUND CAR PARK, @RUSKIN HOUSE, OFF STAFFORD RD, WA4 1GR	Richard Silverman (Loc Manager)
Location: PROLOCK BUILDING, 23-25 BRIDGE STREET, LONDON, EC4 3HY	Tom White (Unit Manager)
	Jamie Smith (Locations Assistant)
Weather: Partly cloudy, sunny spells	Helen Howard (Prod Co-ordinator)
Temp: High 11°C, Low 3°C	ADs Office
Sunrise: 0703	
Sunset: 1714	

UNIT NOTES:
1. PLEASE NOTE THIS LOCATION IS A PARTICULARLY COLD ONE – IT IS ADVISABLE TO WRAP UP WARM
2. PLEASE DO NOT STRAY FROM DESIGNATED AREAS – THIS BUILDING IS OLD AND DELAPIDATED
3. PLEASE NOTE CHANGE IN SCHEDULE FROM FRIDAY 5TH FEBRUARY

SC	SET/SYNOPSIS	D/N	PGS	CAST (Crowd)	PAGE
1/12A pt	INT STUDENT HOUSE Lisa on phone to Hannah, Tom appears	D9 1130	1	6. 10. (none)	White
1/27	INT STUDENT HOUSE LISA'S BEDROOM/ LANDING Tom is angry about Chris being accuse of cheating	D14 0900	6/8	6. 10. (none)	White
1/50	INT STUDENT HOUSE – TOM'S BEDROOM Lisa's ipod and watch alarms are activated	N15 2300	2/8	6. (none)	White
1/50A	INT STUDENT HOUSE Tom wakes on hearing a noise and looks down corridor	N15 2302	2/8	10. (none)	White
1/50B	INT STUDENT HOUSE The front door is open. The minder is missing.	N15 2303	1/8	10. (none)	White
1/50C	INT STUDENT HOUSE – CORRIDOR Tom is grabbed by two men and carried passed Lisa's room	N15 2304	2/8	10. (stunt x2)	White
1/50D	INT STUDENT HOUSE – LISA'S BEDROOM Lisa is listening as they pass her door	N15 2305	1/8	6. (stunt x2)	White
1/50E	INT STUDENT HOUSE – STAIRS Lisa comes out and sees the men. Runs back as one man chases her	N15 2306	3/8	6. (stunt x2)	White
1/50F	INT STUDENT HOUSE – STAIRS Lisa whacks kidnapped number one	N15 2307	2/8	6. (stunt x2)	White
1/50G	INT STUDENT HOUSE – DOWNSTAIRS Lisa hits the other man and they run for it	N15 2308	3/8	6. 10. (stunt x2)	White
1/51	INT STUDENT HOUSE – STAIRS & BASEMENT Lisa and Tom run full pelt down the stairs	N15 2309	2/8	6. 10. (stunt x2)	White
1/51A	INT STUDENT HOUSE – STAIRS One of the kidnappers sets off after Lisa and Tom	N15 2309	1/8	- (stunt x2)	White
MOVE					
1/52	EXT STUDENT HOUSE – STREET Lisa and Tom make a getaway in a car	N15 2310	2/8	6. 10. (stunt x2)	White
		Total pages	4 3/8		

DV UNIT SHOOTING TODAY DEPARTS FROM CLAPHAM @ 0900

SC	SET/SYNOPSIS	D/N	PGS	CAST (Crowd)	PAGE
1/93 pt	INT AIRPORT TERMINAL Passengers walk through the terminal about to board the plane	D18 1830	2/8	(Robyn and Dave Grey, John Barry and family)	White

ID	CAST	CHARACTER	S	D/R	P/UP	M/UP		COST	TRAVEL	LINE UP	ON SET
6.	CARLA FINE	LISA	W	1	0815	0900	F	0945	AS REQD	1000	1000
10.	CRAIG LOWE	TOM	W	2	0830	0945	F	0930	AS REQD	1000	1000

STUNTS		FOR	CALL	M/UP & COST		ON SET
	SIMON THOMAS	COORDINATOR	1000	AS REQD		AS REQD
	JAKE ROBINSON	ASSAILANT 1	1000	AS REQD		AS REQD
	TED JAMES	ASSAILANT 2	1000	AS REQD		AS REQD

STAND-INS		FOR	CALL		ON SET
	JANE LAKE	UTILITY	1000		AS REQD

CROWD c/o CASTING COLLECTIVE – TOTAL 6			CALL	M/UP	COST		ON SET
DV unit	Robyn Grey	CALL TO CLAPHAM FOR 0830	0815	0830	0830		AS REQD
DV unit	Dave Grey	CALL TO CLAPHAM FOR 0830	0815	0830	0830		AS REQD
DV unit	John Barry and family	CALL TO CLAPHAM FOR 0830	0815	0830	0830		AS REQD

Call sheet

TOP TIP

Always check where 'your' unit base is located. Plan your trip prior to filming to ensure you are there in plenty of time. Check where your car is to be left.

Every night the crew gets a call sheet, put together by the first assistant director, informing everyone of what scenes are being shot the next day, how many actors are working, where to go and what time to be there. Other information is on the call sheet, such as department requirements, e.g. 'Make-up department blood for fight scene 2', collection times of actors from their hotels, arrival times for make-up, hair and wardrobe, and times they are expected on set.

Extras, or crowd artists, stand-ins and doubles have call times, plus catering and the general crew. If the call sheet has 'closed set', it means no visitors.

Every day the second assistant director (AD) arranges call times for the following day with the make-up, hair and wardrobe heads for all the actors, according to how long is needed. The first AD works out the order to fit in with the general shooting schedule and emails the call sheets to everyone.

Delegating the make-up work

The designer divides up the work, briefing the team on which actors they are to look after, with advice, reference pictures and notes. The lead actor is made up by the designer, who also takes total responsibility for all the make-up done by everyone on the production. The senior make-up artist is usually given responsibility for the main actors, and the assistant make-up artists are given supporting actors.

On large-scale productions, with big crowd scenes, a make-up artist is often given responsibility for supervising the crowd calls, hiring the daily make-up artists, briefing them on what needs to be done and which products to use. The assistant make-up artists are given supporting actors to look after, and the trainees will be expected to help with the crowd artists' make-up and hair, run errands, make coffee and check stock whilst learning the business.

After filming

On completion of shooting, the packing-up includes returning hired wigs, completing a budget breakdown of money spent and giving it to the accounts department.

Who does what on a film?

Production

Title	Responsibilities
Producer	Finds the money for the film
Executive producer Producer's assistants	Handle the business side of the film
Production manager	Works for the producer, responsible for the daily running of the film
Director	Has complete charge of the film, the cast and crew

Title	Responsibilities
Casting director	Finds the right actors for the parts
Script supervisor	Works closely with the director, marks the daily action of the film. Responsible for continuity
Assistant director (1st AD)	First AD responsible for the shooting of the film. He assists the director and commands the set
Assistant directors (2nd and 3rd ADs)	Training to be producers or directors. Responsible for cast and crew to be in the right place at the right time. Responsible for make-up and hair department's schedule
Editor	Edits the film together with the Director
Musical director	Responsible for the music on the soundtrack
Scriptwriters	Make changes to the script

Camera crew

Title	Responsibilities
Director of photography (DOP) or cinematographer	Responsible for all that is seen on the film
Camera operator	Operates the camera, does the camera work
1st assistant camera or focus puller	Responsible for the focus and reloading of the camera
2nd assistant camera (or clapper loader)	Slates the shot and reloads the camera
Digital imaging technician (DIT) or data wrangler	Downloads the cards and takes care of playback and can sometimes even do a fast edit on set during the shoot

Stage or set crew

Title	Responsibilities
Gaffer	Chief electrician in charge of setting up the lights for the DOP
Best boy	The gaffer's assistant
Electricians or sparks	Responsible for moving and changing the lights

Title	Responsibilities
Key grip	Responsible for moving the camera, laying tracks for the tracking shots
Props	Place the furniture on set for the set designer
Set dresser	Dress the set and are responsible for the look as directed by the designer
Designer	Responsible for the building of sets, locations and overall look of the film
Design assistant	Assists the designer
Sound recordist	In charge of the sound, operates the sound equipment
Boom operator	Holds the boom near the actors to record the sound and assists the recordist
Sound supervisor	Responsible for the overall sound continuity, working closely with the director
Stand-in	Someone with the same height and build as the star actor who stands in while the lights are set for the film
Double	Someone who doubles for an actor when the distance is so far that you cannot tell the difference
Stunt double	Someone who does dangerous things that an actor does not do

The cast

Title	Responsibilities
Stars	The principal actors whose names appear above the title of the film
Featured actors	Well-known actors in supporting roles
Crowd artists or extras	Non-speaking or make crowd noises

Wardrobe and costume

Title	Responsibilities
Costume designer	Designs the clothes worn by the cast of actors. Arranges all the fittings
Costume assistant	Assists the costume designer

| Wardrobe supervisor | In charge of organising and dressing the actors, maintaining repairing, washing and cleaning the actors' costumes |
| Wardrobe assistants | Assist the supervisor and dress the actors |

Make-up and hair

Title	Responsibilities
Make-up and hair designer	Responsible for all the make-up and hair needs of the entire cast, plus the doubles and stunt doubles
Assistant make-up and hair artists	Assist the designer
Personal make-up and hair artist	Chosen by the star to do their make-up and hair

The relationship between the make-up artist and camera/lighting departments by Oliver Hickey, Camera Operator

The camera/lighting and make-up teams

Relationships within the film and television industry are vital, from creating a smooth working environment to networking for future jobs. It is important to remember that on a film set, or television programme, the whole team are working towards the same goal.

The camera department can range from one person to a team of ten or more. For more information on the roles of the camera team see the table on page 147.

The camera and lighting teams can be very male heavy but usually all these guys are happy to help all of the cast and crew to get the job done. Lighting and grip teams tend to make friends with make-up and hair and wardrobe on set as the stand-down times tend to be the same – lots of pre-shoot work and then a short break whilst the camera team shoot the beautiful product that has been created. The camera team tend to work separately – usually on set – prepping the camera, rehearsing the shot, shooting the scene and then repositioning for the next shot, so social time for the camera team can be limited within a working day.

The hardest jobs are the one-day bookings when very few people know each other. One day doesn't give you any time to connect as a team so these can be the most nerve-wracking jobs to do. One-day jobs on commercial or corporate work are fine as everyone is in the same boat and by lunchtime everyone is getting along as friends!

The nicest jobs are the long shoots – working on a feature film or television series where you get the time to make lasting friendships and connections. Film and television folk are a rare breed and need to be around people who understand their work and stresses.

Checks on set

One of the hardest things for the make-up, hair and wardrobe department is doing checks on set. The make-up trailer or dressing room is a safe and organised environment, but once on set these teams are mobile and working out of bags and sometimes it feels like, no matter where they position themselves, they are always in the way. This is not true of course, as vital members of the production, make-up, hair and wardrobe must be cool and confident and remember their important place in the well-oiled machine.

The camera/lighting and grips teams don't always notice the hard work and early call times that make-up artists have to get the talent ready . . . not every actor is naturally radiant and wrinkle free!

The monitor

It is worth having friends in the camera department as they can ensure make-up artists have access to a good HD large monitor so that they can see what the make-up actually looks like on screen.

Times have changed, and digital cameras and editing software can alter the look of a shot drastically – scenes can be made to appear bluer and colder or orange and warmer with the application of a few buttons – so make-up artists really need to see what is being done and have a feed on a monitor so they can do a check with the actor in situation.

The monitor should be receiving the picture so that the make-up artist can see colours and shot size. The first AC can be a great ally in finding stray hairs and glaring pieces of netting without flagging it to all on set, as they have a good eye and know exactly where the point of focus will be in any given shot.

Shot and lens changes

Always listen to the camera team's calls on shot sizes and lens changes – if they are changing a lens (swinging a lens) the first assistant will normally call that out. The general rule is the lower the number, the wider the shot. For example, if the team has been shooting on a 35 mm lens and then the DOP swings to an 85 mm, the make-up will need checking as this is likely to be a head and shoulder shot.

> **TOP TIP**
>
> If you hear a 135 mm or 300 mm, watch out as that will be an ECU (extreme close-up) which means eyeliner will be noticeable if it is not perfectly applied and equal on both sides of each eye.

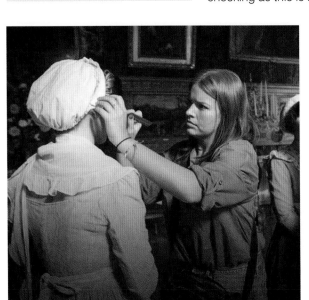

Stacey Holman on set on *Death Comes to Pemberley*

Working on set

The words 'stage', 'set' or 'floor' mean the place where filming is going on. The first AD is responsible to the producer and runs the floor or set. He will call 'Checks' or 'Final checks', which means the make-up and hair artists may move in to check their work and do last-minute finishing touches. Such work can be powdering shiny faces, re-sticking the lace on a beard or wig, or applying fresh lipstick when needed. Time is always allowed for essential work such as blood in a fight scene, or tears and sweat at the appropriate moment. Too many people on the set is considered a nuisance, so very often there will be only one or two make-up artists **standing by** on the set. No-one should get too close to the camera so as not to crowd the camera crew. A monitor is usually nearby to watch the action of the film.

The section on pages 149 and 150 was written by Oliver Hickey.

Time management

In television and film, time is valuable: any delays on set hold up the shooting schedule, and are noted by the first AD who will call out, 'Waiting on sound' or 'Waiting on make-up'.

A production report is written each day, which includes: logging the delays; the number of scenes shot; accident reports; and the working times of cast and crew.

How much time should be spent on each make-up?

All complex make-ups, such as those involving prosthetics, bald caps or detailed body painting projects, should be tested prior to filming. On television programmes such as chat shows, news, weather, interviews, etc., there is very little time for more than general grooming, i.e. powdering shiny faces, correcting under-eye shadows or dark beard lines, applying lipstick and tidying hair. On Sky News the announcers are airbrushed by the make-up artists, but that is an exception to the general rule, and does not apply to the other news channels.

TOP TIP

Remember to switch off mobile phones before going on set.

Approximate time for make-ups – a rough guide

Type of make-up	Time allowed
Corrective, grooming with tidy hair	10 mins–30 mins
Beauty make-up and hair	1 hour
Period make-up and facial hair	1 hour
Fantasy make-up and wig	1 hour
Black eye, bruise, simple cut or scratch	15 minutes
Ageing make-up, bald cap, wig and old-age stipple	2 hours
Ageing make-up with wig and old-age stipple	1 hour 30 minutes
Ageing make-up using bald cap and prosthetics	2 hours

Working as a daily

When a production needs help on a busy crowd scene the various departments engage extra people to work on a daily basis – hence the name. This could be for a day or several weeks, until the scenes are in the can (successfully finished).

On large television or film productions there will be a make-up supervisor, who assists the designer by taking responsibility for all the crowd work. They will have a list of make-up artists to call, offer the work and book the number of extra help allowed by the producers. The supervisor will give the daily information on the rate of pay, the location of the shoot and arrival time for the day. The make-up artists generally ask what to bring with them, and the supervisor will provide information on the scenes they will be working on and the period it is set in. According to the type of make-ups they will be required to do – a street scene, a battle scene, a 1920s' ball scene, a Venetian carnival, etc., the daily make-up artists prepare their kits. This should include outdoor clothing, if it is an exterior scene, appropriate for the climate. The supervisor takes responsibility for preparing the work environment, often in a marquee or a village hall on location. Tables, mirrors and lights are hired for the number of make-up artists, and extra materials supplied, plus wigs and facial hair if needed.

Some make-up artists always work as dailies, going from one production to another, which is hard work. Crowd days are always long, 12–15 hours is usual. The variety of work is interesting, modern pretty make-ups one day, followed by blood, dirt and facial hair or 1940s' make-up and hair on days for other productions.

Many experienced make-up artists do dailies in-between designing and supervising on other projects. This is also how trainees and work experience students start to learn the business and get noticed by the more experienced make-up artists. It is essential to work efficiently, as there are often hundreds of people to make up and every make-up artist must pull their weight in fairness to their colleagues. Most make-up artists bring their basic make-up kit, plus hair kit if required, a set-bag and set-chair or stool. Set bags are individual choices but usually make-up artists prefer a lightweight, waterproof, shoulder-type sports bag, suitable for all weather conditions – hot, cold or wet. For indoor sets a larger size may be used. Transparent cosmetic bags are useful for holding actors' individual items such as lipstick, mascara, powder and powder puff, etc. Transparent plastic zip lock bags are also suitable. The actor's name can be marked on the bags for quick recognition when needed. For general purpose in-crowd work it is best to have a set-bag with the following items:

Set-bag contents

Tools & equipment

- anti-bacterial hand gel
- baby wipes or wet wipes
- box of sticking plasters
- brush bag and brushes – assorted sizes
- brush cleaning wipes
- cleansing milk
- cotton buds
- disposable mascara wands
- disposable shavers
- electric shaver
- eyebrow tweezers
- eyelash adhesive
- eye pencils – black, brown and red

- FX palette – Skin Illustrator or preferred brand
- large box of tissues
- lip balm, Carmex, lip balm with sunscreen
- lipstick palette – assorted colours
- nail polish removal pads
- palette of neutral-coloured matte eyeshadows – black, brown, grey, taupe, white, cream
- palette of skin tones – Skin Illustrator or preferred brand
- powder puffs
- shaving creams
- small scissors
- sponges
- sunscreen SPF 40

If the supervisor asks the daily make-up artist to bring specific items, the kit bags will be adjusted to suit the tools needed for that day. You may have a call sheet emailed to you with all the instructions on how to get to the location and where to report for work. The supervisor will check the night before and help with queries if it is a difficult place to reach or if parking is not allowed. On the day the supervisor will give general instructions when you set up your workstation. The number of make-up artists working with you depends on the number of crowd (background artists), which can range from 10–500 depending on the scene. When everyone has been made up, hair and costumes done, the second AD will lead them to the set or place nearby and the make-up, hair and costume assistants will follow with their set-bags.

Dos and don'ts for dailies

Dos

- ◆ Do stay well away from the camera – there is only space for the key personnel.

- ◆ Do stay out of the way of doorways and entrances. The camera crew and riggers need all the spaces for doing their work.

- ◆ Do follow the supervisor's instructions, such as removing nail varnish or lipstick (even if the crowd artist does not want it done).

- ◆ Do stay away from the main make-up trailers, unless invited in. The lead actors do not like people crashing in on them while being made up.

- ◆ Do ask the second AD for anything you need to know such as the whereabouts of the washrooms, toilets, catering van, etc.

- ◆ Do remember to switch off your mobile phone at work, especially close to the set.

- ◆ Do remember that the crowd artists you made up in the morning remain your responsibility for the rest of the day. Keep an eye on them for touch-ups, especially after meal breaks. Renew lipstick if necessary. If they should not be wearing lipstick, make sure they haven't applied any – if so, remove it.

- ◆ If you are a trainee, do ask the experienced daily make-up artists for advice. Listen to their conversations, as you will learn a lot about on-set behaviour, techniques of make-up and the latest products in use.

Don'ts

- ◆ Don't talk when the AD calls for silence – you will miss what is going on and prevent others from hearing the information.

- ◆ Don't approach the lead actors, or speak to them unless they speak to you first.

- ◆ Don't get in the eyeline of actors when they are working. They find it distracting.

- ◆ Don't speak to the producer or director: they deal with the department heads.

- ◆ Don't ever touch a main actor's make-up or hair. If they approach you for help go and find their make-up artist immediately. Only their own make-up artist will know their continuity requirements.

- ◆ Don't touch any make-up or hair that you are not responsible for. It will not be liked, even if you are trying to be helpful.

◆ Don't give any opinions about costume details to an actor, even if asked directly. Stay on good terms with the costume department.

◆ Don't enter a trailer without calling, 'Coming in' or 'Stepping up', as trailers bounce, and someone may be applying an eyeline at that moment.

◆ Don't trouble the make-up designer with problems or questions, as the supervisor has been assigned to deal with anything related to the dailies.

◆ Don't spend time flirting or talking to other departments, as everyone will notice. Keep it for wrap time (finish time).

◆ Don't flash your business cards around to everyone too publicly, be discreet.

◆ Don't wear provocative clothing – definitely no high heels or low-cut dresses. Be professional.

These rules are not written down, but everyone knows them. The hierarchy on a film set is pretty rigid, but you would never outwardly see it if you didn't know. Actors have their own politics regarding the best trailers and other things dealt with by their agents. This is a gathering of talented, creative people and their egos are large. Everyone has to know their place in the scheme of things for it to be a well-oiled machine working towards a common goal.

One other rule – a trainee should never be seen sitting down, doing nothing. There are always things to do, and an offer of help to another make-up artist is appreciated, even if it is just getting a tea or coffee or cleaning someone's brushes when they are busy working next to you. That way you will make friends, and word will get around that you have 'the right attitude'.

CASE PROFILE: NIKKI HAMBI, MAKE-UP ARTIST

How long have you been working in the industry?

I started in 1986, in the fashion industry, and have been working in television since 1989.

How did you get into the industry?

I originally trained as a beauty therapist, before moving to London and getting on the books of a model agency, as one of their hair and make-up artists. Deciding fashion wasn't for me, my mission became to get into the BBC, where I was then fortunate enough to get taken on, in 1989, as a trainee. This involved being trained at the then, BBC Make-up School at Elstree Studios, and then continuing into the department, where I stayed until we all went freelance in 1996.

Did you have a lucky break or turning point?

I feel my lucky break was getting the BBC post, although it did involve hard work and dedication for a few years before achieving this goal. The training and progression into the

make-up department, learning from the best in the business, and working on the huge variety of programmes being made there, such as period dramas *House of Eliot* and *Pride and Prejudice*, to cult comedy show, *Absolutely Fabulous*. Most of my contacts there, have led to the work I am doing now.

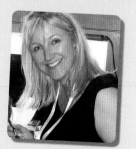

What has been your most significant project?

I have had many memorable jobs, but for me the most exciting was going on tour with Dame Shirley Bassey, which involved huge concerts in all the major UK cities, ending up at Wembley Arena. I have also been involved in numerous publicity events and various album covers for her. I seem to do a lot of live events such as Royal Variety Shows, Comic and Sport Reliefs, Children in Need,

Live Earth, Proms, Fashion Aid, amfAR Cannes, Baftas and Brits, among others, all of which are incredible to be involved in.

What do you enjoy most about the job?

The fun! The people! The creativity! The variety! I could never have had a desk job! I love the fact that every week is different. I may be doing something completely glamorous with celebrities, such as chat shows from *The Paul O'Grady Show*, to Graham Norton or *Jonathan Ross Show*, to something more reality-based like *The Apprentice*. Or I could be doing a daily on a film, such as *Burton and Taylor*, recreating 1980s looks, or testing wigs for the film *Gravity*.

What do you enjoy least about the job?

I absolutely hate the night before the first day of filming. I cannot sleep for fear that I won't wake up at 4 a.m.! Re-running the route to the location all night in my head, and whether I have forgotten anything that I may need in my kit (which is why I am notorious for always bringing too much!). I also hate some days of filming where it's cold, wet and the hours hideously long! That's when the teams you work with come to the rescue, and you all try to find ways to keep yourselves upbeat and amused!

How has the television and film industry changed during your career?

Dramatically. I almost can't believe the days at the BBC when we had a stockroom to help ourselves in, people to transport our kits, and a salary whether we had work or not! Days, long gone. Today, it's all about more hours, and fighting for good pay. Also, sadly, too few productions seem to value our skills, believing that the looks can be achieved in half the time, creating stressful and unrewarding environments. Positively, though, it's still such an amazing job to do, and steps are being made in improving conditions.

What advice would you give to a new make-up artist starting out?

I would say, stay positive, if you want something badly enough, you'll get it. Work will not come to you though, initially, so get out there, and get as much work experience as you can, because you never know what may lead on from one contact. You do need to be enthusiastic, be prepared to work extremely hard, without complaining, be a good team player, perfect your time management and be reliable. Your social life will take second place, your work life will be your social life! If work is quiet, keep your confidence up by continuing to practise your skills. You've chosen such an interesting career path, it will all be worth it.

REVISION QUESTIONS

1 What is a 'script breakdown'?

2 When would a daily be employed?

3 What is involved in pre-production planning? Outline the stages.

4 Explain the principles of continuity.

5 What times will be given for period make-up and hair?

8 Wigs and hairpieces

LEARNING OBJECTIVES

This chapter covers the following:

- Working with wigs and hairpieces.

- How to make a pattern, how to make a foundation and how to knot the wig.

- Different types of hair used in wigs and pieces.

- How to cut, style, place, fit and dress a wig.

- How to remove, clean and **block** a wig.

- How to use temporary colours and 'breaking down effects' to create a desired effect.

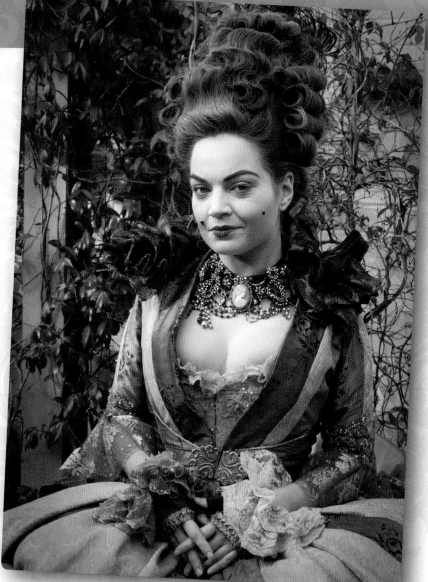

KEY TERMS

Block

Blocking pins

Breaking down

Double knotting

Drawing mat

Dressing out a wig

Foundation

Human hair

Knotting hooks

Wig stand

UNIT TITLE

◆ Prepare and apply wigs and hairpieces to change performer's appearance

◆ Oversee fittings for wigs and facial hair

INTRODUCTION

This chapter will help you with Level 3 hairdressing qualifications such as wig services and how to make and style hair additions. It will discuss working with different wigs and hairpieces. You will explore different types of hair used in making wigs and hairpieces and understand the different stages of working with a wig, including cutting and styling, fitting and placing. The importance of removing, cleaning and blocking a wig or hairpiece correctly will also be covered.

When working with hair, additional hair services may also be required to enhance the design or style. This could be with the use of temporary hair colours or different 'breaking-down effects'. Having knowledge of working with wigs and hairpieces is essential for a make-up artist. These skills can be applied to many areas of the industry including period dramas, films, character changes and photo shoots.

Wigs and hairpieces

As well as working with the actor's own hair, the make-up artist uses wigs and hairpieces to achieve the look of the period, the age, and the character, according to the director's vision.

On a large-scale production there may be numerous wigs and hairpieces: a character ageing may need several wigs from youth to old age. When stunt doubles are used duplicate wigs are often required.

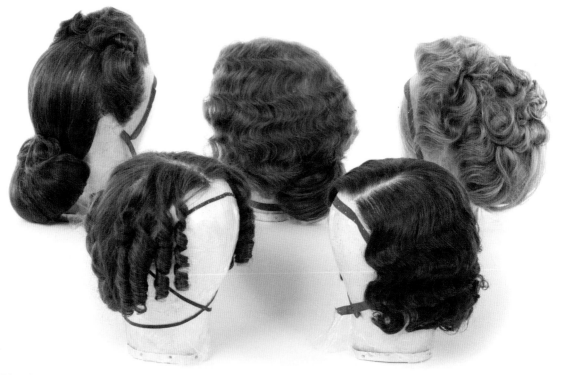

Wigs dressed and ready to be attached to the head

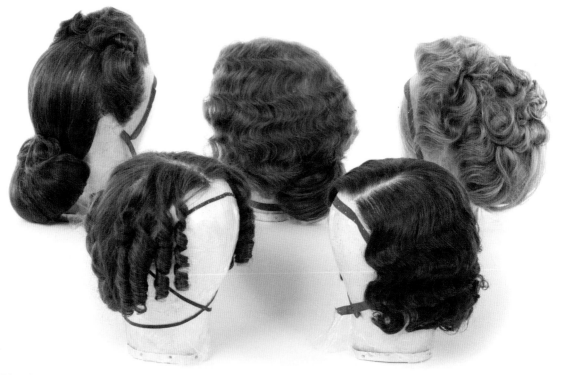
See CHAPTER 7 Working in television and cinematography, developing the design.

Make-up and hair artists do not make wigs (which is a full-time, specialist job), but an understanding of HOW they are made is important in order to oversee the hiring or making of wigs from a good company. Several wig companies should be contacted to find the one that offers the best workmanship and price. Once a company has been chosen the actor would have to go there, to have their head measurements taken before any work can begin. There will be several fittings and the designer briefs the wigmaker on the required style, providing drawings, reference pictures and verbal descriptions. The designer oversees the wig-making process, and makes sure that it is delivered to the studio before shooting begins.

During production the wigs are cleaned and redressed at the end of each day, ready for use the following day.

Working with wigs

The process of making a good quality wig involves knotting small bunches of real hair onto a **foundation** base of gauze or hair lace, using special **knotting hooks**. Hand-made carpets and rugs are made in a similar way, only using wool. Actors often refer to a toupee or wig as their 'rug'.

WIG CHART

NAME: ....

CHARACTER: ....

DATE: ....

MEASUREMENTS TAKEN BY: ....

ARTICLE ....

PERIOD OR TYPE OF WIG ....

WEIGHT OF HAIRPIECE ☐ THICK ☐ THIN ☐ SPARSE

HAIR LENGTH ☐ ins.

COLOUR ....

DRESSING ☐ CURLY ☐ WAVY ☐ STRAIGHT

DIRECTION OF COMBING ....

REMARKS ....

NOTE – WHEREVER POSSIBLE SUPPLY SKETCH OF THE STILLS OF THE ARTIST WITH THIS FORM.

WIG MEASUREMENTS

1. CIRCUMFERENCE AROUND HEAD ☐ ins.
2. FRONT TO BACK ☐ ins.
3. TEMPLE TO TEMPLE AROUND BACK OF HEAD ☐ ins.
4. EAR TO EAR OVER CROWN ☐ ins.
5. NAPE OF NECK ☐ ins.
6. TOP OF EAR TO NAPE OF NECK ☐ ins.
7. EAR TO EAR OVER FOREHEAD ☐ ins.
8. TEMPLE TO TEMPLE ACROSS FACE ☐ ins.

PARTING ☐ RIGHT ☐ LEFT ☐ CENTRE ☐ NONE

TOUPEE MEASUREMENTS

1. LENGTH ☐ ins.
2. TEMPLE ☐ ins.
3. CROWN ☐ ins.
4. BACK ☐ ins.

PARTING ☐ RIGHT ☐ LEFT ☐ CENTRE ☐ NONE

Example of a wigmaker's chart

The foundation on which the hair is knotted is the size and shape of the actor's head. This is fixed to a wooden **block** with small nails called block points. The block is held in position by a clamp attached to the edge of a table or workbench. The loose hair used for knotting is held in place using a **drawing mat** or card. The foundation is made from a pattern of the actor's head shape.

Making a pattern for a wig

The wigmaker usually takes a pattern of the actor's head at the first meeting, but the make-up artist can do it if necessary, and send it to the wig company.

1 Prepare the head by brushing the hair back from the face, as close to the head as possible.

2 Wrap cling film tightly around the head, towards the back. A single piece should be enough to wrap the front of the head, leaving two sides to attach at the back. If there is a gap on top of the head, fill in with another piece of cling film.

3 Now secure this shape with lengths of clear adhesive tape. First apply the tape over the top of the head from ear-to-ear, making sure it is not too tight. Next, put adhesive tape along the entire circumference. Cover the whole head in this way, until the pattern is rigid, like a stiff cap.

4 Draw in the existing hairline with the soft pencil: from the front, around the ear and down to the nape of the neck. If the hair is fine at the hairline, draw fine lines.

Repeat on the other side of the head until the entire hairline is drawn on the pattern. Cover the pencil line with adhesive tape to protect it.

5 Remove the pattern from the head by easing it off gently.

Making the foundation

The wigmaker cuts the pattern at the back and places it on the correct-sized wooden block. The block should be approximately 15 mm larger than the pattern (which is the circumference of the actor's head). If the block is too small it will be padded. A cut is made and tissue paper pushed through, then resealed with clear adhesive tape, and further cuts made as necessary, but not too near the hairline.

The foundation, mount or base is now made using net, gauze or silk. Springs, ribbons and fasteners provide extra support and fit. Galloon, a type of silk ribbon, is sewn around the outline of the pattern. The foundation net is sewn onto the galloon, and this forms the shape of the wig base. For a more natural looking frontal hairline, which is more suitable for television and film work, a galloon-less edge is more suitable. Once the wig foundation has been made-to-measure, it is ready for knotting the hair.

Knotting

A make-up artist needs to be able to recognise good workmanship. If the wig does need improving then knotting is a practical way of improving it, e.g. by knotting in extra hairs on a wig to soften and generally improve the appearance of a damaged or poorly knotted hairline.

Tools & equipment

- brush or comb
- clear adhesive tape
- cling-film roll
- scissors – to cut the cling-film and adhesive tape lengths
- soft black pencil

HEALTH & SAFETY

Applying the cling film

Always explain the process to the actor before you begin. Applying the cling film may make the actor feel slightly claustrophobic and warm. Ensure they are kept comfortable in a well-ventilated room and offer them a glass of water.

ACTIVITY

Cling-film activity

Measure and apply cling film to a variety of different heads. This will help to improve skill, speed and technique.

Knotting is a delicate operation, requiring patience and good eyesight. It is best to start by practising on spare pieces of foundation net attached to a block with wooden points, using straight hair, about 150 mm in length. Select a knotting needle to suit the size of the mesh of the net, and secure this firmly into the wooden handle.

Types of knotting

There are many different types of knots. Those generally used in making a wig are described below.

Single knotting

Individual knots of hair are added to the foundation net. This is the most common method of knotting when fine net is used. Different sizes of hooks can be used, depending on the amount of hair needed for each knot.

Double knotting

Double knotting is used to make the hair absolutely secure, but are less easily concealed. Generally they are used on the crown and large parts of the foundation, with single knots for the visible parts of the wig.

Point knotting

Point knotting is single knotting the point ends of the hair. The root ends are cut away, allowing the hair to lift from the piece. This technique is used for men's short-haired wigs, on the nape of the neck, on women's short-haired wigs and on light fringes.

Underknotting

After the piece has been knotted, it is turned out on a malleable block. Single knotting is applied around the edge of the foundation, following the direction of the hair on the other side. Two or three rows of underknotting can be added. The wig is usually pressed when finished, using tissue paper or cloth to protect the hair.

Types of hair used in wigs and pieces

Human hair

This is used solely for wigs and hairpieces, usually from Italy, Spain and Asia. Cleaning and dyeing processes weaken the hair and make it porous. Because the hair no longer has its natural supply of oil, it does not behave as it would on the head: either in its movement or in the way it holds any curl.

When handling a swatch of human hair, it is important to keep the root ends of the hair (the clubbed ends), lying in the same direction to stop it from tangling, and because that is the way that hair grows.

Angora goat hair

Angora goat hair is very soft and fine, suitable for specialised wigs such as period powder wigs. It can be added to other hair to provide softness.

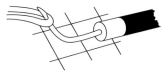

Single knotting – a small quantity of hair is placed in drawing mats with the ends protruding. A few hairs at a time are drawn out and turned over to form a loop held in the left hand; this is dampened. The knotting hook is inserted under one mesh of the lace and one or several hairs are picked up from the loop in the left hand

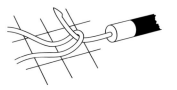

This loop is drawn under and through the hole in the lace

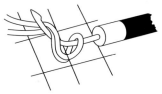

The hook is turned to catch the remaining ends of hair

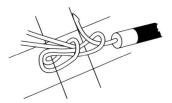

These ends are pulled carefully through the loop on the hook towards the right-hand side

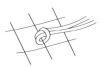

The completed knot is pulled tight so that it is as invisible as possible (dampening the hair at the outset helps this). Care should be taken to ensure that both ends of the hair are always pulled through

Horsehair

Horsehair is stiff and straight, generally used for barristers' and judges' wigs.

Artificial hair

Wigs and hairpieces are available made of synthetic hair, and are much less expensive than real hair (animal or human). They are tough and long-lasting, so are useful for theatre productions. They do not need much maintenance, just immersing in lukewarm water with fabric conditioner, rinsed in cold water and left to dry naturally. However, they are more difficult to dress, as too much heat can damage them.

Lace

The types of hair lace or gauze range from thick theatre lace to very fine laces used by television and film productions. Film and television lace comes in two thicknesses: 30 denier and 20 denier. With HD cameras the lace is getting finer and so less visible than ever before. It takes greater care and skill to knot on fine lace, as it is prone to tearing.

The colour of the lace varies from off-white to darker skin tones, and is usually coloured before knotting.

Cutting and styling the wig

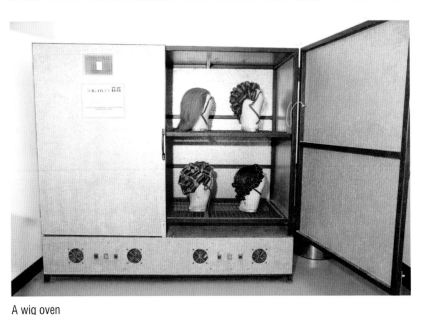

A wig oven

When the wig has been made, it is pinned onto a malleable wig block and the hair is cut and styled in the required shape. The type of setting will depend on the period or fashion. This will have been discussed during the actor's fittings and the wig dresser will have the make-up artist's notes, sketches and design material to hand. The wig is usually wet-set on rollers, secured with a hairnet and placed in a special wig oven to dry slowly for several hours or overnight. Care has to be taken when the hair is being set that the rollers, pins and clips do not damage the foundation net of the wig.

For flat styles, such as 1920s and 1930s, the wigs are finger-waved, secured with nets and placed in the oven to dry in the same way.

Delivery of the wigs

The wigs are sent by the wig company to the television or film studio on the specified date, in large wig boxes. On the lids are labels dating the time of delivery, the name of the actor, the name of the make-up designer, and the name and order number of the production company that bought or hired the items. The wigs are packed with tissue paper, dressed and ready to put on the actors' heads.

From now on, the make-up department is in charge of the wigs throughout the shoot. Their responsibilities include:

1 Preparing the actor's own hair for fitting the wig.

2 Fitting and securing the wig.

3 Dressing the wig on the actor's head.

4 Removing the wig when the actor has finished.

5 Blocking, cleaning and re-dressing the wig.

Fitting the wig

Preparing the head

If the wig has a parting, match the hair to it by parting in the same way.

1 Use grips to pincurl the natural hair – two on the crown and one on either side of the head, forming anchors.

2 Wrap the remaining hair around the head.

3 Put stocking or hairnet on the head; fix with hairpins.

4 Gel or soap short hairs around the hairline.

Tools & equipment

- gel or soap
- hairgrips
- hairpins
- stocking or hairnet

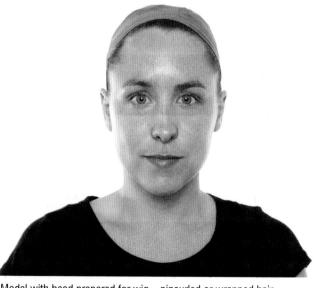

Model with head prepared for wig – pincurled or wrapped hair plus hairnet

Very short hair

If the actor's hair is very short, it is hard to make pincurls. Instead, use tiny rubber bands to secure the natural hair in very small tufts all over the head, at the crown, nape and front hairline. This method is often used on male stunt doubles.

Long hair

If the actor has long, thick hair, it is not possible to pincurl it flat. In this case the hair should be wrapped around the head as flat as possible, then covered with a hairnet or stocking top. Pins and grips can be used to secure it firmly.

Placing the wig

1 Hold the back of the wig with both hands and slide the wig front over the forehead.

2 Place one finger at the front of the lace to hold it in place, then pull down the back of the wig until it fits well on the head.

3 Using the open palms of the hands, holding the wig on each side of the head, slide the wig front back until reaching the desired hairline.

4 Comb back any stray hairs away from the front of the wig.

Attaching the hair lace

Attach the lace to the forehead, just in front of the natural hairline so that the hair growth is in line with the wig hairline.

1 Roll back the edge of the lace a little and apply spirit gum adhesive to the fore-head in three spots.

2 With the tip of one finger, make the gum tacky by tapping it gently.

3 Roll the lace back over the adhesive, pressing the edge onto the forehead with a damp cloth, making sure the lace is flat on the skin.

4 Adjust the dressing of the wig to suit the required look.

Tools & equipment

◆ damp cloth – muslin or silk
◆ spirit gum adhesive – matt

TOP TIP

Prior to attaching a wig, always ensure the actor has had a patch test for the spirit gum.

ACTIVITY

Application, removal and maintenance of a pre-styled lace wig

Working in pairs carry out the following activities:

◆ Prepare the hair for the application of a lace front wig.

◆ Apply the wig.

◆ Photograph all angles.

◆ Safely remove the wig.

◆ Clean the lace front wig.

◆ Prepare the wig for the next application by replacing the wig onto a malleable block.

Removing the wig

Always take great care when removing a wig with hair lace, so as not to damage either the actor's skin or the lace itself.

Tools & equipment

- astringent or toners
- make-up cleansing milk or cream
- mild mastix – removing liquid or cream
- moisturiser
- pad of tissue, towel or wad of cotton wool
- scissors
- small cosmetic brush

1 Loosen the lace by applying a little mild mastix on the brush to the edge of the lace.

2 Hold the tissue pad in the other hand below the lace, so that any drops from the brush trickle onto the pad and not into the actor's eyes.

3 Continue gentle dabbing at the lace where it is stuck down.

4 When the adhesive has softened, the lace may be lifted from the skin at the edges and rolled back to remove any remaining adhesive.

5 Remove the hairpins attaching the wig to the head.

6 Lift the wig from behind, holding it carefully at the sides; pull it gently forwards and off the head.

7 If it is a man's wig, detach the hair grips from the anchor points on the crown and sides; if a woman's, remove the hairnet and then the hair grips.

8 If the natural hair is so short that you used tiny rubber bands as anchor points, cut the rubber bands carefully with scissors.

9 Remove any remaining spirit gum on the face using mild mastix remover.

10 Cleanse, tone and moisturise the skin.

11 Brush through the actor's hair to restore the normal hairstyle.

Wigs without lace – hard-fronted wigs

Attach and remove the wig in the same way – without mastix and remover.

CASE PROFILE: LAURA SOLARI, HAIR AND MAKE-UP SUPERVISOR

How long have you been working in the industry?

I have been working in the industry since 1995.

How did you get into the industry?

I trained at the London College of Fashion between 1989–1991. My first professional job was in the theatre working for a good friend of mine, Wendy Topping. We had been at college together and after several years since leaving college of travelling and doing other jobs she gave me my first wig job on *Oliver* at the London Palladium.

Did you have a lucky break or turning point?

In 2007 the theatrical show I had been working on closed and I was suddenly unemployed for the first time ever. During this time a friend of mine, who worked in film, asked if I was free to do a day's filming on a Sunday. *The Duchess* film needed good hairdressers for a big crowd day at Greenwich. The hair supervisor then booked me on the rest of the film and through the contacts made on that job I became freelance and started working in films.

What has been your most significant project(s)?

Of all the theatrical shows I have done, *Mary Poppins* stands out as I was there right from the start of the design process as a head of department and had a real input into the look of the show, as well as plotting out all backstage plots and making it all happen. The creation period of a brand-new show is unlike any other experience. I am proud to have been a part of that and the friendships I made there are still with me today.

What do you enjoy most about the job?

I loved the immediacy and adrenaline in the theatre and the camaraderie and friendships you build are like family. Now I am in film I enjoy the constant changing, one day I would be creating 1940s' hairstyles and the next day doing pirates. No two days are the same.

What do you enjoy least about the job?

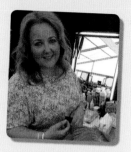

One of the things that I both love and dislike about working in the film industry is constant travel and being away from home. It's exhausting and you miss out on lots of things with family and friends. But it's also exciting and you go to places you would never ordinarily get to see. Also, working as a freelancer can be quite scary as you don't have a regular income and that takes a while to get used to.

How has the theatre/television and film industry changed during your career?

When I first started in the industry, theatre was all about hair but once Disney got involved things really changed, as they focused on every detail and the make-up became as important as the hair. This has opened up a lot of opportunities for new make-up artists.

What advice would you give to a new make-up artist starting out?

The most important thing of all: smile. Your social skills are every bit as important as your practical knowledge. Our jobs as hairdressers and make-up artists require a large degree of diplomacy and you need to be able to get along with a wide variety of people. This aspect of the job is every bit as important as your talent. Also, learn some hair skills – you will struggle to get anywhere without them. Every aspect of this industry requires some knowledge of hair, so practise.

A lot of students think that once qualified they will know everything and will be snapped up to work on the next Hollywood film. But these skills take time to acquire. So be patient, be ready to start at the bottom making tea. Your college course is just the beginning.

Cleaning and blocking a wig

When the wig has been removed from the actor's head, the hair lace will need cleaning to remove the spirit gum and make-up. Surgical spirit will do the job, using a brush to stipple onto a paper towel.

1 Pour the spirit into a bowl.

2 Place the hair lace part of the wig onto a clean towel, covered with a paper towel or tissue.

3 Dip the brush into the spirit and tap it gently onto the wig lace, forcing the dried-up mastix and make-up to go through the lace and onto the towel below. Use a gentle, firm, tapping motion: not too harsh as the lace is delicate and must not tear.

4 When the lace is clean, place the wig on the block, ready for blocking and setting.

Blocking the wig

1 Set up the malleable block and **wig stand**, and carefully centre the wig in position on the block.

2 Make sure that the hairline at the front is in position. Check that the hairline in front of the ear position is level with the other side.

3 Use large blocking pins – t-pins – to secure the wig at the ear sections and both corners of the nape area at the back of the wig.

4 Cover the lace front with galloon to reinforce the hair and protect the lace from being torn. Use small pins, known as 'short whites', to minimise stress on the lace. Place the pins in a triangular pattern along the tape. Run the tape or ribbon around the front hairline from ear to ear. Do not place any tension on the lace, only on the tape. Fold the tape to suit the shape of the hairline.

5 If the wig still feels loose, add long pins at the back of the wig until it feels secure on the block. The wig can now be set and dried – or if it needs cleaning, now is the time.

Tools & equipment

- small bowl, glass or enamel – never plastic as it can melt
- small brush – toothbrush, sable make-up brush or stipple brush
- surgical spirit or acetone
- towel, tissues or paper towels

Tools & equipment

- blocking pins – t-pins
- galloon tape
- malleable block and stand
- 'short white' pins

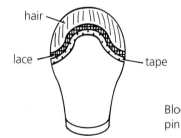
Put wig on from front to back: make sure that it is central

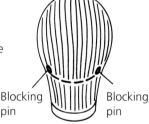
Attach the tape from ear to ear and secure it with T-pins at the two corners at the nape area

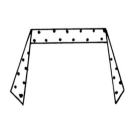
Tape down the lace, securing the tape with small pins in this pattern

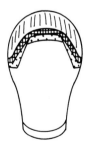
The wig is blocked and ready to be dressed

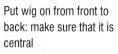

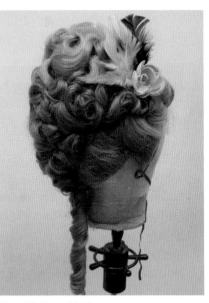

Dressed wig on block

Cleaning a wig

At some point on a long shoot there comes a time when the wigs begin to feel in need of cleaning. This is done when the wig is securely blocked, and before being set and dried. Fill a basin or sink with warm water and a squeeze of fabric conditioner. Dip the wig (still on its block) into the bowl, but do not rub or pull the hair around. Dunk the hair several times, rinse in a bowl of clean water without letting the hair become tangled. Stand the block and secured wig upright on a wig stand. Use a large detangling brush or comb, with hair conditioner if necessary, to comb the hair straight. The wig can now be set and dried in a wig oven or warm place.

Dressing a wig

Tools & equipment

- brushes – bristle, vent, half-round, round
- clips, various sizes
- crimpers
- flat irons
- galloon tape
- gels
- grips – various colours, matte if possible
- hairbands
- hairdryers – hand and hood types, or wig oven
- hair combs – tail, setting, clubbing
- heated rollers
- malleable wig blocks and stands
- mousses
- scissors
- setting rollers
- spirit gum – mastix
- tongs
- water spray

STEP-BY-STEP: VICTORIAN WIG

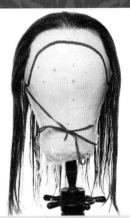

1 Block the wig.

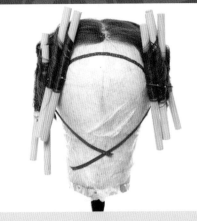

2 Set the wig on dowling, to create ringlets, and leave to dry.

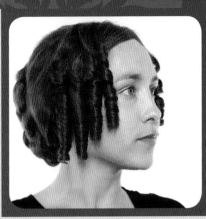

3 Dress out the wig and attach to the head with natural make-up look.

STEP-BY-STEP: EDWARDIAN WIG

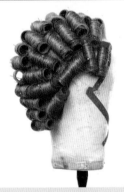

1 Block the wig, then set it with rollers and leave to dry.

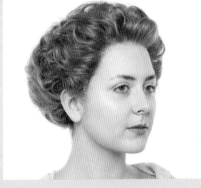

2 Attach the wig to the head, with natural make-up.

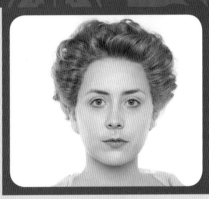

3 Front view of the finished look.

STEP-BY-STEP: 1930S WIG

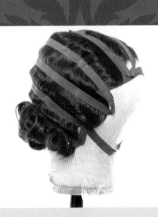

1 Make reverse pincurls at the occipital bone area. Secure the finger waves with wig tape across the dip of the waves ready for drying.

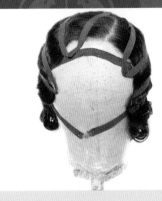

2 Front view of wig set.

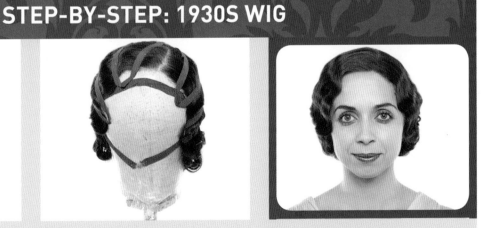

3 Dress out the wig and apply to model with 1930s make-up.

STEP-BY-STEP: 1940S WIG

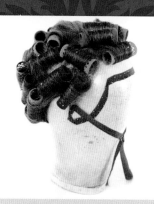

1 Block the wig, then set it on rollers, ready for drying.

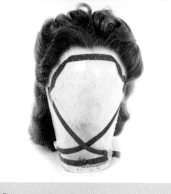

2 Dress out the wig.

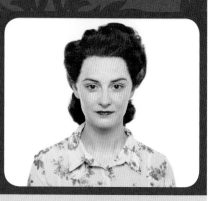

3 Attach the wig to the person, with 1940s make-up for final look.

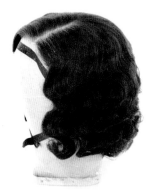

Dressed out 1930s finger waves

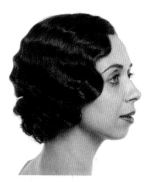

1930s finger waves' final look

Finger waves

Finger waves were fashionable in the 1920s and 1930s. The technique of finger waving is moulding the wet hair into S-shaped movements using the fingers and a comb. Finger waving a wig is carried out as follows:

1 Block up the wig in the usual way and spray down the hair without getting the lace and malleable block too wet. Make a straight side parting.

2 Keeping with the root direction of the hair, make the first wave of the hair by combing the hair from the roots.

3 Pinch the 'crest' of the wave between two fingers and comb the rest of the hair in the opposite direction.

4 Move your fingers down to pinch the next 'crest', then comb the rest of the hair, again in the opposite direction. Try to keep the waves an even width. Use fingers as a guide – two fingers are approximately 30 mm.

5 Work in circles around the parting, taking the waves around the head until you reach the occipital bone. At this point, continue with reverse pincurls, barrel curls or pincurls set into the centre.

6 Secure the finger waves by applying wig tape across the 'dip' of the wave. Use a little tension and insert pins along the tape.

7 Place in a warm place to dry thoroughly. It will help if you remember the following tips:

◆ The hair should be combed thoroughly to get rid of any tangles.

◆ Use warm water to wet the hair and comb it on the slant backwards.

◆ Keep the hair wet (but not dripping) during the waving process.

◆ Take care with the parting. It must be perfectly straight. Pin a tape along the parting to keep it neat, but do not place pins through the parting.

◆ For short hair, make shallow rather than deep waves.

◆ For a soft, natural look, it is best to avoid deep waves as these can look hard.

◆ Short hair at the front of the wig can be curled separately. This gives a soft effect around the face and forehead.

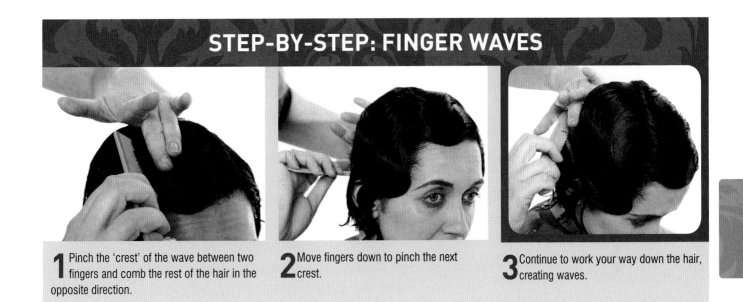

STEP-BY-STEP: FINGER WAVES

1 Pinch the 'crest' of the wave between two fingers and comb the rest of the hair in the opposite direction.

2 Move fingers down to pinch the next crest.

3 Continue to work your way down the hair, creating waves.

Complete **dressing out a wig** as follows, when dry.

1 After removing the block from the oven or warm place, allow it to cool for a few minutes.

2 Using a tail comb, lift up a thin layer of the hair along the parting. Backcomb the hair strongly near the roots, gradually lessening the backcombing as you work towards the points.

3 Continue making divisions and backcombing until the entire wig has been worked on.

4 Comb softly over the top to smooth the hair down and push or press the waves into position. Try not to comb out too much of the backcombing.

5 Use one or two large pins to hold the waves down at the edges.

6 Leave the hair at the parting raised: hair on the head does not grow flat from the parting.

7 Adjust the final shape, place a hairnet over the wig and return it to the oven or warm place for about 30 minutes.

8 Do not comb out the wig afterwards or it will look too flat. The very top layer of hair can be combed smooth.

ACTIVITY

Finger waves research

Research different hairstyles that contain finger waves. Produce a mood board with images from your research and photos of styles created on your models.

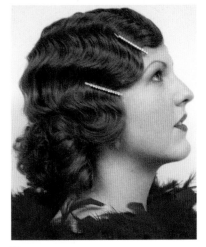

Finger waves

Tools & equipment

- hairgrips
- hairpiece
- hairpins

TOP TIP

Always ensure the hairpiece has been colour matched prior to application. Good quality photographs may be used before the event to gain the best results.

Tools & equipment

- hairpins
- parting piece or toupee
- toupee tape – tape that is sticky both sides

Hairpieces

Hairpieces add length and fullness to a hairstyle.

A pincurl base is made by curling a small section of hair close to the head and securing it with hairgrips crossing over one another to form a cross.

1 First assess the size and weight of the hairpiece.

2 Make a pincurl base, as above, on the natural hair or the wig, as appropriate.

3 Attach the hairpiece to the pincurl base with hairpins. Hook a hairpin through the loop of the hairpiece, pinching the pin together as you do this, so that when you let it go it springs out and grips the surrounding hair.

4 Secure the piece with more pins, making sure that they grip into the pincurl base.

5 Dress the piece to blend with the natural hair or wig.

Parting pieces and toupees

A parting piece or toupee is attached at the centre of the head. Always look at the piece first, placing it on the head in different positions to find out where it looks best.

1 Make pincurls on the head with the natural hair. If there is no hair, as on a balding man, toupee tape can be used.

2 Attach the piece with hairpins, weaving them in and blending them with the natural hair.

3 Style the hair as required.

Hard-front wigs

Hand knotted wigs of human hair with hair lace are used in television and film because they can stand up to camera close-ups. They are very expensive to buy, rent, repair and maintain.

Hard-front wigs cost less and are more hardwearing. They have no lace fronts and provide a full head of hair without the need to blend the make-up. They are easy to put on, and are used in theatres, low-budget films, and background shots in television and film crowd scenes. Made with human hair, they are dressed in the same way as hair lace wigs. To hide the hard front edge, some front hair on the actor's head can be pulled forwards and then combed back to cover the edge.

A temporary hair colour can be sprayed on the real hair to blend with the wig.

CASE PROFILE: JO NEILSEN, WIG SUPERVISOR

How long have you been working in the industry?

I left college in 2000, but was fortunate to start working within the industry in the previous year.

How did you get into the industry?

I was a student at the London College of Fashion and there I found an advert for work experience in theatre. At the time I had no industry experience and so I applied. I was so fortunate to get the placement. The job turned out to be a 'swing' for the wig department on *Oklahoma* at the Lyceum in the West End as it moved from The National. I couldn't believe my luck.

Did you have a lucky break or a turning point?
I wouldn't say I had a lucky break but I was so very lucky with the people above me on that job. They absolutely carved my career by teaching me what was right and what was wrong. I was lucky to have mentors who helped me make the right choices in future work and still do to this day.

What has been your most significant project?
It would have to be *Wicked*. The show has taught me so much and continues to do so. It has transformed my views on theatre. It was the first show I supervised and I owe it a lot.

What do you enjoy most about the job?
We do something different every day. We meet new people with different ideas every day and consequently we learn something new every day.

How has the theatre industry changed during your career?
When I first started, to me there were very much groups of make-up artists that stayed within their industry boundaries. Now I see people in theatre working in film, fashion people in theatre and television people in fashion, etc. People are crossing from group to group. It's fantastic. Everybody learning from each other, sharing tips, stories and helping with situations that we would otherwise be none the wiser about.

What advice would you give to a new make-up artist starting out?
Don't pre-judge anybody.

Weft work

Wigs and hairpieces

Weft work is the weaving of hair in making wigs and hairpieces. The hair is interwoven onto silk, cotton thread or wire, interweaving at the root ends and forming lengths of weft. The weft is folded, spirally wound, or sewn onto a mount or base.

Wigs made in this way are known as weft wigs, and many other hairpieces use woven or weft work.

Weft wigs and pieces are less expensive than hand knotted ones, but the quality of the finish is not as good. Weft pieces are useful for adding to natural hair to provide bulk and length in period hair work.

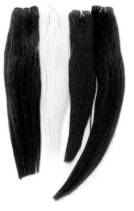
Hairpieces

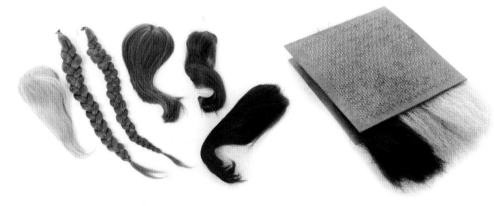
Wefts   Hackle

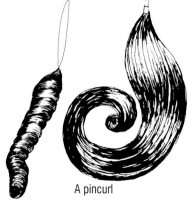

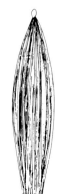

A pincurl

A ringlet

Other hairpieces

Extra can be added to a wig or the natural hair.

◆ **Chignons** Knotted or wefted hairpieces attached between the crown and neck. Good for adding fullness, height and shape.

◆ **Marteaux** Pieces of weft folded together, attached to the hair with combs or sewn loops. Good for adding a wave.

◆ **Switches** Lengths of weft wound spirally around a tailcord. They can be coiled, plaited and twisted in a variety of ways.

◆ **Pincurls** Small pieces of weft sewn into curl shapes. Good for adding to a dressed hairstyle.

◆ **Swathes** Made from two marteaux, sewn end to end. Good for encircling the head.

◆ **Torsades** Coiled pieces of hairwork added to the hair.

◆ **Bandeaux wigs or cape wiglets** Can be knotted or wefted hairpieces. Good for turning a short hairstyle into a long one. Held in position by a band, leaving the real front hair showing. They can be any length at the back.

◆ **Transformations** Hairpieces, either wefted or knotted. Worn to add length or bulk to the existing hair. Often used on men for period work.

◆ **Semi-transformations** Smaller pieces also used to add length to the existing hair.

◆ **Fringes or frontal pieces** Wefted or knotted, used on the front of the head.

◆ **Double loop clusters** Wefted hairpiece, made by winding and sewing onto a card, finished with loops at each end.

◆ **Hidden comb** A bunch of curls attached to a hidden comb; the technique is also known as top knots. These may be knotted pieces, but are usually wefted. The weft is made on two silks and a wire which, when folded and sewn, forms a very pliable foundation piece.

See Cleaning a Wig section on page 168 for how to clean the hairpieces.

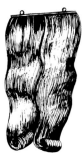

A switch

A coiled switch

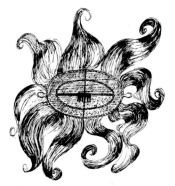

A marteau with hoops

Temporary hair colours

Temporary colouring is often used in television and film to alter the colour of the hairpiece, wig or natural hair. It can be used to cover white or grey to make actors look younger, or to paint in white and silver to make them look older. They are also used to create vibrant fashion effects.

Types of temporary hair colours that wash out easily

◆ **Coloured hair lacquers** Available in many colours and used by spraying onto the dressed hair.

◆ **Hair colour sprays** Liquid or powder, sprayed onto dressed hair.

◆ **Hair colour setting lotions** Applied to towel-dried hair.

A chignon: view from underneath to show the foundation with loops and a comb to attach the piece to the head

◆ **Cosmetic hair colouring liquids** Packaged in bottles or wands for painting onto the hair with a brush.

◆ **Hair colour crayons** Used directly on the hair when dressed. Good for colouring hair at the temple areas or filling in a bald patch on the head.

◆ **Gels and mousses** Used directly onto the hair, they colour and condition the hair and give extra 'hold'.

◆ **Hair glitter** Available in loose form to sprinkle in the hair for a sparkling, glittering or twinkling effect.

◆ **Hair gel glitter** Comes in tube form in iridescent colours. Gives strong effects under lights.

◆ **Hair colour creams** Packaged in small pots, the pinks and yellows can be painted onto individual hairs to neutralise dark hair before applying the chosen colour. They are generally used before painting streaks of white, cream and silver at the front hairline.

'Breaking down' effects

Very often a scene may require an actor to look dirty or wet, including the hair. The type of dirt – dusty or muddy – must be considered for the effect to be realistic looking.

Products for dirtying the hair

◆ **Powders** Dark brown, grey or black for dry-looking dirt. Fuller's earth is also useful.

◆ **Greasepaint or creams** Gives a greasy, matted effect.

◆ **Coloured hairsprays** In dark colours for **breaking down** blonde hair.

Making the hair look wet

Use a spray bottle filled with water and used before each take. Be mindful of continuity, because sets and locations are so expensive, the order in which the production is filmed hardly ever follows the storyline.

When filming rain scenes, always take photographs of the actor's hair. When the character comes in from the rain the interior scene may be shot weeks later.

'Breaking down' effects add to the realism of the story. For casualty effects, any blood on the hair should be a washable, non-staining product.

> **TOP TIP**
>
> Glitter can sometimes shed after application. This can cause problems with photographers, as loose glitter can drop on the model's face and need editing after the photoshoot.

> **TOP TIP**
>
> Never use products made for the hair on an actor's skin. Always follow the manufacturer's instructions for use.

REVISION QUESTIONS

1 How would you maintain artificial hair?

2 How would you wash and style a lace front wig?

3 How should a make-up designer store and care for a wig?

4 State the differences for removing a lace front wig and a hard front wig.

5 What is a 'short white'? And what is its purposes?

6 What is the purpose of galloon tape?

7 When pouring cleaning solvent into a container to clean hair lace, why is it wrong to use a plastic bowl?

8 How would you protect the actor's face when applying solvent to the lace in order to remove a wig?

9 Period make-up and hair

LEARNING OBJECTIVES

This chapter covers the following:

◆ Researching and designing period make-up.

◆ Make-up and hair worn by people in different eras including the Egyptians, Greeks and Romans.

◆ Make-up from different periods including the Middle Ages, and the sixteenth, seventeenth, eighteenth, nineteenth and twentieth centuries.

◆ How to choose the right look for a period.

◆ Adapting fashion make-up to period styles.

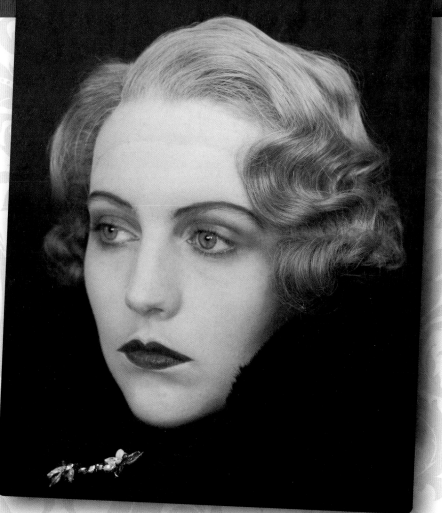

UNIT TITLE

◆ Prepare and apply wigs and hairpieces
   to change the performer's appearance

INTRODUCTION

This chapter covers different period make-up looks and different historical eras, from the Middle Ages through the sixteenth, seventeenth, eighteenth, nineteenth and twentieth centuries. You will understand how to choose the right look for specific periods and how to adapt fashion make-up to period styles. This research will help you to develop your Level 3 fashion and photographic work, and understand how to create an accurate look to reflect a specific period. A sound knowledge of period make-up and hair is invaluable for various different areas of the industry, especially period dramas and historical films. Iconic celebrities that epitomise different eras are used as examples to help you to develop your knowledge of different period looks.

Period make-up

Many productions are made within a specific time period in the past. Researching the period in which the story is set is one of the most interesting parts of a make-up artist's job. The history of the times that people lived in, how they dressed their hair and what make-up they wore are always fascinating to research. How authentic the final look you choose depends on the job you are working on. Sometimes the style will be softened to suit current fashion; at other times it will be accurate to the last detail. When planning the make-up and hair, the age, type of person and environment should be taken into account as well as the fashion of the day.

Research and design

All areas of the media are subject to research and design in period make-up and hair. The script, type of production and director's wishes are the main thing, followed by other departments' decisions, e.g. using certain colours. Then there are the views of the actors themselves. The setting of the story, culture, climate and period all guide the make-up artist in finding the right information and inspiration for the production.

Following are some basic guides for period fashions in make-up and hair based on vintage photographs, magazines, old films, paintings and sculptures. The time periods are measured in decades which provide a quick reference, but the beginning of each decade will be strongly influenced by the previous one, so more detailed research will be needed in many cases.

Prehistoric people

The Natural History Museum in London has evidence of prehistoric people in reconstructions, as well as pictures and books on anthropology. Early cave drawings also provide visual information and are the earliest known drawings by human beings.

The earliest drawings of Neanderthal men show a receding forehead with a broad flat nose and a heavy powerful jaw. The neck was thick, the eye structure projected forward and they were very hairy.

Films set in this period have used prosthetics and dentures to achieve the look.

The Egyptians

The Egyptian civilisation, founded around 3000 BC left plenty of material recording their culture. It is known that Egyptians shaved their heads and wore wigs made from the hair of animals, humans and vegetable fibres. They wore plenty of make-up and were probably the first people to use black kohl around their eyes. Vegetable dyes, red clay and white lead were all used to adorn the faces of both sexes. The hair colour was usually black, but the wigs were sometimes dyed in bright shades of green, blue and red with the eyeshadow often matching the wig.

The eye make-up has become well known through archaeological evidence following the uncovering of buried tombs. The famous black lines drawn around the eyes from the inner core and extended outwards in a straight line 3 cm beyond the outer corner is the classic Cleopatra style. The eyelashes and eyebrows were blackened and

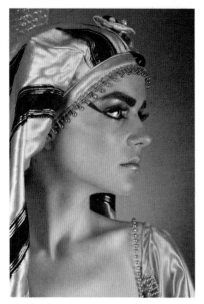
Cleopatra

the brows extended outwards. The cheeks and lips were reddened with carmine and the natural brown skin tone was often whitened with lead and oil foundations.

The Greeks

The Greek civilisation around 350 BC offered the ideal of the perfect face, which was accepted for many years. A painted marble head, dating from 350 BC and found in a Greek temple, depicts a fashionable lady with full make-up. The eyebrows are painted black, the upper eyelids are reddish-brown, and dark green is painted in the eye sockets. The same green is used as a strong eyeline on the eyelids close to the upper lashes and extended at the outer corners. The lips and cheeks are rouged a brownish-red colour. The women had long hair and dressed it in elaborate styles, incorporating ringlets. Combs and jewels were used to decorate the hairstyle.

The men did not wear wigs. Soldiers were clean-shaven and had their hair cut short and curled; many statues exist which show the curled hair brushed forward. Some men dyed their hair blond or red and many of the elders had beards and moustaches.

The ideal of the perfect Greek form of physical beauty relied on the proportions of the female face – large eyes, short nose – heart-shaped face, etc., and the legendary athletic men racing with flaming torches, which led to the Olympic Games today.

The Romans

A statue of a Roman beauty from the first century AD shows heavily darkened eyebrows, rouged lips and cheeks. Most of the information about the use of make-up in those days comes from the objections in writing during the early Christian period. In the fourth century, St Ambrose called women, 'harlots' for whitening their faces, necks and breasts, blackening their eyebrows and dyeing their hair. The fashionable colours for hair were blonde and red.

Pictorial evidence shows that the average Roman man had short hair and was clean-shaven. The older men, intellectuals and philosophers had long hair and flowing beards.

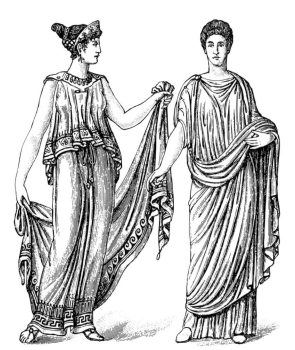

Greek woman (left); Roman woman (right)

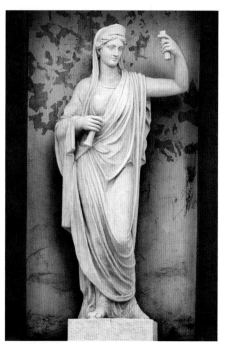

A Greek statue

The Middle Ages

The Middle Ages span the period AD 400–1500. Medieval women used white lead to achieve a pale complexion, as the fashion for pale skins continued throughout Europe. A fourteenth-century sculpted Madonna from Spain shows plucked, painted eyebrows, rouged lips and cheeks, and black-lined eyes.

Many Dutch and French paintings dating from 1447–75 show plucked eyebrows and high, shaved foreheads. The women wore headdresses and removed any hair showing at the hairline. When not covering their heads, their hair was long and dressed close to the head. The fashionable colours for hair were blonde and black, but not red.

Medieval men had long hair with flowing beards. By 1509, when Henry VII of England died, men's hair was being worn shorter, with the facial hair trimmed. Hair had become less elaborate than earlier in the century.

ACTIVITY

Use books and the Internet to research Holbein paintings or pictures of Henry VIII at court to gain an accurate understanding of the fashion, hair and make-up worn in the Middle Ages.

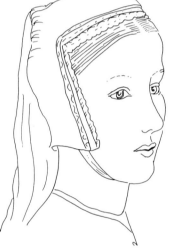

The sixteenth century

The sixteenth century

The Renaissance is the name given to this period of history because of the revival of arts, literature and science, bringing in a new style of architecture and decoration to succeed the Gothic style.

In England, Queen Elizabeth I (reigned 1558–1603) favoured red hair, which became fashionable. She also favoured heavy cosmetics, which became heavier the older she became. During her reign the influence of the Renaissance became strong, and the dress, speech and manners of Italy became fashionable at her court.

White lead was still being used for a pale skin colour, and artists' pigments used for painting the face. No attempt was made to extract colours from natural plants because this was the new scientific age. There are many portraits of Queen Elizabeth and society ladies of that era for reference material.

ACTIVITY

Use books and the Internet to research portraits of Queen Elizabeth I and Francis Drake to gain an accurate understanding of the fashion, hair and make-up worn in the sixteenth century.

Queen Elizabeth wore wigs when she became old and the style was hair dressed high on the head, often decorated with pearls or other jewellery. Large ruffles were worn around the neck by both sexes, so men had short hair with neat beards and moustaches.

The seventeenth century

The French and English make-up and hair became similar when Charles I of England (reigned 1625–49) married Henrietta Maria, the sister of Louis XIII of France (reigned 1610–43). It is important to remember that cosmetics were used only by sophisticated society living in large cities. Country people used little or no paint and had healthier lives.

As the fashionable ladies of the English and French courts used more make-up, they started putting patches on their faces. The patches were shaped in stars, half moons and round shapes, cut out of black taffeta, Spanish leather or gummed paper. The patches

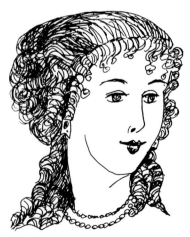

The seventeenth century

became useful for hiding scars or skin afflictions, becoming more excessive in use. Famous portraits dating between 1670 and 1685 show that the fashionable look was a wide, fleshy face with a double chin, prominent eyes, full red lips, dark eyebrows and dark hair.

The Cavalier men wore their hair shoulder length and curled. Their moustaches were curled, trimmed and waxed. Beards became shorter and neater.

Puritan men cut their hair short and round with no facial hair. They were called Round-heads. Louis XII started the fashion for men's wigs in France and Charles II popularised black wigs. The men were also using make-up. Judge Jeffreys, Lord Chancellor of England in 1678, was notorious for his extravagant use of make-up.

In Asia and Africa the make-up was different. According to writers of the early seventeenth century (1603–25) we learn that many Moorish women were observed with tattoos on their faces, and bodies were decorated with henna.

CASE PROFILE: SALLIE JAYE, MAKE-UP DESIGNER

How long have you been working in the industry?

Thirty-four years.

How did you get into the industry?

I did a City & Guilds in Ladies' Hairdressing at Kingston College and then joined the BBC as a trainee for two years. I then became a member of the department and stayed for 12 years.

Did you have a lucky break or a turning point?

My lucky break came when I got employed as make-up designer on *The Wings of the Dove*, which was my first feature film, for which I was lucky enough to win a Bafta for Best Make-Up.

What has been your most significant project?

Gosh, that's a difficult one. Every job I do is significant as I never stop learning and everything I do adds to my experience.

How has the industry changed during your career?

The industry has changed a lot recently with the advance in digital viewing, as opposed to the old film rushes on a big screen. Also the huge advance in visual effects, with so much now able to be adjusted in post production.

What advice would you give to a new make-up artist starting out?

My advice to anyone joining the industry now would be to only do it if you really love doing make-up and hair, as it is a really tough job.

The eighteenth century

The ladies at court continued to use heavy make-up, whitening their faces with lead pant and applying rouge heavily. They also powdered their shoulders and accentuated veins on the bosom with blue. By now there was publicity about the danger of using white lead paint, but the fashion still continued in England, and even more excessively in France from where most of the cosmetics came.

The gentlemen also wore face paint and rouged their cheeks heavily. The fashion of powdering the hair or wig was very popular. White powder or flour was used by the nobil-ity and soldiers. Moustaches and beards were out of fashion. The hair was still worn in a pigtail (or queue), using either the natural hair or a wig.

Military men did not have facial hair at this time. By 1768 the men at court were blackening their eyebrows and reddening their lips. Women's eyebrows were plucked and redrawn

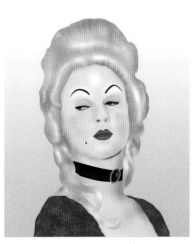

The eighteenth century

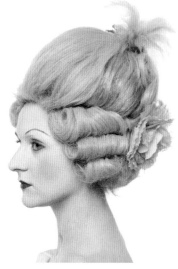

The eighteenth century look

high and curved. The lips were painted red in a small rounded 'beesting' effect. By the middle of the century rouge was being placed in a round shape, low on the cheeks in a bright pink colour. Patches were still being worn. During Queen Anne's reign (1702–14) patches became a political symbol, with Tories wearing their patches on the left side of the face, and Whig supporters on the right.

The wigs became larger and more fantastic until a tax on hair powdering was introduced in 1759. The excesses of this period were worst in France, and it all came to an end with the French Revolution.

ACTIVITY

Eyebrows

Research different eyebrow fashions over different historical periods. Include research information and eyebrow styles you have applied yourself. Compare the changes in different periods.

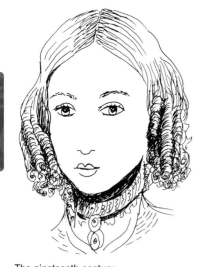

The nineteenth century

The nineteenth century

After the French Revolution anything associated with the aristocracy went out of fashion. Powdered wigs were not used, and most men had short hair. They grew sideburns and moustaches, and by the middle of the century beards came into fashion. Wigs were only used in the courts for official legal occasions.

Women used cosmetics very discreetly. When Queen Victoria came to the English throne (reigned 1837–1901), there was a reaction against the use of painting the face. Cosmetics were still used, much of it home-made, and used lightly. Officially, powders, creams and lotions were all that ladies used to preserve their looks. Only stage performers and courtesans openly applied face paints.

Women's hair was long, and dressed high on the head in rolls and curls, with ringlets at the sides of the face, and centre partings.

The men cultivated large handlebar moustaches with carefully curled ends.

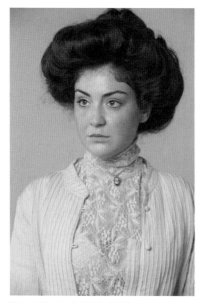

Edwardian look 1901-1914

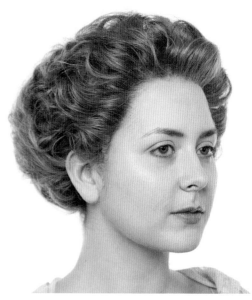

Edwardian look 1901-1914

CASE PROFILE: STACEY HOLMAN, MAKE-UP ARTIST

How long have you been working in the industry?

Four years.

How did you get into the industry?

Whilst at Delamar Academy, I was lucky enough to do work experience with some of the tutors, Tracey Lee on *Episodes* and Lorraine Hill on *Outside Bet*. I have worked for Lorraine on many projects, and she gave me my first paid job on a low-budget feature called *Get Lucky*.

I got some work experience days on *Dancing on Ice* which let to me being paid as a trainee on the hair designer's next job *Popstar to Operastar* and then again on the next series of *Dancing on Ice*. To support myself financially, I worked in a makeover studio whilst doing student films and low-budget features. Doing student films during your study time is essential. It gives you the basis of set etiquette and a great foundation of putting everything you learn together.

What has been your most significant project?

Being the trainee on *The Muppets – Most Wanted* was an amazing experience. I hadn't worked on a big-budget feature and it was eye opening. As there was no crowd supervisor in charge of the crowd room, I was the only permeant fixture, which came with a whole load of paperwork and organisational skills I didn't realise I had. Every day was a challenge, and the hours were extremely long, especially when the crowd room was moving, I would have to be there when the boxes arrived in the morning and to set the new crowd room up – this had to take place most days before 5 a.m. Luckily for me, there wasn't much else being filmed in London, so we had many of the top designers and make-up artists in the crowd room. It was amazing to get my name out there and break into the big-budget film work. After *The Muppets*, I had many job offers from people I met in the crowd room, and was very lucky to get onto *Game of Thrones* in Croatia as a result of working on *The Muppets*.

What do you enjoy most about the job?

I love that I'm constantly learning, you will never know everything as it's always changing and there is so much to know. I am always looking for different courses and ways to widen my knowledge.

Traveling is also a part I love, whether it be the Yorkshire dales or a castle in Croatia. I have been very lucky to visit to the places I have filmed in. On *Death Comes to Pemberly* we shot in the most beautiful manor houses of England, and I have seen places I never would have visited otherwise. I love travelling and with this job you get to see everything!

What do you enjoy least about the job?

The hours are the hardest part about the job, they are early, long and late! The key is to never moan though! Everyone else is doing exactly the same hours as you. You don't want to be known as the moaner and it brings down the mood on the make-up truck. Just make sure you get enough rest on your days off and try to keep yourself as healthy as possible. Take multivitamins and, even though it's hard to eat healthy on set, it really does make a difference if you reach for an apple instead of chocolate.

What advice would you give to a new make-up artist starting out?

Don't give up, and don't be afraid to ask questions.

There were many times in the first two years that I was close to quitting and getting a 9–5 job. But something was always holding me back from doing that. I now know there is nothing else I would rather do, and it's so rare to love your job so much that it doesn't feel like a job! I know money can be an issue when you are first starting out, if you need to get a part-time job, try to do something with make-up or hair, such as working on a counter or makeover studio, that way you can still practise your skills.

The twentieth century

Make-up continued to be used discreetly. The hairstyles for women were still long and dressed on top of the head in a looser style, such as the 'pompadour' (see photograph).

The outbreak of World War I (1914–18) changed society in England forever. During those years there was a shortage of manpower in the country, and women took on many of the traditional male roles. The women's suffrage movement had been ignored, but women

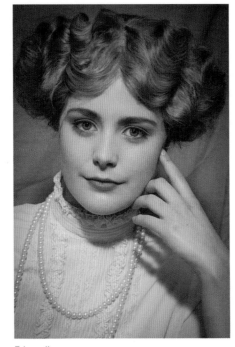
Edwardian

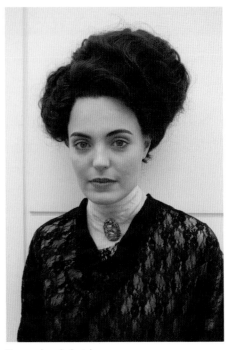
Pompadour hairstyle

were continuing to demand the right to vote. It was not until 1928 that women over the age of 21 were granted the same voting rights as men.

After the war the younger women started ditching their long bustle skirts, corsets and long up-swept hairstyles. The skirts and hair became shorter, and a new look was created for the new era.

The 1920s

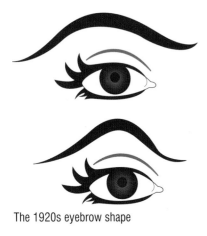
The 1920s eyebrow shape

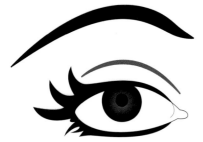
The 1930s eyebrow shape

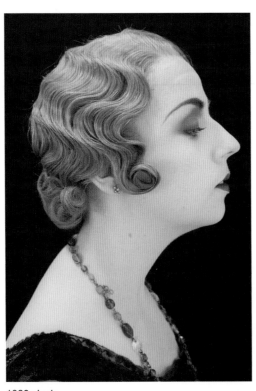
1920s look

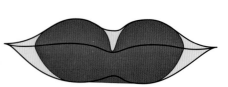
Cupid's bow lips

The new short hairstyle was called the 'bob' and a new make-up style complemented it. By 1925 the fashion was pale powdered skin, red lips in a 'cupid's bow' shape, plucked eyebrows redrawn in a thin arch sloping downwards at the ends. The eyes were heavily shaded with smudgy soft eyeshadows in greys, blacks and blues. The short hairstyles were set in finger waves, with tongs or rag curlers.

The advent of films shown in picture houses created a new breed of movie stars. One of them was Clara Bow, and her look was copied by many women. Other role models were Joan Crawford, Claudette Colbert, Greta Garbo, and, for men, Clark Gable, among others.

Men were shaving off their facial hair, and any moustaches were neatly clipped. Their hair was always short, neat and dressed with hair oil or cream.

The 1930s

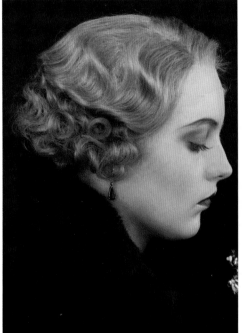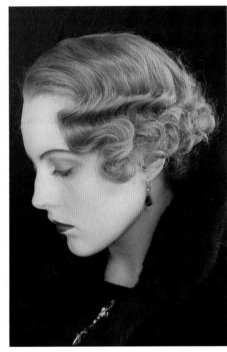

1930s make-up and hair

During this decade the make-up and hair became a bit softer. The face was still heavily powdered and rouge was applied lower on the cheeks than before. Eyeshadow was blended from the eyelids to the eyebrows in subtle smoky blues, violets and greys. The eyebrows were not plucked so heavily – only at the ends – but were still pencilled elegantly. Lipstick was still red but the shape was wider and more natural looking. The film industry had grown in popularity, continuing to provide role models who were widely copied by everyone. These included Jean Harlow with her platinum bleached hair, Norma Shearer, Greta Garbo, Joan Crawford, Marlene Dietrich, Ginger Rogers and Vivien Leigh. While the male stars included Fred Astaire, Laurence Olivier, Spencer Tracy and Clark Gable.

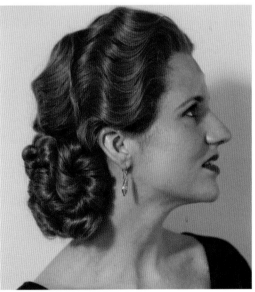

1930s make-up and hair

ACTIVITY

Use books and the Internet to research pictures of Jean Harlow, Greta Garbo, Joan Crawford, Marlene Dietrich, Ginger Rogers and Vivien Leigh to gain an accurate understanding of the fashion, hair and make-up worn by women in the 1930s.

ACTIVITY

Use books and the Internet to research pictures of Fred Astaire and Spencer Tracy to gain an accurate understanding of the fashion, hair and make-up worn by men in the 1930s.

ACTIVITY

Use books and the Internet to research pictures of Lauren Bacall and Veronica Lake to gain an accurate understanding of the fashion, hair and make-up worn by women in the 1940s.

Men's moustaches were popular, but beards weren't. Their hair was usually curly, and short. Nail varnish was used in bright or dark colours by the women.

The 1940s

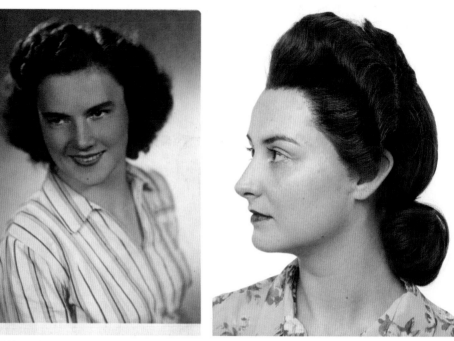

1940s make-up and hair

From 1939, World War II in Europe meant there was a shortage of cosmetics. The only make-up produced was a red matte lipstick which the government allowed to be made to raise women's morale. Once more women were doing men's jobs: driving buses, working in factories and ploughing the fields. Long hair became a symbol of their femininity, along with the red lipstick.

The Americans did not join the war for several more years, but their films continued to provide entertainment in the cinemas, and the theatres did well as people looked for escapism in musicals and love stories. Favourite film stars included Lauren Bacall, Gene Tierney, Vivien Leigh, Joan Crawford, Marlene Dietrich, Veronica Lake and Norma Shearer.

The fashionable look in make-up and hair became stronger than the doll-like look of previous decades. Not much eye make-up was used; it was generally long hair, up or down, strong eyebrows, full red lips. Padded shoulders and knee-length skirts or dresses, which contributed to the empowering look.

The film star Veronica Lake wore her hair long in soft waves falling across one side of her face: a style which many girls copied. Although glamorous, this was a health hazard when operating machinery, so women working in factories had to roll it up in a scarf or snood to avoid accidents.

Another hairstyle was long at the back and turned under, with the sides pulled up and secured to the top of the head. Curls were rolled up at the front or sides of the forehead. There was no hairspray available, but women used sugar and water.

The men had moustaches but no beards. Brylcream and other products were used to keep their short hair shiny and in place.

The 1950s

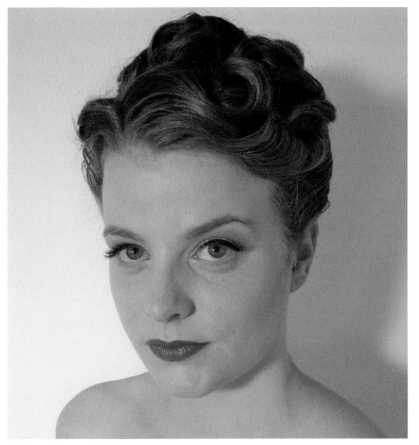

1950s make-up and hair

ACTIVITY

Use books and the Internet to research pictures of Elizabeth Taylor, Grace Kelly, Doris Day, Deborah Kerr, Audrey Hepburn, Cary Grant, James Dean, Elvis Presley, Burt Lancaster to gain an accurate understanding of the fashion, hair and make-up worn in the 1950s.

ACTIVITY

Use books and the Internet to research pictures of Gina Lollobrigida with an Italian cut to gain an understanding of this hairstyle.

ACTIVITY

Use books and the Internet to research pictures of Jackie Kennedy with a bouffant to gain an understanding of this hairstyle.

The war was over in Europe, and the mood was optimistic. This was reflected in women's fashions. There was a choice of products and colours, as make-up was being manufactured and imported again.

The new look was clean, bright and girlish. The eyebrows were beautifully shaped and filled in. The eyeshadows were on the eyelids only in muted blues, greys, greens and browns. Lips were fully painted in not just red, but coral, pink or orange. Rouge or blusher was not obvious in this look. What was different was the eyelines on the top eyelids painted close to the eyelashes and flicked up at the outer corners. The skin tone was still pale and powdered.

The hairstyles became shorter, fuller and curlier. Blonde was still a popular colour; in films it was often platinum blonde. As the cinema was more popular than ever, the stars continued to inspire the trends – actors such as Marilyn Monroe, Vivien Leigh, Elizabeth Taylor, Doris Day, Grace Kelly and Audrey Hepburn. The role models for the men were Clark Gable, James Stewart, Cary Grant, James Dean and Elvis Presley.

European films influenced fashion. In 1953 the Italian film stars started a trend in hairstyles called the 'Italian cut'. This was a short, shaggy-looking style which was popular for a while. Another was the bouffant: a thick pageboy style, full at the sides and heavily sprayed with lacquer to hold it in place.

In the mid-1950s the 'Mandarin' look arrived from Paris. The outer ends of the eyebrows were plucked, and redrawn in an upwards stroke. The eyelines were also drawn upwards at the outer corners. Red lips, no cheek colour, pale powdered skin completed the look. The hair was pulled up in a chignon or short and curled.

The men's hair was short back and sides, with long hair at the front in a tuft or wave. Crew cuts were also popular.

TOP TIP

Many different eras have influenced eyeliner styles. Practise, practise, practise to help perfect different lengths, flicks depths and angles.

Always stretch the skin around the eye area to help achieve your look.

Try different mediums including kohl liners, gel pots, cake liners, pens and liquid liners.

The 1960s

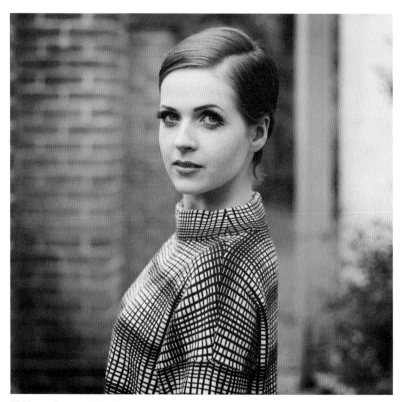

1960s make-up and hair

The ladylike look of the 1950s gave way to a different generation of people seeking changes in art, music, theatre, film, literature and fashion. There were many different trends, each more bizarre than the last.

For women, eye make-up dominated the decade. In 1962 the Egyptian look was fashionable, with heavy black eyelines and strong eyebrows. In 1963 the lips were played down, with no colour, as attention was focused on the heavy eye make-up. In 1965 the eyebrows were played down (or hidden by heavy fringed hairstyles), as were the lips. The heavily made-up eyes included false eyelashes. This was a very theatrical look, using a pale neutral colour on the lids, dark shading in the eye sockets, pale colour on the brow bones with painted eyelines on the top and bottom lids. Sometimes false lashes were worn on the bottom lids as well as the top. Eyelash curlers were used to curl the natural eyelashes before applying the false ones, and mascara to brush them together.

Any lipstick used was frosted pink or chalky colours. Another look was to outline the lips lightly with a brown pencil and use Vaseline on the lips.

TOP TIP

When applying false eyelashes always get your model/actor/client to look away from you. Ensure they are not staring directly into the light as their eyes will water and make the eyelash application difficult.

Skin tones were no longer pale, as everyone travelled and suntans were fashionable. Freckles were sometimes dotted across the nose to look like freckles on a tanned skin. Blusher or rouge was placed under the cheekbones to contour the face.

Hairpieces were popular for making the hair fuller and longer. A style called the 'beehive' consisted of a basic French pleat at the back of the head, with the rest of the hair back-combed strongly and combed smoothly on top. Fringes were popular, with short layered hair, cut with a razor for an uneven effect.

A model called 'Twiggy' became the face of the 1960s from 1966–70, with an angelic face, big eyes and short straight hair.

Brigitte Bardot, a French film star with long blonde, tousled hair and pouting lips, inspired a new look which was copied by many.

A new brand of clothing and cosmetics called 'Biba' was a big trend, with new colours in browns and beiges for the eyes.

Hairdressers, such as Vidal Sassoon and Leonard, became stars for creating new haircuts. Photographers like David Bailey were famous for their work, discovering models and making them icons in the fashion world.

Men grew their hair long. Sideburns, moustaches and beards were fashionable with students, artists, pop singers and designers. Short hair was still de rigeur in the police force and civil service. Towards the end of the 1960s, straight hair was fashionable and ironing long hair on an ironing board was the only way to do it, as straightening tongs had not been invented. Heated Carmen rollers were used by most women to style their hair.

The world of pop music grew in popularity, as did television, which promoted pop stars on programmes such as *Top of the Pops*. Of the numerous singers and groups, the most successful were The Beatles and the Rolling Stones. London's street fashion became famous and Carnaby Street a mecca for tourists. It soon became known as 'Swinging London'.

The general look for young women was mini skirts, tights, knee-high boots and heavy theatrical eye make-up. Hair could be short or long, straight and glossy, or layered and curly. Plenty of fringes, false eyelashes, played down lips and eyebrows.

For men, the general look was tight jeans, silk shirts, colourful T-shirts with slogans, fitted velvet jackets, cravats, long hair and lots of facial hair.

The 1970s

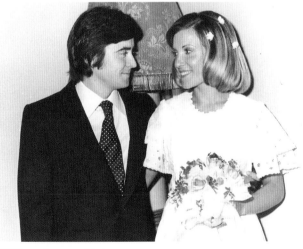

1970s make-up and hair

The effect of the 1960s was still changing society in the early 1970s: freedom of expression through music, fashion, art and literature. Most men had hair below the collar, with sideburns and moustaches still popular.

Women's make-up and hair became more natural looking, with hairpieces and false eyelashes no longer in fashion.

A movement called 'Flower Power' that originated in San Francisco, America, had come to Britain in the late 1960s, and its followers were protesting against the war in Vietnam. It gradually grew in numbers among the young, who called themselves 'hippies'. They rebelled against the work ethic and many travelled around India in search of enlightenment. The men had long, scruffy hair with a central parting and they grew beards and moustaches. The women had similar hair, sometimes adorned with flowers, and wore very little make-up. The movement lasted in England until 1975. Its 'Make Love, Not War' slogan directed against the invasion of Vietnam was a message from the younger generation. There was more unrest when women began to demand rights in the workplace, with Germaine Greer publishing a book in 1970 called *The Female Eunuch* urging women to 'get out from behind the hoover'.

This was a colourful decade, with frosted soft blues, greens and brown eyeshadows, and brown or black eyelines around the eyes plus mascara, but not in a heavy way. Lipstick colours were soft, shiny corals and reds or pinks and oranges.

The men's sideburns became larger as they spread down their faces, complete with moustaches of different shapes. They wore flared trousers and jeans with platform shoes.

In 1975 Malcolm McLaren, (who ran a vintage clothes shop in the Kings Road, London during the 1960s, with his wife Vivienne Westwood), founded a group called The Sex Pistols featuring a singer called Johnny Rotten. The music was aggressive and anti-establishment, but full of enthusiasm and raw energy. Their followers called themselves Punks. The men partially shaved their heads, with the remaining tufts of hair dressed upwards in spikes, dyed in fluorescent shades of pink, orange, green or red. They stuck safety pins in their noses to appear menacing. The women went for the same look with black eyelines and dark eyeshadows. The Punks were tolerated on the streets, becoming a tourist attraction. Soon there were picture postcards of them being sold in shops alongside postcards of other London sights.

The anger in Punk music was reflected in the general mood of the country. There were strikes in the public sector resulting in electric power cuts, and uncollected rubbish piling up on the streets. There was also an economic recession with many people out of work.

In 1979 the country voted in Margaret Thatcher and the Conservative Party to run the country and sort it out. The Punk look gave way to a Gothic look, with white faces and dark eye make-up.

The 1980s

This was the decade of "Greed is Good", and corporate excess. Designer clothes with wide, padded shoulders became the look for the 1980s. The make-up and hair became stronger in style. Every feature of the face was emphasised: eyebrows, eyes, cheeks and lips.

Eyeshadow was used on the eyelids in shades of purple, grey, brown or rust, with a highlight colour on the brow bones. Eyeliner and mascara were brown, blue or black. The eyebrows were strong and filled in with pencil. Blusher was used on the cheeks, and under the cheekbones to contour the face. The top of the cheekbones was highlighted. The

ACTIVITY

Use books and the Internet to research pictures of Punks to gain an understanding of the fashion, hair and make-up in the 1970s.

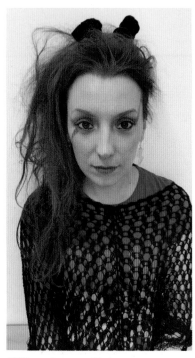

1980s make-up and hair

lips were painted in red, fuchsia, purple, pink or rust. An American television soap series, *Dynasty*, starring Joan Collins was popular, and epitomised the look. The hairstyles were big and curly to balance the wide shoulder pads.

Men's hair was short, with 1950s styles in fashion and no facial hair.

Waves of styles for women were based on previous decades, such as the 1940s. One trend was the fashion for heavy, ungroomed eyebrows: a look started by an actress called Brooke Shields, who had naturally heavy eyebrows.

There was also a trend for pink eyeshadow.

The 1980s became 'boom' years, with young business people called 'Yuppies' tending to be materialistic, spending their money on clothes and grooming. Madonna, "The Material Girl" came onto the scene and her beautifully made-up face was the 1980s look.

The boom years finished with the decade, followed by a recession.

The 1990s

The Grunge look was popular on the streets, with unmade-up looking faces and casual hair.

For the fashion enthusiasts there was a trend towards nostalgia, adopting and revamping styles from previous decades. The models on the catwalks showed a 1960s revival, and false eyelashes were back in fashion. This was followed by looks reminiscent of the 1930s and 1950s, with hairstyles ranging from waved bobs, elegant upswept chignons and braided plaits. There was also a new trend for large, full lips, with models overpainting their mouths, and using silicone injections to give a swollen look to the upper lip.

Organic skincare products became popular, and cosmetics using pigments extracted from plant extracts. The interest in homeopathic medicines was responsible for natural-based products.

Film stars popular in this decade were Angelina Jolie, Julia Roberts, Winona Ryder, Russell Crowe, John Cusack and Robert Downey Jnr.

In the music world, there was Beyoncé, The Spice Girls, Coldplay and Liam Gallagher. Madonna caused a sensation with her conical bra and provocative performances.

ACTIVITY

Use books and the Internet to research pictures of Joan Collins in *Dynasty* to gain an understanding of iconic fashion, hair and make-up in the 1980s.

ACTIVITY

Use books and the Internet to research pictures of Madonna in the 1980s and 1990s to gain an understanding of iconic fashion, hair and make-up from the eras.

ACTIVITY

Use books and the Internet to research pictures of Angelina Jolie, Julia Roberts, Russell Crowe and John Cusack to gain an understanding of iconic fashion, hair and make-up from the 1990s.

CASE PROFILE: HELEN SPEYER, MAKE-UP DESIGNER

How long have you been working in the industry?

This is my twentieth year – it's gone so fast and I still love it!

How did you get into the industry?

I wanted to be a make-up artist since I was 14. I was advised to train as a hairdresser first, which I did, and worked as a hairdresser for several years before going back to college full time to train in media hair and make-up.

Did you have a lucky break or turning point?

I didn't know anyone in the industry, so while I was at college I took every opportunity to get as much work experience as I could, making

as many contacts as I could. When I left college I had met and worked with make-up designers who were willing to take me on as their trainee assistant.

What has been your most significant project(s)?

It is great to have worked on films and television dramas that have ended up winning awards, but you're only as good as your last job! I still love the job and love the fact that every job you do is creative in different ways.

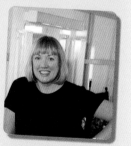

What do you enjoy most about the job?

Travel and meeting a huge number of interesting people. I have had the amazing opportunity to live and work while filming in many countries in Europe and Africa. I also really enjoy the fact that every day I get to be creative.

What do you enjoy least about the job?

I'm not a big fan of getting out of bed to the alarm going off in the morning at a time starting with the number four or three in it!

How has the television and film industry changed during your career?

HD cameras have changed filming a great deal. The camera picks up everything which means our work has to be adjusted so the camera can't see what you have done, especially things like wig lace and prosthetics' edges. The other big change which effects make-up and hair is the ability to computer edit work after the filming process. This has brought computer effects into make-up and hair work like never before.

What advice would you give to a new make-up artist starting out?

Come into make-up with some other skill to offer – it could be an art background, hairdressing or beauty. Take every opportunity you're given while at college to get experience – it's not just about doing make-up it's the whole package: you need to be a team player, self-motivated, creative, hard-working, have a lot of stamina and good health, and enjoy meeting people. The ability to look on the sunny side of life is always going to be helpful!

ACTIVITY

Period research

Research three different period dramas or films from different eras. Create a mood board of the hair, fashion and make-up from each historical period of your choice and include images to showcase the looks. Re-create one of these looks and take photos of your project.

Choosing the right look for the period

Fashion trends do not happen immediately. The end of each decade overlaps into the next by several years. Magazines and commercials promote fashions for people to buy into, but not everyone follows a trend straightaway.

People in the country adopt a look much later than those living in cities such as London, Paris, Rome and New York.

It is important to pin down the exact year of the action of the script. Take into account the characters, their environment and age, (older people do not always change their style). Wealth and the class system are deciding factors in the centuries that precede the rapid communication of the twenty-first century.

Adapting fashion make-up to period styles

Some faces adapt easily to period styles. You will often hear a make-up artist remark that a certain actor has a period face.

It is not always possible to reproduce faithfully the 'correct' historical look. The effect may be too distracting or considered unattractive relative to the current fashion. Sometimes it is necessary to indicate the period by conveying the feeling of the look. For example, in the seventeenth and eighteenth centuries, a fashionable lady at court would have used white lead paint on her face. You can use white cream-based products and white powder for an authentic look, but a pale liquid foundation would be more attractive-looking on a cinema or HD screen. It is often better to use a softer version of the period, unless it is for a theatre production.

The Victorian period is easy because no one should look as if they are wearing make-up, so it can be very natural and pretty. The look is set by the women's hairstyles, and facial hair on the men.

Actors must be comfortable in their roles. In the 1940s not every man had a moustache, but if he is playing an RAF pilot he will be more believable with a moustache because there was a trend at the time among aircrew to grow one.

When the characters in a story are based on normal people – office workers, teachers, nurses, shop assistants, mothers on the school run – the best sources for research are vintage photographs and film or television documentaries of the era.

The make-up and hair should be as varied as today: with some people in fashion, some not. There should never be the same look for everyone on a period production, even for a crowd scene.

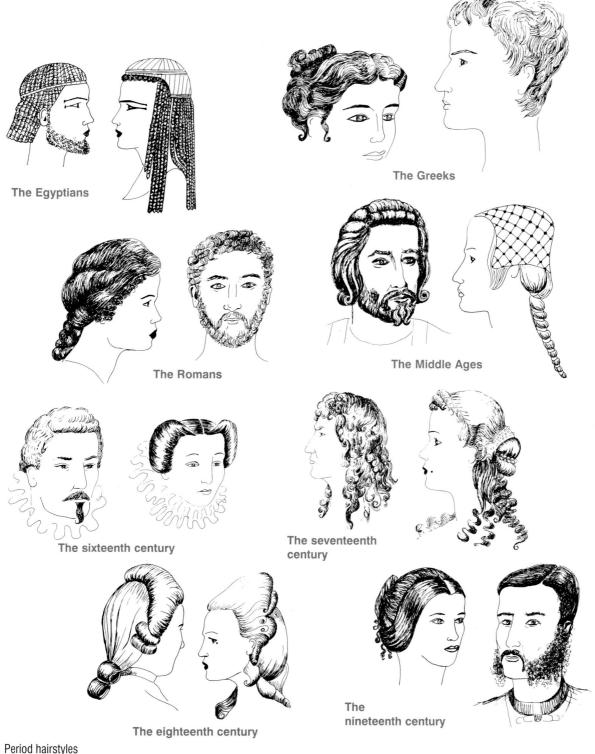

The Egyptians

The Greeks

The Romans

The Middle Ages

The sixteenth century

The seventeenth century

The eighteenth century

The nineteenth century

Period hairstyles

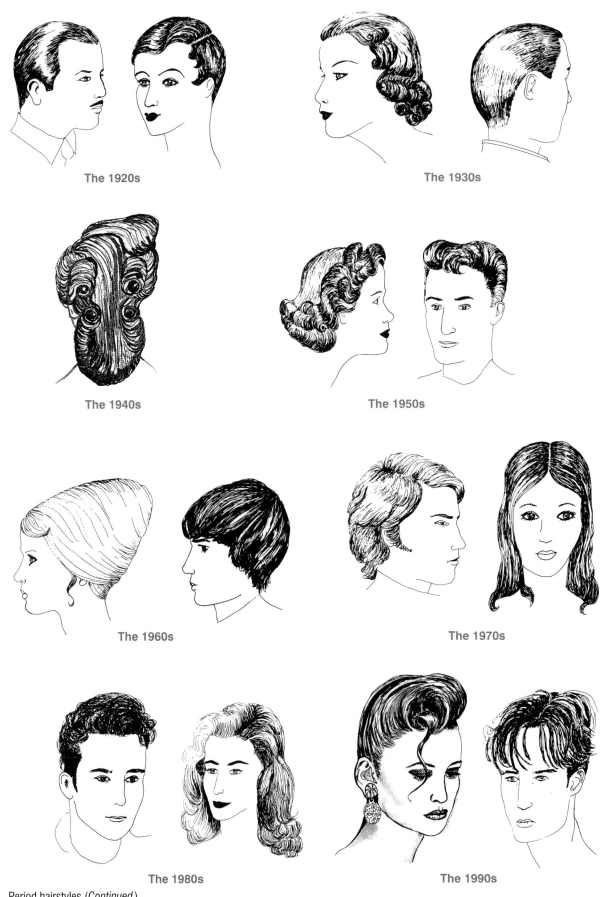

The 1920s

The 1930s

The 1940s

The 1950s

The 1960s

The 1970s

The 1980s

The 1990s

Period hairstyles (*Continued*)

CASE PROFILE: LORRAINE HILL, MAKE-UP DESIGNER

How long have you been working in the industry?

I have been in the industry for about 17 years.

How did you get into the industry?

I started my career as a hairdresser but I always knew I wanted to expand my skills. Learning to do make-up was the best way of achieving this and still be able to create a vision, whether it be a character on a period film with a beautiful wig, enhancing somebody's natural beauty, or transforming someone's appearance into a character. It was learning to achieve a full look.

Did you have a lucky break or a turning point?

I don't really think I had a lucky break or a turning point. I've had a natural progression and worked my way up the ranks. Starting from being the work experience girl, working for expenses only, to eventually becoming a hair and make-up designer. It's taken a long time but I feel I've learnt a lot more working this way.

What have been your most significant projects?

Every job you work on is totally different in its own way. Sometimes the most gruelling jobs can visually be the most rewarding. Other jobs you can be in fits of laughter with the cast in the make-up truck every day. I try to get the most out of every project I work on.

What do you enjoy most about the job?

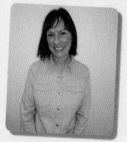

There are so many things about the job I enjoy. I think I like doing the research the most for a period production – it can almost be like a history lesson.

What do you enjoy least about the job?

Most of the time you have to forget about having any kind of social life whilst filming as you just don't have the time or energy. However you do know once the job ends you can get it all back again when you have your time off.

How has the film and television industry changed during your career?

The biggest change for me has been switching from the old digi beta and super 16 film to HD. It was a change for all departments but the make-up department had to completely alter the way make-up was applied.

What advice would you give a new make-up artist starting out?

Don't give up! It's not the easiest industry to break into but the rewards are massive. Keep pushing forwards and eventually you'll get there. The hardest times are when you're not working but eventually your contact list will grow and the times when you're out of work will get less and less.

REVISION QUESTIONS

1 What historical period is referred to as the 'Renaissance'? Give a brief description of the look.

2 In what year did the 'bob' become a fashion trend?

3 Briefly describe iconic make-up looks for the 1960s.

4 Explain why make-up was very limited in the 1940s. What product was sold to help develop moral?

5 In what era did the 'beehive' become fashionable?

10 Facial hair

LEARNING OBJECTIVES

This chapter covers the following:

◆ Making facial hairpieces.

◆ Making templates and patterns for facial hairpieces.

◆ Applying and removing facial hairpieces.

◆ Hand-laying facial hair.

◆ Dressing out side whiskers.

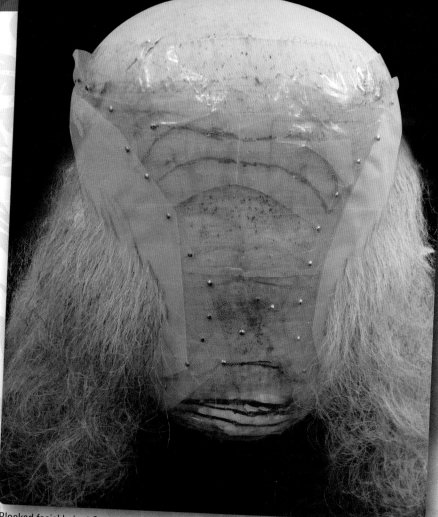

Blocked facial hair at Sarah Weatherburn's workshop

KEY TERMS

Laying a beard

Laying on hair

Moustache waxes

Tong heater

Stubble

Yak hair

UNIT TITLE

◆ Prepare, apply, remove and clean facial hair to change the performer's appearance

◆ Oversee fittings for wigs and facial hair

INTRODUCTION

This chapter will help you with Level 3 hairdressing qualifications such as wig services, and making and styling hair additions. You will use knowledge gained from Level 2 cutting units to advance further techniques that are discussed in this chapter. The knowledge gained in this chapter will help when beards, moustaches and sideburns are required to enhance or change an actor's appearance. Making the templates or patterns will also be outlined and you will understand how to apply and remove facial hairpieces in a safe manner. Continuity is very important to a make-up artist working with facial hair. Having knowledge of working with facial hairpieces is essential for a make-up artist. These skills can be applied to many areas of the industry including period dramas, films, character changes and photo shoots.

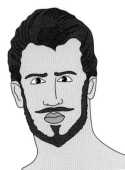

Facial hair

Throughout history, facial hair has been important in men's appearances. The practices of trimming, shaving or partially shaving the face have had an importance beyond vanity or habit. Across the world, shaving or not shaving has at times taken on superstitious, religious or political significance.

Facial hair plays a key role in changing a man's appearance, particularly in ageing and period make-up work, whether it is a beard and moustache, sideburns, eyebrows or just a moustache.

The hair is knotted onto lace: thicker for the theatre, very fine for television and film. As a make-up artist you will not be expected to make facial hairpieces, but you need to understand the process in order to assess the quality of the work when commissioning it from specialists. Students should learn how to knot a moustache, as the skills learned will be useful one day.

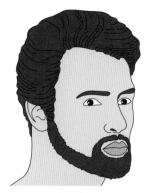

Facial hair cannot be hired, for reasons of hygiene, and because it has a short life. It must match or tone in with the actor's own hair or wig, so samples are taken from the top of their head and the nape of the neck.

Making facial hairpieces

A moustache

To begin, you will need to make a template or pattern of the actor's upper lip, take hair samples from his own hair or wig and take a picture of the moustache design.

Making the template or pattern

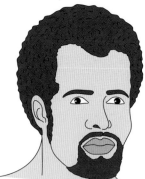

Tools & equipment

◆ clear adhesive tape
◆ cling film
◆ eyebrow pencil – brown or black
◆ scissors
◆ the actor – seated in front of the mirror
◆ wet wipes or make-up remover and tissues

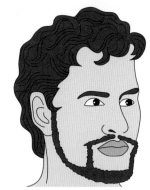

Method

1 Place a piece of cling film on a flat surface. Cover it with adhesive tape to make it more solid. Cut out a V at the top, to allow a space for the nose.

2 Put this pattern on the actor's face, in the moustache area. Press firmly, and draw the required shape, with the eyebrow pencil, onto the pattern.

3 Go over the pattern with more tape, to protect the pencil line. Set aside ready to attach to a beard block.

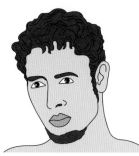

Examples of beard shapes

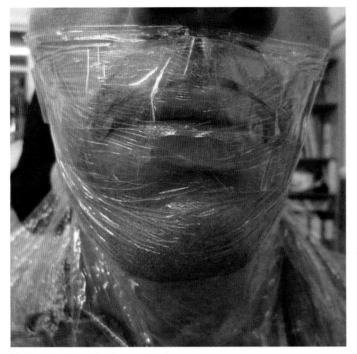

Making the pattern for the moustache

Making facial hair

Tools & equipment

- beard block
- block pins
- clear adhesive tape
- cradle – a wooden box in which the beard block rests while you are working

- drawing mats – to hold loose hair
- hair lace
- knotting hook and needles
- loose **yak hair**

- small bowl of water – to slip the hair into
- tongs and **tong heater** – for dressing the hair

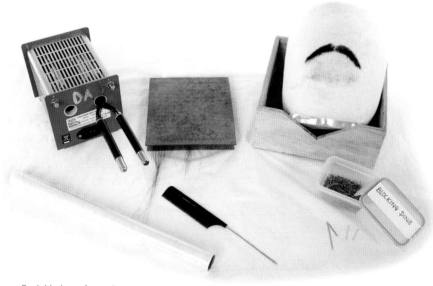

Facial hair equipment

TOP TIP

You can use a wig clamp that will clamp to worktops or tables or a freestanding wig stand that you can change the height and adjust the angles, so that you can work comfortably.

Attaching the moustache pattern and lace to the block

1   Use adhesive tape to attach the moustache pattern to the block.

2   Place a piece of lace across the pattern and secure it around the edge of the shape, using the small block pins.

3   Pin the lace as tightly as possible over the pattern. This makes it easier to apply pressure on the hair whilst knotting and helps to achieve tight knots. Stretch the lace evenly so as not to distort the direction of the line of holes.

4   The moustache pattern should be clearly visible through the lace. Make sure it is not off-centre on the block. The moustache pattern should be dead straight.

5   Place the block in the wooden box so that you can work on it comfortably.

Knotting the hair

1   Use a knotting holder and hook to knot the hair. Be careful with these hooks as it is easy to hook them back into your skin.

2   Use yak hair for the moustache. Place the hair between two mats to keep neat. The mats have teeth on them; these should be turning towards you.

TOP TIP

Be very careful that you do not get the hair mixed up. It is important not to mix the root and tip of the hair. If the hair gets mixed up or put in upside down it will not sit right. All the hair cuticles need to be in the same direction (known as root to tip). Label the drawing mats, by putting a mark on the mats to indicate the root end of the hair to ensure the hair does not get inserted upside down.

3   Lay the hair over the teeth and push the mats together. As you pull the hair out, a bit at a time, the teeth will separate it.

4   Fold the hair in half and dip the doubled end in water. Continue to do this as you work.

5   Decide which way you want the hair to lie. If you want the hair to lie downwards, then knot upwards.

6   When you have completed the knotting of the moustache, trim the lace and hair to size and curl it with moustache tongs into barrel curls.

7   Dress out the moustache to the finished style.

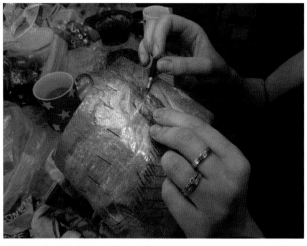

Knotting facial hair

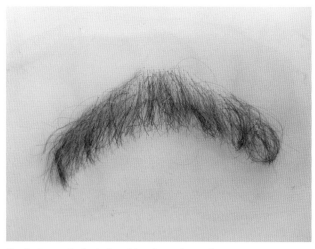

Knotted moustache before it has been dressed

CASE PROFILE: SARAH WEATHERBURN, FACIAL HAIR PIECE SPECIALIST

How long have you been working in the industry?

I have been working in the industry for 30 years.

How did you get into the industry?

I trained as a hairdresser and after working in hairdressing salons I started an apprenticeship in the wig department in Stratford Ontario Festival Theatre. This was a fantastic opportunity and I loved my time in Canada.

Did you have a lucky break or turning point?

When I came back to London I started work for Sarah Phillips' facial hair-making company. After six years I left to work in theatre again, working on *Phantom of the Opera* and *Joseph*. Maminda Harkness and I then bought Sarah's company. It was a huge learning curve for both of us, but as we had both already worked for Sarah Phillips we knew a bit of how the business worked. Seventeen years ago Maminda left and the company became 'Sarah Weatherburn & Co.'. I've never thought about the next step, I have been very lucky and my career has evolved naturally.

What has been your most significant project to date?

I have really enjoyed many films that we have worked on – *Elizabeth*, all the *Harry Potters*, *Lord of the Rings* and *The Hobbit* (which I went to New Zealand for). Almost every project teaches me something new – technically or creatively.

What do you most enjoy about the job?

I get very excited when I get a telephone call from a make-up designer asking us to make facial hair for a project – I will never take that for granted.

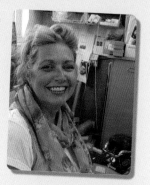

It's great seeing your work on the screen – the best thing is when an actor is wearing a piece of our facial hair that nobody thinks is not his own. The pieces have to be made beautifully, and the make-up artist has to skillfully apply them.

What do you enjoy least about the job?

The deadlines – casting is often very late and we have to make pieces quickly, which puts a lot of pressure on everyone. Delivering on time is a crucial part of the work. I also don't like to see badly applied facial!

Has the television and film industry changed during your career?

It's constantly changing. HD means we all have to up our game – very fine knotting and film lace which is closely colour matched to the actor's skin tones, for example. Also prep time seems to get shorter, so we very often have to work intensely to get things done. Online media – with companies like Netflix and Amazon moving into production – is increasingly important to the industry.

The British film industry is booming right now and television drama has never been such high quality, or had such high production values. It's a great time to be involved.

What advice would you give a new make-up artist starting out?

Try everything – theatre, film, television. You never know where it will take you. Be enthusiastic, helpful, make tea and coffee, ask questions when it's appropriate and watch everything. It's a fascinating world, with some very clever, creative people to learn from.

A beard

Taking a pattern for a beard follows the same procedure as for a moustache. When taking the pattern for a theatre production, particularly for an opera singer, the mouth should be open. For television and film the fitting must be exact.

HEALTH & SAFETY

When using knotting hooks, be sure to store them in a safe place or in a small box, as they are very sharp. Some wigmakers use a finger guard, when working (which looks a bit like a thimble).

Making a pattern for a beard

1 Using the eyebrow pencil, follow the actor's beard line, drawing the entire outline on his skin.

2 Put cling film across and under the mouth and up to the temples. Leave the nose uncovered so that the actor can breathe. Make sure the pencil line is covered.

3 Cover the cling film with clear adhesive tape under the mouth.

4 Add tape underneath the chin.

5 Add tape from the sideburns to the mouth.

6 Check that the tape is tight around the chin.

7 Repeat the procedure – two or three layers of cling film and tape are enough for a firm pattern.

8 Trim any excess cling film.

9 Use the eyebrow pencil to draw the beard shape, following the previous line on the actor's skin.

10 Cover the pencil line with clear tape to protect it.

11 Cut out the beard pattern above the pencil lines, leaving about ½ inch (12.5 mm) spare.

12 Remove the beard pattern from the actor's face and place on the beard block.

13 If necessary, pad the block to the shape of the pattern.

14 To make sure of a good fit, shape the lace for the beard into at least four pleats underneath the chin. 'Whip' or tack it into place with nylon thread, using a hook.

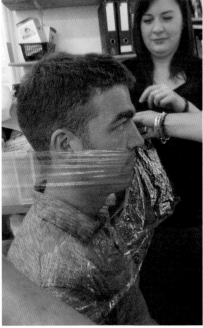

Apply the cling film

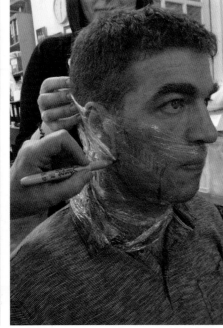

Draw the beard and moustache shape onto the cling film

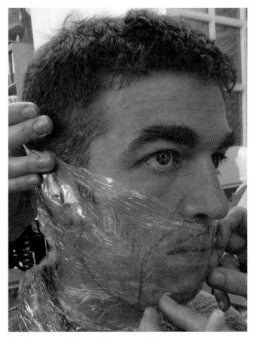

Make sure the cling film is a good fit

Alternative method of taking measurements for a beard

To make sure of the measurements, use a soft tape measure and send the details, as well as the pattern, to the facial hair specialist. The measurements should include:

◆ The width of the sideburn.

◆ From the bottom of the mouth to the neck.

◆ From the sideburn to the point of the jaw.

◆ From the centre of the chin to the point of the jaw.

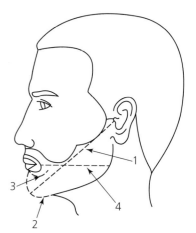

Measuring a beard: the dotted lines represent the measurements taken; the numbers show the sequence

The facial hair workshops

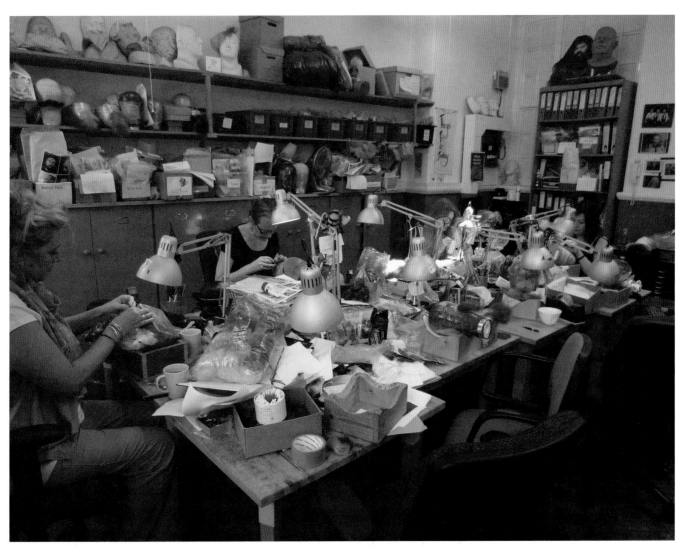

Sarah Weatherburn's facial hair workshop

CASE PROFILE: EMMA JONES, WIG AND FACIAL HAIR MAKER AND DRESSER

How long have you been working in the industry?

I have been working in the industry since 2004, when I got my first proper job in the industry at the Royal Shakespeare Company [RSC], in Stratford-upon-Avon.

How did you get into the industry?

My way into the television and film industry came from working at Sarah Weatherburn and Co., knotting facial hair for screen and stage.

Did you have a lucky break or turning point?

I feel like there have been three major lucky breaks in my career. The first is getting my first job in the industry, as wig assistant at the RSC in Stratford-upon-Avon. I am still amazed that I got that job with the little experience I had at the time. It was from the RSC that I got my second lucky break, when a fellow wiggie put me in touch with *Les Miserables* in London's West End. I was welcomed on to the *Les Mis* wig team in 2005, and as well as working on many other shows over the years, I am still at 'my home' in *Les Mis*. I feel proud to be part of such a prestigious show, and I am thankful for the lucky breaks I received so early on in my career.

My third break came in 2006 when I joined Sarah Weatherburn and Co. as a knotter of facial hair. I jumped at the chance to work for such a well-known company and have been there ever since.

What has been your most significant project?

To date, I think my most significant project has to be working on *The Hobbit* while at Sarah Weatherburn and Co. Each of us chose a dwarf character and then knotted every piece of facial hair needed for that particular character. This included a large

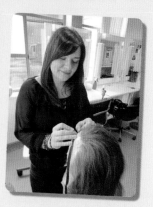

number of duplicate beards for the actual character, spanning over three films, and all the facial needed (with duplicates) for that character's stunt doubles. It was an enormous project for us and it was hugely exciting to be part of something so iconic.

What do you enjoy most about the job?

I really enjoy all my jobs. Working in the theatre has an enormous buzz about it, sometimes it doesn't even feel like you are at 'work'. Working for Sarah Weatherburn and Co. as a knotter, is just as enjoyable but on a totally different level. It's a great mix of seeing your friends while working on major blockbuster films, it's all about concentration and precision rather than, rushing to the next quick-change. I am very lucky to be able to feel that way about my places of work.

What do you enjoy least about the job?

Knotting also has its downside, although the thought of sitting down all day doesn't sound too strenuous, when you are sat in the same position for long periods of time knotting, it can soon create aches and pains. Neck and back problems are common complaints amongst knotters.

What advice would you give to a new make-up artist starting out?

When you are starting out apply for everything! Whether its work experience or your ideal job, go for it! The more people you meet, the more doors will be opened to you.

ACTIVITY

Period hair research

Research different postiche styles for different historical periods. Research television period dramas that have used facial postiche. Produce a timeline to showcase different period of fashions in facial postiche.

Applying and removing facial hairpieces

Applying a moustache

Method

1 Make sure that the skin is grease free; use a wet wipe or astringent if necessary.

2 Using a brush, place a thin layer of matte adhesive spirit gum onto the actor's moustache area. Stipple with your finger until tacky.

   Apply another thin layer and using your finger, stipple again.

3 Place the moustache in position on the adhesive.

4 Use the tail end of your comb to press the lace down firmly, in-between the hair, at the base of the lace. Make sure the edges of the lace are glued down firmly. When the spirit gum is dry, gently comb the top layers of the moustache into shape.

Tools & equipment

- matte adhesive spirit gum
- metal hair comb
- two brushes
- wet wipes or astringent

TOP TIP

All equipment and materials should be prepared before your artist arrives for the facial hair application

HEALTH & SAFETY

Patch tests should be carried out at least 24 hours prior to application. Sometimes this may not always be possible, as you may be working on supporting artists and you may not get to see them until the day you will be applying the postiche. You can use barrier products in these instances, so the adhesive does not make direct contact with the skin. There is a variety of different makes available in liquid and mousse form in professional make-up shops.

Adhesive must not be applied to broken skin. Ideally, you should contact your actor prior to application, to ensure they have clean-shaven skin prior to application.

Removing the moustache

Method

1 Dip a clean brush into the mastix remover and stipple the edges of the moustache lace to loosen it.

2 Slowly work around the edges with the brush until the moustache can be gently eased off.

3 Use remover to clean the rest of the gum from the actor's face. Check the actor's skin for any redness and provide after care advice. Put the moustache aside, ready for cleaning.

Tools & equipment

- mild mastix spirit gum remover
- small brush

Applying a beard

1 Position the beard on the actor's face before applying the mastix spirit gum.

2 Apply the mastix thinly with a small brush to the skin on the chin area. Tap the gum with your fingertips until tacky.

3 Apply another thin layer and tap lightly as before, until tacky.

4 Adjust the position of the beard for the actor's comfort, before pressing it down firmly.

5   If a full beard, turn back the beard at the side of the face, and apply mastix in the usual way.

6   When securing the beard in front of the ears, lift up the actor's own hair with your tail comb and stick the lace underneath.

7   Use the tail of your comb to press down onto the lace, in-between the hairs, all over the beard.

8   Comb down the actor's own hair at ear level to hide the join. Use a toning colour to blend the beard into the hair.

Applying sideburns

Use the same method as you would when applying a beard – that is, sticking the lace under a small section of hair. On long production shoots with big close-ups, some make-up artists cut or shave a small section of the actor's own hair after first lifting a section, which can be allowed to blend over the adhered lace. Discuss with the actor, and ask permission first.

There should be no visible gap between the sideburns or beard and the natural hair. Tattoo colour, such as Reel Hair palette is useful for blending the colour difference between the actor's hair and false beard or sideburns.

Cleaning facial hairpieces

Tools & equipment

◆ lintless towels
◆ small bowl or plate
◆ small brush
◆ surgical spirit and acetone

TOP TIP

When you have cleaned the facial hair, always place it back on to the appropriate chin block, correctly labelled with the actor's name, ready for the next application. Apply moisturiser (if wanted) to the actor after cleansing as the removers can dry out the skin.

HEALTH & SAFETY

When working with chemicals always remember to replace lids and store in the correct place. If you are using chemicals in bowls, they must be clearly labelled. Wear PPE when necessary. Ensure there is proper ventilation; use extractor fans and open windows.

When the actor's face has been cleaned, the hairpiece you have removed needs also to be cleaned and dressed, ready for using again. The matte adhesive on the hair lace can be cleaned off with surgical spirit and acetone. Brush cleaner will remove make-up from the hair.

Method

1   Pour surgical spirit and acetone into bowl or plate – just enough for lace to be covered.

2   Place the facial hairpiece lace down into the mixture, which should not cover the hair. Leave for cleaning fluid to work: 2–3 minutes.

3   Remove from fluid. Place lace down on a lintless towel.

4   Use brush dipped in cleaning fluid to gently tap down on lace so that the glue goes onto the towel.

5   Move the hairpiece to a clean area of the towel and continue stippling the lace with the cleaning fluid. Use brush cleaner to clean off any make-up.

6   Allow the facial hairpiece to dry thoroughly before pinning it on a beard block, ready to be dressed.

A quick way of cleaning hair lace that is used in theatres, is to make a pad from cheap muslin folded around a flat wad of cotton wool which has been soaked in acetone. The hair lace used in theatres is thicker than television or film lace, so it can take a more robust method of cleaning. Toothbrushes are also used for removing spirit gum from lace.

The hair lace for HD television and film is extremely fine and delicate because HD shows every detail. It is often dyed in skin-tone colours before the knotting process. Large beards are often made in sections to allow the actor more movement of the face.

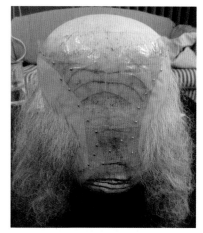

Facial hair on a block

HEALTH & SAFETY

Consult with your actor prior to the removal so you are both aware of the procedure. Ask your actor to assist you by holding a tissue to protect them from any removers going in their mouth.

TOP TIP

A small piece of silk can also be used to press areas of the lace to the skin.

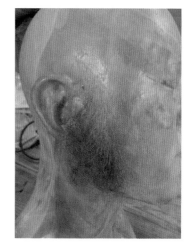

Sideburns on a block

Hand-laying facial hair

Instead of using hair knotted onto lace, another way of creating facial hair is to apply it directly to the face. This is an old method that veteran make-up artists used to employ, and has been updated over the years, using different adhesives.

The skill involved in the process remains the same. It has several advantages. When the hair is laid directly onto the actor's face there is no lace edge to conceal. Also, with sufficient expertise the make-up artist can create any style at a moment's notice, when there is no time to commission or make a piece. Also, the overlaying of hair at the edges of hair laces to change the shape of a piece, or to soften a hard-looking line or hide the edge, is very useful when working in HD.

HEALTH & SAFETY

When working with chemicals always remember to dispose of any unused products correctly, as they can be highly flammable.

Tools & equipment

- acetone
- brush
- comb
- curling tongs – no. 1 moustache irons
- electric tong heater
- eyebrow tweezers

- hackle
- loose hair – yak in black, dark brown, blonde, red, white
- matte mastix spirit gum
- scissors
- tissues
- Vaseline

HEALTH & SAFETY

When working with curling tongs or moustache irons, make others aware of this by labelling the equipment 'caution very hot'. Make sure the area you are working in is safe. Sometimes you may be working on make-up buses, where there will not be much space to work. Position yourself in a safe place, or schedule styling of postiche when you have less people around.

TOP TIP

Always test moustache irons on a tissue first before using them to style a postiche. Secure a tissue to a block using a wig pin or t-pin and test the temperature of the moustache irons on the tissue. If the irons are too hot they will burn through the tissue and can catch alight. As the temperature drops, the irons will make a light brown/yellow tone on the tissue. Repeat this test a few times to ensure the temperature of the irons has dropped. If the irons are too hot they will burn the postiche hair.

Preparing the hair

The hair should be texturised, as it is difficult to spread evenly when straight. Crimp the hair with the no. 1 tongs.

Hackling the hair

1   Draw the crimped hair through the teeth of the hackle to separate the different lengths.

2   Place these in the teeth of the hackle in order of the colours, very much like paint on a palette.

HEALTH & SAFETY

Be very careful when working with a hackle, take precautions to ensure your safety and others. A hackle is like a small bed of nails and is very sharp. Always store hackles correctly. Some hackles have a wooden protective box that fits over the top for safe storage.

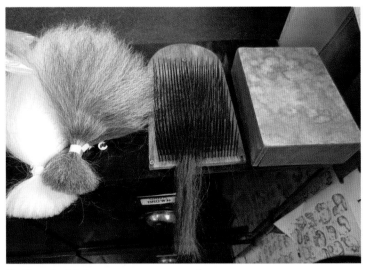

Hackle and yak hair

Mixing the hair

To achieve a natural effect with facial hair you need to mix several colours together. Never lay a one-tone beard or moustache as it will not look realistic.

By mixing hair carefully you will be able to imitate any of the colours and tones that occur in natural facial hair. Take care not to overmix the hair or you will make a nondescript colour – much like overmixing paint.

Laying the hair to create sideburns

1 First place a fine cutting comb under the actor's own sideburn and lift it upwards to expose the skin underneath. Secure the comb in position by placing it over the top of the actor's ear.

2 Using the brush, paint a thin layer of matte adhesive onto the skin in the shape you want.

3 Wipe the scissors with acetone to remove any adhesive and then wipe them with Vaseline to coat the blades lightly. This helps to prevent the build-up of adhesive on the blades and should be repeated frequently during the process of the laying.

4 Now draw the hair from the hackle, holding it between the thumb and forefinger of the left hand if you are right-handed, or the right hand if you are left-handed. Tap the spirit gum to make it tacky.

5 Taking the scissors in the other hand, spread the hair onto the sticky area by rolling the hair between the forefinger and thumb, and lightly tap the ends of the hairs so that they stick to the adhesive. Cut these hairs to the required length.

Note that you lay hair starting from the bottom and working upwards.

Dressing the sideburns with heated tongs

Method

1 Heat the tongs. Test the temperature on a tissue. If the tongs singe the tissue, wait until the correct temperature is reached.

2 Use the hot tongs to dress the hair. Rest them on a comb held in the other hand to avoid touching the face with the tongs. Start at the roots and using the tongs, shape the sideburn.

3 Turn the underneath layers upwards.

4 Trim and style the sideburn to the shape you want. Bring hair down to cover any gaps.

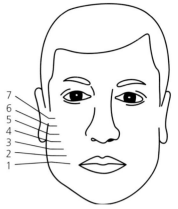

Order of laying hair for sideburns

Tools & equipment

◆ comb
◆ scissors
◆ tissues
◆ tong heater
◆ tongs
◆ tweezers

HEALTH & SAFETY

When drawing hair from the hackle be very careful as the nails are very sharp.

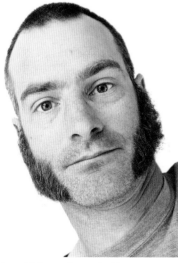

Laid on sideburns dressed with tongs

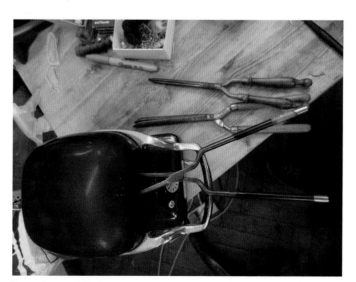

Tongs in a tong heater

Laying on the hair to create a beard and moustache

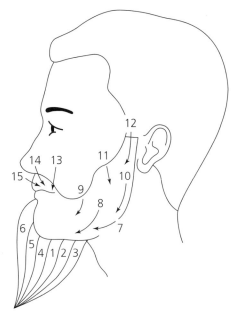

Beard and moustache direction of growth; numbers show the position and sequence of application

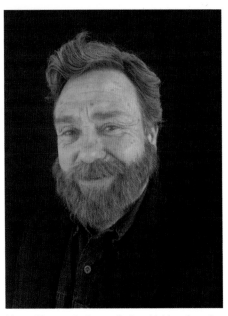

Man with moustache applied and laid on beard

For a beard the process is similar. Soft edges are produced by thinning out, and by using lighter-coloured hair. Never make an actor look bland or dull by using one colour. With black beards, add a little white or red to give colour, life and interest to the character.

1 Apply matte adhesive under the chin in the desired shape. Tap to make it tacky.

2 Draw the prepared hair from the hackle, applying it to the face as described for the sideburn. Use the darkest colours underneath, fanning out the hair with the forefinger and thumb.

3 When it has stuck, cut the hair to the required length.

4 Mix in a lighter colour and keep applying a small section at a time. Always mix some light into dark hair.

5 Work up towards the mouth, adding the lightest colours.

6 When a fairly large area has been covered, use a towel to press onto the hair firmly (for extra pressure, gently use your thumbs). This secures the hair and gets rid of extra gum and odd loose hairs.

7 Start to apply the moustache, section by section.

8 As you work up the side of the jaw, start thinning the top hairs out and use a lighter hair colour.

9 When finished, use a large-toothed comb to gently comb through the beard and moustache.

10 Cut the hair into the shape you want. Use eyebrow tweezers to remove unwanted hairs.

Dressing out the beard and moustache

The laid on beard and moustache should be styled as described for dressing out the sideburns.

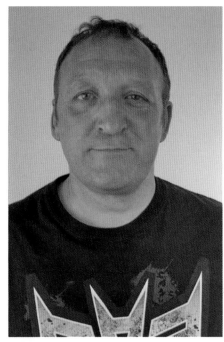

Before application of facial hair

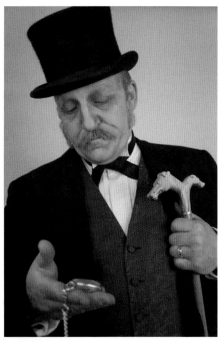

After application of facial hair

ACTIVITY

Beard and moustache styling and dressing

Research beard and moustache products and techniques for facial postiche.

Include:

- Blocking on of facial hair.
- Styling facial hair.
- Dressing out with **moustache waxes**.
- Practice techniques on styling and dressing postiche.
- Photographs before and after.
- Evaluation of your work.

REVISION QUESTIONS

1 What type of block would you style and dress facial hair on?

2 What products are used to clean facial hair?

3 What would you use to secure a block with when styling and dressing facial hair?

4 What is used to test the heated irons temperature?

5 What test is required on electrical equipment?

6 How often do you need to have electrical equipment tested?

7 What is used to mix hair?

8 What is used to secure hair when making postiche?

11 Casualty effects

LEARNING OBJECTIVES

This chapter covers the following:

◆ Planning and researching casualty effects.

◆ Working with different products, such as blood, gelatine, wax and pro bondo moulds.

◆ Creating different casualty effects such as bruises, burns, sweating, scars, scratches, cuts and grazes.

◆ How to create different scenarios such as stab wounds, gunshot wounds, fight scenes, slit wrists and a slit-throat effect.

◆ How to make your characters look ill and shocked, dirty, vomiting or addicted to drugs.

◆ Using prosthetics for casualty effects.

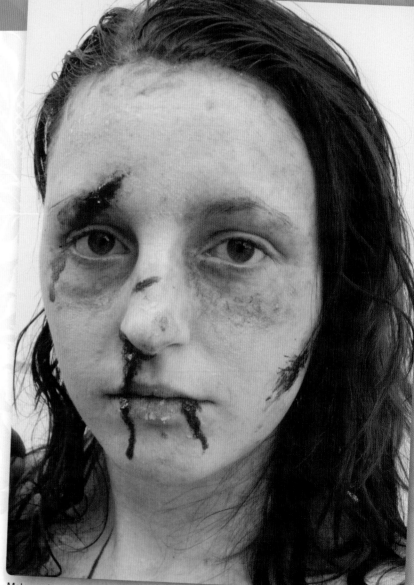

Make-up by Giorgio Galliero

KEY TERMS

Glycerine

IPA (Isopropyl Alcohol)

Plastic

Plastic scar material

Pro bondo

UNIT TITLE

◆ Apply make-up to change the performer's appearance

◆ Apply special effects to change the performer's appearance

INTRODUCTION

This unit will help you develop your skills to apply to all character work you will complete in Level 2 and Level 3 media units. You will be introduced to different effects that may be required for television, film and theatre. This chapter covers step-by-step application techniques and the products and equipment that will be required to complete casualty effects. When applying casualty effects you may need to use the skills you gained from basic make-up application Level 2 and fashion and photographic Level 3. These basic make-up elements will be the foundation for casualty effects. Hair may need styling to complement the casualty effect, with dirt, vomit or blood applied to enhance the finished results. You will use a variety of techniques from Level 2 hairdressing or Level 3 style and dress hair to create casualty effects.

Casualty effects

Casualty effects are frequently called for in theatre, television and film, and sometimes in fashion, on models. In theatre, from Shakespeare to grand opera the stories are full of bloodshed. In television, the dramas, police series and hospital soaps feature casualty effects. Most films have bloodthirsty scenes for dramatic effect.

The traumas range from bruises, scratches, cuts, old and new scars, knife and shotgun wounds, burns, diseases, illness, disease and death. Also blood, sweat and tears.

These effects have a strong visual impact in helping to tell the story, so it is important that they look realistic to the audience, whether on stage or through the camera lens.

Choosing which products to use, and how to achieve the look depends on careful research and preparation.

Planning and researching

Everything starts with the script, and a description of the action in the story. Whether it is a battle scene, a fire, car accident or crime scene, the script will reveal some details of how it looks. The next thing to consider is how to achieve the look to match the action. Plan what to do by studying medical books, collect real photos of injuries from newspapers and journals, get advice from doctors, soldiers, nurses, armourers and the Internet for all the information you need. Take notes, download pictures and make sketches.

The next stage is to take your research material to the production planning meeting to hear what the director expects. They will have a visual idea of how the injury should look. Other departments will be involved. In a car crash or police crime scene the props department usually supplies the blood that is splashed around the set, while make-up is responsible for the blood used for the wounds. The costume department is involved if clothes are bloodied in the action, often needing duplicate costumes for each take, and will be keen to know if the blood is stain-proof. These and other questions will be raised when the make-up artist shows their research work and offers ideas for consideration.

It is easy to get carried away when doing casualty make-up. Over-enthusiasm can result in 'over the top' effects and ones that are difficult to repeat. It is important to be in control, and suit the effect to the production's needs. The producer will have a say in how much blood there is in a scene, because of television and film ratings, and the stunt co-ordinator will also be involved.

Preparation week on the television series Casualty

Make-up artist Sharon Anniss describes working on the British television drama series Casualty.

As a designer, of an episode of *Casualty* you usually get three weeks preparation time for two one-hour episodes, which is standard for an ongoing series, and four weeks to film both.

The script

The first thing to do is read the scripts, which are more often than not draft ones, so they are mainly a guide and a lot could change as the prep goes on. It is important to get some idea of what might be involved, so firstly you should make notes about each character and what happens to them:

◆ How should they look, i.e. smart, scruffy, glamorous, etc.?

◆ Is the story set on a wet windy day, i.e. do they need to look wet and windswept (as you'll very rarely film in the correct season to which the story is set)?

◆ What injuries are sustained and how are they changed throughout the episode? Do we see them actually happen?

◆ Do we see them get treated, i.e. stitched, operated on, blood spurts out, etc.?

From this, you can then work out if there will need to be stunt doubles and if wigs will be needed etc. to look like the actual actor.

Prosthetics

Now you would start to work out what prosthetics need to be made and how many repeats of each piece will be needed, so that the director can have a few takes of the shot. From this, you will know if you need to take actual casts of the real actor's limbs/body/face so that close-up shots (for example, of stitching a wound) can be done with no danger to the actor. First, you would research the injuries in the story, to get a true image of what it should look like, and then start to sculpt the wounds or look through old stock of moulds to see if anything will match the particular injury.

Meetings

In amongst all of the above there will be meetings with the director and production meetings.

A production meeting consists of all heads of departments looking through a shooting schedule and sorting through the details of how, where and when the scenes will be shot, particularly as the scenes are rarely shot in order, so it will flag up any problems like major make-up changes. For example, if the schedule states that the aftermath of a car crash is due to be shot and the next scene is of the character driving the car before the crash, there would be a long make-up change to get the actors cleaned up and remade for that scene. So in the production meeting the person responsible for doing the schedule may shuffle the scenes around to reduce the time in-between scenes.

You would also have a meeting with the director to discuss how they see each character looking and what detail they want to see for the injuries, etc. It's useful to have some research to hand to show a director what a certain injury should look like.

Continuity

Eventually you will get a shooting script, which you can go through to do the script and character breakdowns whereby you write down each scene that each character is in, so you can work out their continuity (where they were last seen and in what state). This is essential when filming as you very rarely film in the order of the story. You then need to go through the schedule and note when certain injuries/prosthetics are needed, stunt doubles and when you'll need extra help.

Brief your team and get your make-up kits, continuity files, prosthetics, etc. ready to load on a make-up truck, as there is always a part shot on location. The designer is also in charge of working out the times of the call sheet, which basically tells everyone what's happening each day. It is the designer's responsibility to work out who is doing each character's make-up and what time they need to come in to get made up.

Things can change from day to day and you have to be ready for anything, be able to think on your feet and always be flexible, even when at times things can be very fraught and frustrating.

Preparation week on the television series Casualty, pages 214 and 215 was written by Sharon Anniss.

Blood

Blood is always red, but the colour tone used on a production will depend on how it looks under lighting and film processing conditions. On a dimly lit set, a dark colour does not register well, so a brighter tone may be needed. On a brightly lit set with light surfaces, such as a bathroom or kitchen, a darker colour can often look more realistic.

Arterial blood is bright red, vascular blood is dark red; both types can form in clots, and then scabs when the blood dries.

The director will probably ask how much time you will need to do the make-up, and this might be a major consideration. A trial make-up might be necessary, and sometimes a lighting test on the blood is done to establish the colour tone.

STEP-BY-STEP: REAL CUT TO THE HAND CAUSED BY WORKING WITH HEAVY MACHINERY. HEALING STAGES OVER THREE MONTHS

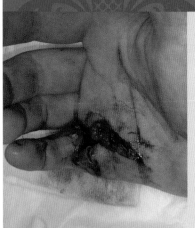

1 Fresh cut to hand.

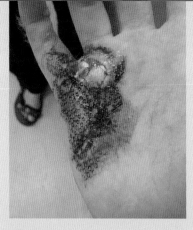

2 Cut has been stitched up, starting to heal and is producing pus.

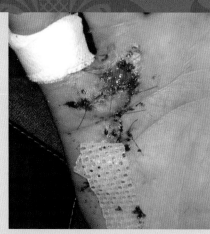

3 Cut starts to crust over.

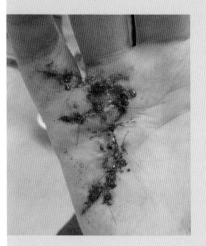

4 Scabbing.

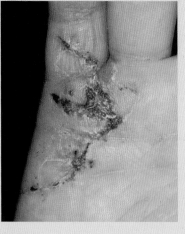

5 Scabbing and peeling skin.

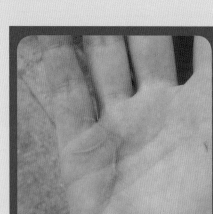

6 Cut has healed and left a scar.

Stab wound

A stab wound will show a deep, penetrating hole in the flesh, the depth and shape depending on the instrument that caused it. When it has healed, a knife wound might form an even or irregular scar, which would protrude in a line across the skin surface.

Questions to ask

1 How obtrusive is the wound to be?

2 What caused it?

3 How will it heal?

4 How can I repeat it?

Gunshot wound

Depending on the type of gun, and distance of the shooting, the wound is usually small and neat with blackened edges, and the exit wound is larger and messier, with extensive damage.

Questions to ask

1 What calibre was the gun?

2 From how close was the shot fired?

3 Is the victim dead or alive?

Bruises

A bruise should always look as if it has worked from the inside of the skin outwards, and not as if it has been painted on. The fresher the bruise the redder it is, becoming yellow and brown as it ages. The stages of a bruise are: red – reddish blue or dark purple – brown – paler brown – yellowish – green – yellow in the last stages of healing. A bruise is caused by broken blood vessels under the skin. Apart from the discoloration it is shiny on the skin surface.

> ### TOP TIP
> For successful results establish whether the entry wound or the exit wound will be visible. Make yourself familiar with the differences.

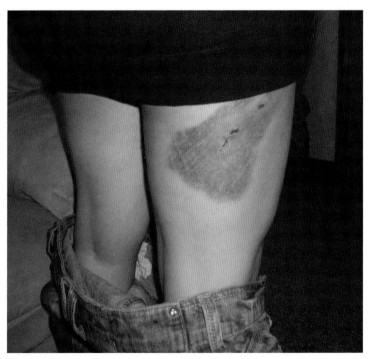

Real dog bite injury

Questions to ask

1 Where are the bruises to be positioned?

2 How old are they?

3 What caused them?

A black eye

The symptoms are swelling and bruising, plus scratches or grazes. At first it is black and blue, followed by green and yellow as it heals.

Questions to ask

1 How old is the injury?

2 Was the attacker wearing a ring?

3 If the attacker wore a ring, how many cuts would be inflicted on the victim?

4 Would the eye be bloodshot?

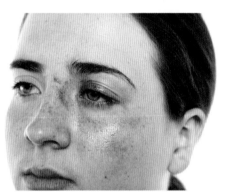

Fresh bruise

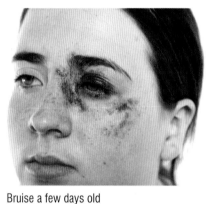

Bruise a few days old

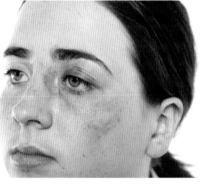

Old bruise

Burns

◆ **First degree burn** Slight, causing redness and sometimes a blister.

◆ **Second degree burn** Causes severe blisters, with redness on the surrounding area of skin.

◆ **Third degree burn** Causes much more severe damage. The flesh will be charred and black. Around this area there will be second degree burns and, towards the edge, first degree burns.

Questions to ask

1 What caused the burns?

2 Would the eyebrows and hair be singed?

3 How old should the burns be?

Stages of sunburn

1 Prep any 'strap' marks with masking tape.

2 Apply sunburn colour to area using Illustrator palette, the shade and depth depending on the skin tone you are working on. It needs to look sore (first degree burn).

3 Apply blisters with gelatine. A bottle with a nozzle works well as you can achieve blisters in various sizes and in clusters – apply to the areas that have been burnt the most (second degree burn). You can also add 'Duo' eyelash glue to achieve blisters.

4 A peeling effect can be created by sponging on latex and rubbing it with your thumb/fingers just before it is dry.

5 Remove the masking tape to show a paler skin that has not been burnt.

STEP-BY-STEP: STAGES OF SUN BURN

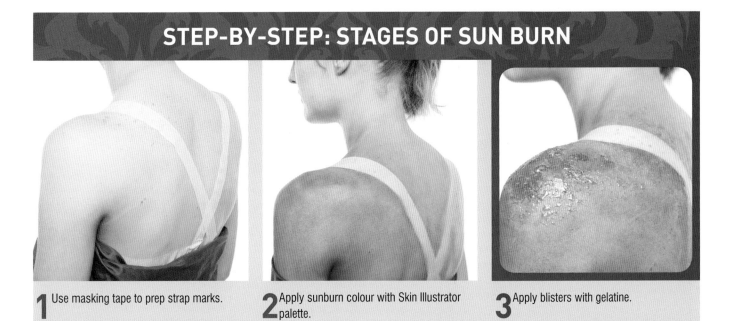

1 Use masking tape to prep strap marks.

2 Apply sunburn colour with Skin Illustrator palette.

3 Apply blisters with gelatine.

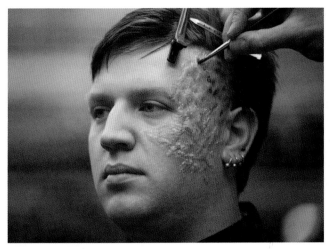

Close-up of burn make-up

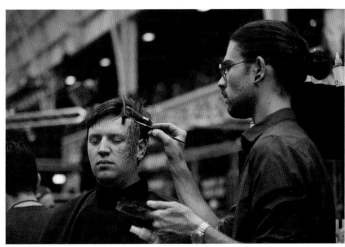

Colouring a burn make-up

Sweat

◆ **First stage** A red, shiny face.

◆ **Second stage** Droplets of sweat on the forehead and upper lip.

◆ **Third stage** Sweat all over the face, with wet hair. Wet areas on chest, back and under arms.

Fight scene

The stunt co-ordinator is in charge of choreographing a fight scene. Whether it is fencing, boxing, knife fights or fisticuffs he will dictate the type of wound, and when in the action to apply bruises, cuts, blood and sweat.

A broken nose

The nose will look crooked on the bridge bone. The surrounding skin will be heavily bruised. Depending on the action, the whites of the eyes might be bloodshot. Cuts and scratches could be present if the attacker was wearing a ring. Lighting and shading the nose can create a crooked effect.

Scars

Scars can be new or old, inverted, protruded or contracted. Crucial to the type of scar is what caused it.

Illness and shock

For both illness and shock the face is usually drained of colour. The skin is pale with shadows under the eyes – blue or mauve on light-coloured skins – brown or black on dark skin tones. When feverish there will be blotchy, red patches on the nostrils and eyelids, with sweat to indicate a high temperature.

The exact look of a particular disease should be researched in advance of applying the make-up.

Scratches, cuts and grazes

Surface injuries to the skin, superficial scrapes or cuts that heal quickly are injuries that do not last long, perhaps for one scene only. A palette knife or coarse stipple sponge used to apply blood to the area works well. As usual, the shape depends on what caused the injury.

Drug addict

Pale skin tone, dark shadows under the eyes, bruising around the veins used for shooting up on the inner wrists, arms or around the ankles. Track marks, tiny black dots on top of red needle marks. There are old and new bruises. Users have unhealthy looking, sweaty skin.

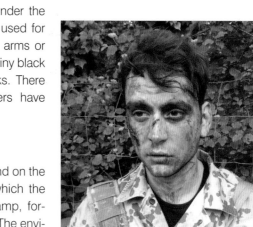

Dirtied-down and wounded soldier

Dirtying down

The materials and colours depend on the type of dirt of the location in which the action takes place: desert, swamp, forest, street, coalmine and so on. The environmental conditions will dictate the look, e.g. sand sticking to sweaty skin, mud running down a face in the pouring rain.

For worn-in dirt it should include the back of the neck, neck creases, around and under the nails, and in the creases of the knuckles.

Vomiting

There are products that are made for holding in the mouth, but mashing up fresh, ripe strawberries or other red fruits is more pleasant for an actor to eject from the mouth and an effective result.

Water sprays

A spray bottle with a fine nozzle, filled with water is useful for refreshing blood on wounds during fight scenes. It can also be used on the hair to refresh hair gel and reactivate it during the course of a long day's shoot.

For heavy fight scenes the spray can be filled with half water and half **glycerine** for providing perspiration. If you put a fine layer of petroleum jelly on the actor's forehead first, the sprayed mixture will stick to the skin and not dry too quickly.

HEALTH & SAFETY

Health & safety checklist

◆ The materials used must be safe for use on the skin and appropriate to the actor's skin type.

◆ The actor must be seated comfortably, suitable for the length of time to complete the work.

◆ Protection must be sufficient to prevent damage to the actor's hair and clothing.

◆ Preparation of the actor's skin must be thorough and suited to the materials to be used.

◆ Any adhesives used must be suitable for the skin area, the tenacity of adhesion required and the intended removal technique.

◆ Application must observe all health and safety legislation and procedures, and avoid any contact to the inside of the eye, or cross-contamination.

◆ Any likely contraventions to health and safety regulations must be notified promptly to the production department, and steps taken to ensure that a qualified practitioner is present to take responsibility.

Prosthetic casualty effects

If an effect is needed that is three-dimensional and covering a large area, it is best to use prosthetics. They can be applied every day and, provided the edges are skilfully hidden, are easy for continuity. The effect must be made in advance, either by the make-up artist or commissioned by a specialist workshop ready for the make-up artist to apply.

This is shown in CHAPTER 12 Prosthetics

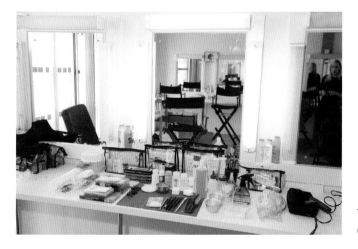

Tools and equipment for casualty effects

How to succeed

◆ The degree of the effect must be achieved on and/or off the set, within the allocated time appropriate to the type of production.

◆ The degree of the effect must be suitable given the watershed (television) or certificate (film) and production requirements.

◆ The final effect must look realistic and natural on camera.

◆ The materials chosen must achieve the desired effect.

◆ Techniques must be suited to the materials and achieve the desired effect on screen.

◆ Actors must be seated comfortably; the process carried out so as to minimise discomfort to them, and a good relationship maintained at all times to ensure their continuing co-operation.

See CHAPTER 12 Prosthetics for more on working with pro bondo and silicone.

Working with pro bondo

Pro bondo moulds can be made by a prosthetics artist to order, or moulds can be bought from specialist professional make-up shops.

Tools & equipment

◆ blood
◆ brushes
◆ fixer spray
◆ IPA (Isopropyl Alcohol)
◆ mixing palette or tile

◆ palette knife
◆ pro bondo
◆ pro bondo moulds
◆ Pro Clean
◆ release and seal

◆ Skin Illustrator palette
◆ Vaseline
◆ washing-up liquid

The pro bondo comes in various colours to match the skin tone – olive, pink and brown.

Filling the moulds

1 Clean out the mould with IPA on a brush, ensuring you remove all dust, grease and fibres, then leave to dry.

2 Add a very small amount of Vaseline to your finger and rub over the mould, giving it a very light coating of Vaseline. Make sure your fingers are clean – you can wipe them with IPA.

3 Paint some release and seal onto the mould with a paintbrush, only where the piece needs filling, with a very light edge – you don't have to fill the whole piece, just the edge of the piece you are making. Be careful not to fill with too much release and seal. It should be lightly painted on and not swimming in product.

4 Fill the mould with your chosen pro bondo with a palette knife, making sure the surface is smooth.

5 Leave to dry in a warm temperature for six to eight hours.

Application of a pro bondo piece onto the skin

1 Clean the skin with IPA, where the mould will be placed.

2 Place the mould on the skin and push hard.

3 Peel back the mould to release the pro bondo.

4 Clean around the edges with a very small amount of IPA.

Colouring

The injury can be sealed with a fixer spray, if necessary. Sometimes blood slides off silicone and pro bondo. To prevent this you need to use a very small amount of washing-up liquid on the piece, then add the blood and it will prevent the blood from beading.

Use a dark thick-clotted blood, wound filler or scab first. Make sure the wound edges are clean of blood so they are highlighted.

If you need the colour to stay for a long time, then apply IPA first before the colour. When using the Skin Illustrator palette, use washes of colour like water painting so the colour doesn't look too heavy and stick to the pro bondo. Work with a wash of colour mixed with IPA.

STEP-BY-STEP: APPLYING THE PRO BONDO PIECE

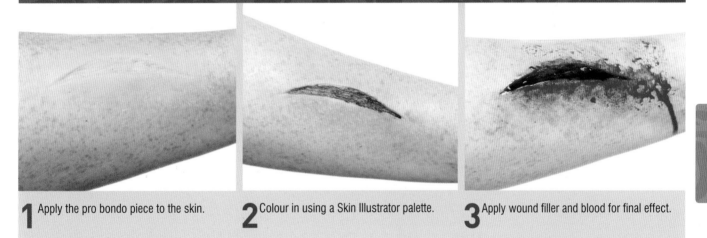

1 Apply the pro bondo piece to the skin.

2 Colour in using a Skin Illustrator palette.

3 Apply wound filler and blood for final effect.

Removal

Pro bondo pieces can be removed from the skin by using Pro Clean. Baby oil and olive oil also work on smaller pieces. Then wipe the skin clean, first with IPA, then with toner.

It is important to clean the mould properly – remove all bits of product and clean with IPA.

Working with silicone

Applying silicone directly to the skin

Silicone can be applied directly to the skin, using products such as Third Degree. Mix the parts A and B together on a tile or palette, then apply to the skin to create the required effect. Make sure you use a separate spatula for each, to avoid cross-contamination, as this will make the silicone harden and become unusable.

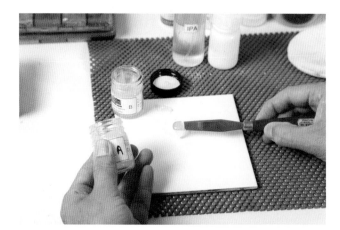

Mixing A and B Third Degree together

STEP-BY-STEP: CREATING A BULLET HOLE WITH SILICONE

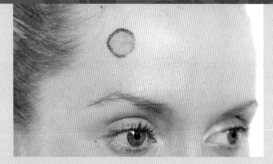

1 Mark out the injury design.

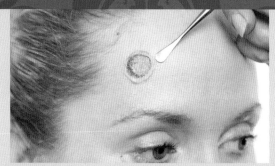

2 Having mixed equal parts of A and B together, apply to the skin and blend.

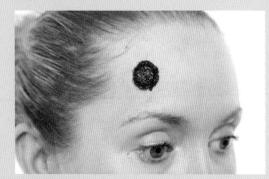

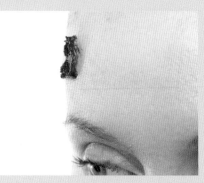

3 Colour the skin and wound using the Skin Illustrator palette. Build up layers of colour in the wound for depth, and add wound filler.

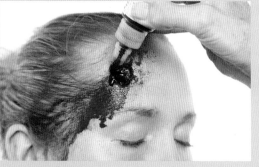

4 Add blood.

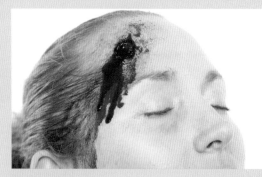

The final look.

CASE PROFILE: BRIAN KINNEY, MAKE-UP ARTIST

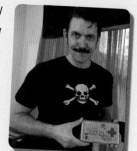

How long have you been working in the industry?

Fifteen years.

Did you have a lucky break or turning point?

My first real job, *Band of Brothers*, was a game changer. I was very green, and it was a baptism of fire ... Every day was a new challenge. Set etiquette and techniques I learned there are with me to this day.

What has been your most significant project?

Band of Brothers showed me the business at its best, with an international crew pulling together to create a groundbreaking work of impeccable detail. Once I returned stateside, *CSI: NY* showed me everything else. Over the course of eight years I went from an assistant in the SFX make-up department, to a daily hire make-up artist, to a full-time personal make-up artist for the show's lead actor. Politics come into play in every career, make-up included. It was not always an easy path, but every experience there, good and bad, prepared me for every job since.

What do you enjoy most about the job?

I enjoy the creative challenges that come up on the job. You might not always have ideal preparation or materials, but there's nothing like the feeling of creating a successful make-up under pressure. Collaborating with colleagues to bring an idea to life is always rewarding and fun.

How has the television and film industry changed during your career?

Faster cameras mean details are now clearer. Make-ups must now be cleaner in design and adjusted to compensate for colour discrepancies. Also, in a relatively short span of time, I've seen continuity pictures literally go from polaroids to digital images.

What advice would you give to a new make-up artist starting out?

Once you commit to being a make-up artist, never give up! Strive to be a great make-up artist by honing your craft every day.

About 'Hurt Box'

While working on location doing special effects make-ups, I was often sculpting, pouring moulds, and running prosthetics in kitchens, hotel rooms and trailers. To aid in making quick wounds and appliances, I created a series of silicone moulds that could travel with ease. I passed a few onto colleagues and the Hurt Box was born. Eight different-themed moulds exist, with more on the way. From scars to cuts, bullet holes to blisters, each mould is coloured and labelled with distinctive flair. A variety of materials can be used to cast up quick appliances, including cap plastic, silicone gels, pro bondo, gelatine and more. I've even made custom moulds for departments on shows like *Sons of Anarchy*. Hurt Boxes are currently available at make-up stockists in North America and Europe and at www.fullslap.com.

Improvisation

It is not always possible to plan in advance if a director wants an effect on the spur of the moment. The unexpected is part of the fun of the business. Every make-up artist has had to improvise and come up with what is needed at the last minute. Some directors are a continual challenge to the make-up artist's ingenuity.

If there isn't time to make prosthetic pieces there are many ways to improvise effects at the last minute, using wax and gelatine.

Gelatine

Gelatine is very useful for creating casualty effects directly onto the skin. It can be coloured red to produce a good artificial blood, which doesn't run. It is harmless to the skin and provides fast, effective results. Not to be confused with the professional gelatine for filling moulds in prosthetic work, this gelatine is in powder form and is available from food stores. It is mixed with glycerine (available from pharmacies or chemists), with water and cosmetic and food colouring. This is an easy way to create an effect in the kitchen or classroom.

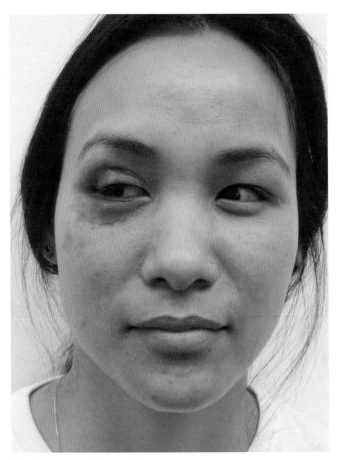

A swollen eye made from gelatine

Tools & equipment

- ◆ colouring – food colouring, cosmetic powders, etc.
- ◆ gelatine powder
- ◆ glycerine
- ◆ modelling tools

- ◆ saucepan or microwave dish
- ◆ spirit gum – for very firm hold
- ◆ stove or microwave
- ◆ water

Basic recipe for direct application of gelatine

1   Use equal amounts of gelatine powder and glycerine, plus water and colouring. Mix the gelatine and glycerine together, while adding a small amount of water at a time (it is easier to add water gradually than to add gelatine).

2 Heat the mixture in a saucepan on a stove or in a microwave. Heat gently until the mixture has clarified.

3 When clear, add the colouring. Add a little more water until you are happy with the texture.

4 Test by putting some on a plate and then applying it to the back of the hand. Be careful not to burn yourself. The mixture should be warm enough to be liquid when it is applied, yet cool enough to be harmless and thick enough to set quickly.

Colouring effects The gelatine can be coloured in advance, to give a flesh-coloured effect, for use as blood which stays in place, or using additional colour for use as a burn effect. For blood, mix red food colouring to the gelatine mixture. It is also easy to colour the gelatine once it has been applied to the skin and become firm to the touch. Painting with water-based make-up and powders produces a good effect. Other substances can be mixed in for textural effects – dirt, gravel, even splinters or glass fragments. (Don't use real glass – smash a clear, boiled sweet.) It will all wash off with soap and water. Gelatine is easy to apply using sponges, brushes, spatulas or modelling tools. For a really firm hold when it must last a long time, e.g. stage work for an entire scene, you can use spirit gum on the skin before putting gelatine on top. The beauty of using gelatine is that it is completely harmless to the skin and gives a lovely translucent effect.

Blood recipe

> 2 oz/62 g gelatine
>
> 2 fl. oz/57 ml water
>
> 2 oz/62 g glycerine
>
> Red and brown colouring
>
> Breadcrumbs
>
> Rice Krispies
>
> Cornflakes

Mix together and gently heat the ingredients until all have dissolved. Add a few drops of red food colouring, or add brown for a darker colour. Keep in a thermos flask for use later. A few seconds in a microwave oven will soften it up. It can get very hot, so never put it on an actor's face without first testing it on yourself. Breadcrumbs, Rice Krispies and Cornflakes can be added to the blood for different effects.

Wax wounds

As well as changing the face shape or feature, e.g. a nose, wax can be used for building up an area, which can then be cut into for a deep cut or wound.

1 Spread the wax thinly and blend edges.

2 Cut into the wax with a palette knife to make the incision you want.

3 Apply three coats of sealer. Allow to dry between each application.

4 When dry, colour the area to match the surrounding skin. Stipple to camouflage the waxed area using red first, powder, then skin-tone colour. Put red into the wound and a trickle of blood.

HEALTH & SAFETY

Always check the temperature of the blood prior to applying it to the skin. This will prevent causing contra-actions to the skin such as burning.

Tools & equipment

- ◆ 'blood'
- ◆ colouring
- ◆ palette knife
- ◆ sealer
- ◆ wax

Slit wrists

1 Apply wax and sealer as before, this time on the wrists, and disguise with camouflage make-up and matching skin-tone colours, then powder.

2 Slice the cuts with a palette knife.

3 Paint the areas with bruise colours: blue, purple, red and yellow.

4 Place fake blood into the cuts.

Slit throat

Before starting, think what was used for the wound – smooth or serrated edge knife. Think about the length, depth and shape of the cut.

1 Apply wax and sealer as before, build up the wax in the centre of the wound for depth. After several coats of sealer, paint pink or red make-up, stipple it gently with a piece of torn-up sponge or orange stipple sponge. Add skin-tone colours, blend edges.

2 Using a palette knife, slit through the wax with a smooth sweeping movement. Gently pull back areas of the wax for torn effect.

3 Fill the wound with dark and light wound fillers, or 'blood' and coffee granules.

4 Add flowing blood for photograph or shoot – but not too much or it will hide the wound.

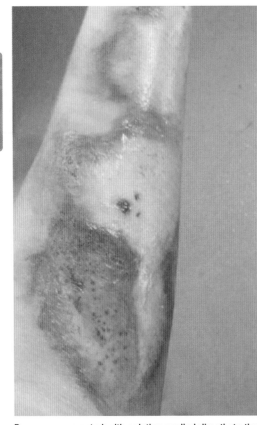

Burn on arm created with gelatine applied directly to the skin, with a film of Vaseline

Burns

Kitchen gelatine powder and glycerine are good for directly applied burn effects. Providing you check that it is not hot, but just comfortably warm or tepid, you can apply it safely around the eyes or anywhere else. As always, plan the effect. How did it happen? What caused the burn?

◆ A first degree burn is slight, usually causing redness and sometimes a small blister.

◆ A second degree burn causes severe blisters, and is surrounded by a first degree burn.

◆ A third degree burn will cause much more damage; the flesh may be charred and black. Around the third degree burn will be blisters and redness.

Use the basic recipe for direct application of gelatine

For creating blisters in a second degree burn, simply drip the gelatine so that it forms blisters where you want them. You can use a dropper from a medicine bottle or the end of a make-up brush. Layers of gelatine can be coloured on top with make-up, and black painted on for a charred, third degree burn effect. The gelatine can be torn back to look like damaged skin.

Alternative techniques for severe burns

Tools & equipment

- artificial blood
- basic recipe gelatine mixture – in plastic bag
- black hair-colouring spray
- brush
- cotton wool
- handheld hairdryer

- latex
- modelling tool
- palette knife
- palettes of grease and watercolours
- tissues – separated into single layers, torn in pieces
- Vaseline, KY jelly

Latex third degree burn

This is a very theatrical-looking burn effect, suitable for stage and long-distance shots. It would not stand up to HD digital cameras in close-ups. It is, however, good practice work for classroom, kitchen, student films and amateur dramatics because it costs nothing. It is also fun to do.

1 Paint latex along someone's arm.

2 Place torn-up pieces of tissue across the latex while it is still wet. Do not use scissors to cut the tissue – we want the torn edges. Cover the tissue with another layer of tissue pieces.

3 For a charred flesh effect, add a small amount of cotton wool. Apply another layer of latex. You can use the hairdryer to speed up the drying process – use the cool setting.

4 When the latex is dry, spray the area with black hair colouring.

5 When dry, peel this back in irregular bits to reveal the real skin below.

6 Put the prepared gelatine in its plastic bag into a bowl of hot water. When the gelatine has melted (test that it is not too hot), apply it to the blackened area to give a blistered shiny effect. Let the gelatine drip from a brush or tool to form droplets around the burn.

You can apply make-up over all these products. Where the real skin is exposed after pulling back the latex paint, paint the skin bright red and add 'blood'. Vaseline, KY jelly or glycerine can be used for shine on the surfaces.

Latex built up in layers, gelatine, and scar material can all be used for burn effects. Scar material can be spread roughly and punctured when dry, with 'blood' pushed into the material. Latex gives a shrivelled effect; clear gelatine on top gives a watery, blistered effect. The most severe part of the burn should have the greatest depth. Around this the effect should fade away with blisters and redness surrounding the area.

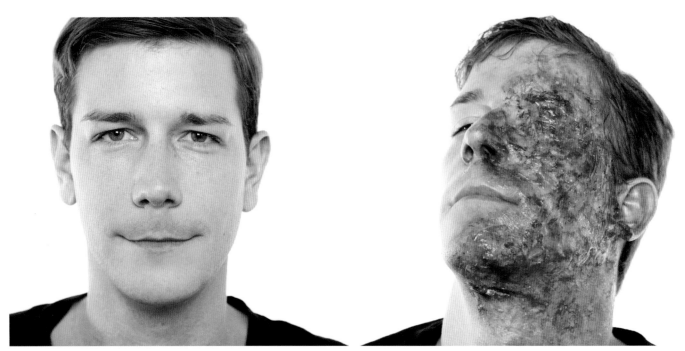

Before

Third degree burns

Fire burn make-up

1 With a 'trauma red' colour from an illustrator palette, mark out the position of the burn make-up. If covering the eye, find out which one is more comfortable to keep closed while the non-burnt eye is open. Apply Vaseline to any hair that may come into contact with the gelatine, i.e. eyebrows, eyelashes and the hair-line. Melt the clear gelatine in its bottle in a baby heater or melt it in a bowl in the microwave for a few seconds. Check the temperature of the melted gelatine on your arm or hand before applying to the face that you are working on. (You do not want to cause any real burns!)

2 Apply a layer of gelatine with a modelling tool to create an uneven texture, spreading and lifting it up in places to create a blistered and burst blister effect. Tear small shapes of tissue (do not cut with scissors as straight edges will not work) and place them onto the wet gelatine. Where you want a peeled skin effect, lift slightly before it is dry to create peeling skin. Apply gelatine above the eyebrow and around the eye. Tear a piece of tissue to cover the area and stick it to the wet gelatine. Apply a thin layer of gelatine over the tissue, making sure that the eye underneath is closed. Apply another layer of tissue and then more gelatine, building up your desired effect. Thin cotton wool fibres can also be applied for more texture. For severe burns, a small amount of blood can be pushed under the blisters. Latex and third degree burns could also be used – latex giving a more shrivelled effect.

3 More red can be added but exposing the skin that you have already coloured should be sufficient with the clear latex. To create a charred look, small amounts of black can be applied with black illustrator, black grease paint or, used sparingly, black powder.

4 KY jelly is applied on burst blisters for a watery, weepy effect.

Scars

Scars can be made with special plastic formulas available in several brands, e.g. Tuplast, packaged in tubes and easy to apply quickly with realistic looking results. Alternatively, latex can be used or even eyelash adhesive which is made of latex. These products are useful for providing a last-minute effect when there has been no time for planning in advance, or the production cannot afford prosthetics.

Creating a scar using Tuplast/scar plastic

Tools & equipment

- barrier cream
- lipstick and eyebrow pencils – crimson lake, scarlet, medium brown
- palette of basic colours
- powder, powder puff, powder brush
- Tuplast – scar plastic
- wooden modelling tool or metal spatula

Tuplast is a more expensive method, as it costs more than latex or gelatine. Do not use scar plastic near the eyes. A skin test should be done 24 hours in advance, on the back of the hand, to test for any reactions.

1 Apply barrier cream, rub in well and powder. Brush off excess powder.

2 Draw a line, on top of the barrier cream, where the scar is going to be, using a red cosmetic pencil.

3 Apply the Turplast along the line and shape it quickly, using the modelling tool or spatula, before it dries.

4 For a new scar, paint crimson lake around the edges in an uneven way. Blend a little scarlet red as well, to make it look sore. Leave it shiny.

5 For an old scar, paint brown around the edges unevenly. Powder all over with powder puff pressed firmly to give a faded effect. Brush off excess powder with powder brush.

Contracted scars

Test in advance for adverse reactions. Do not use near the eyes.

Collodion causes the skin to pucker up, and gives the appearance of a very old scar. The result is subtle and realistic looking, and can be used around burn effects or at the edge of **plastic scar material**.

1 Apply barrier cream where the scar will be.

2 Powder well and brush off excess powder.

3 Paint the collodion, which is transparent, onto the skin and allow to dry.

Tools & equipment

- collodion
- barrier cream
- powder, powder brush

To remove the scar plastic or collodion

All Clear is a product made by Kryolan which safely removes scar plastic, latex and spirit gum from the skin. Apply with cotton wool to the area, and peel off when it is loose, rubbing gently with the All Clear on a cotton bud.

CASE PROFILE: SHARON ANNISS, MAKE-UP DESIGNER

How long have you been working in the industry?

I have worked in the industry for the past 18 years, starting out as a trainee and assistant, working my way up to supervisor and finally, last year, designer. After working as a hairdresser in a salon I always had an ambition to do hair in film and television and when I looked into it I was advised to have make-up as a skill as well, so then set about training in that too.

How did you get into the industry?

Coming from a small village in Devon I had to work very hard after finishing my training. I had four jobs that I would juggle just to keep my head above water so that I could get up to London for work experience, which was always unpaid but essential to learn everything I could about the industry. I learnt how to behave on a film set, my role as part of the team and all aspects of make-up, continuity, even down to knowing the right clothes to wear.

I started working on student films and very low-budget movies and through those productions I met other people starting out in their careers too, who worked in different areas. Between us we'd help each other out by passing on our details to other productions. I would also literally knock on doors. Whenever I saw unit signs I would follow them and knock on the production office door and ask if I could either speak to the make-up designer or at least leave my CV and card.

Did you have a lucky break or a turning point?

I first got my lucky break after two and a half years of perseverance of knocking on doors and working for no money. One day I knocked on a door and it was answered by a make-up designer I had met three weeks before on a day's work experience. She realised she had met me before and thought that by knocking on the door I had been very intuitive as well as bold. On that basis, she told me about a job she had coming up where she needed a trainee. I was offered a month's trial. The job lasted three months and I was on board the whole time and getting paid. I have since gone on to work with that make-up

designer for the past 18 years and learnt a huge amount of valuable knowledge. She also introduced me and recommended me to many other make-up designers who I have worked with on several occasions and still do. But when out of work, I still knock on doors, so it is a lot about who you know but also pushing yourself to get another job and never being blasé as it's a tough industry.

What has been your most significant project?

I would say my most significant project was this job as a trainee, it was a pilot episode of a drama series called *The Inspector Lynley Mysteries* and the following year it was made into a series which was offered to the same make-up team. I ended up staying for three series with the same make-up designer and consequently went on to work with her on many other productions, the longest being five series of *Waking the Dead*.

I have also worked on many other productions for different designers such as *Spooks*, *Holby City*, *Casualty*, *Whiteheat* in television and as a daily hair or make-up artist on films such as *The Sweeney*, *Anna Karenina*, *World War Z* and *Warhorse* to name but a few. I have also worked in theatre and in photographic genres too, but I prefer television and film.

What do you enjoy most about the job?

I most enjoy the variety of work and the research involved in creating something as true to real life as possible, particularly special effects and injury make-ups, but also having hairdressing as a skill too I really enjoy creating period hairstyles. But more than that, I love being part of something that becomes a story for others to enjoy.

What advice would you give to a new make-up artist starting out?

Be prepared to work incredibly hard, don't expect to make it straight away, I gave myself five years and it almost took that long to get regular work. At times I still had to resort back to bar work or hairdressing, but don't give up and always knock on doors.

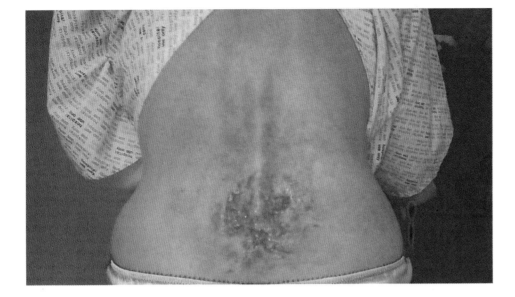

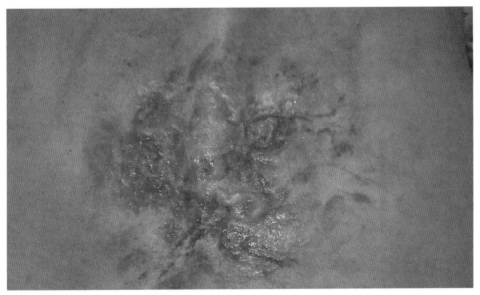

Make-up by Sharon Anniss for television drama *Holby City* – infection of removal of tattoo

REVISION QUESTIONS

1 What colour are the first stages of bruising?

2 What are the different types of bloods available on the market?

3 What is the most suitable blood to use in the mouth?

4 What different techniques will you consider to break an actor down as a drug addict?

5 What products do you mix together to make sweat?

12 Prosthetics

LEARNING OBJECTIVES

This chapter covers the following:

◆ How prosthetics are made.

◆ The materials used to make prosthetics.

◆ Preparing, blending, colouring and removing pieces.

◆ Sectional lifecasting.

◆ Lifecasting application (including preparing the actor and removal of the lifecast).

◆ Health and safety.

◆ Bald caps.

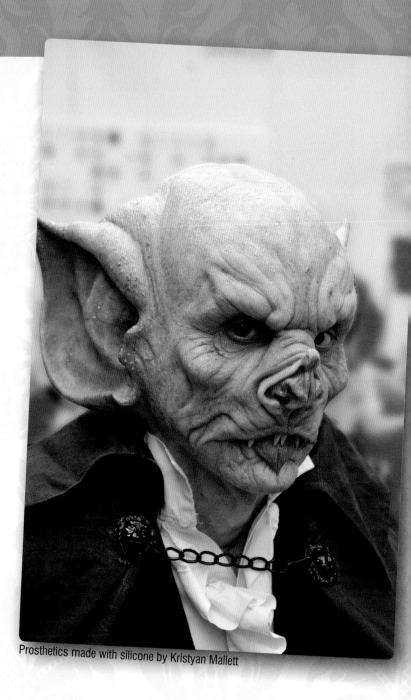
Prosthetics made with silicone by Kristyan Mallett

KEY TERMS

Alginate

Face powder

Flash

Gafquat

Lifecasting

Modelling clay

Plaster bandage

Plaster

Sectional lifecast

UNIT TITLE

◆ Part cast and make small prosthetic pieces and bald caps

◆ Apply, maintain and remove prosthetic pieces and bald caps

◆ Produce original lifecasts for prosthetic pieces

◆ Create prosthetics

INTRODUCTION

This chapter covers the techniques required to make and use prosthetic pieces. You will examine what materials are used to make prosthetic pieces, including: gelatine, foam latex, clay, silicone and plastics. Health and safety is very important when working with prosthetics, which is explained in detail in this chapter. This chapter also explains how to make, clean and use different forms of positive and negative moulds. It will help with Level 3 media courses, including cast and create prosthetic pieces, and advanced media make-up university degree courses.

Prosthetics

Prosthetics are three-dimensional pieces used to change an actor's face or body shape. They are usually made from some form of flexible rubber products that pick up details, imitate the mobility of flesh, without being heavy, and are easy to attach to an actor's face for art working. When coloured and attached they should blend in seamlessly to the natural parts of the face. The most commonly used products are latex, silicone rubbers and gelatine. Small prosthetic pieces such as warts, wounds, scars and diseases do not require a face cast. More complex ones like swollen eye pieces, noses, chins, foreheads and eyebags do need a lifecast – or at least an impression of part of the actor's face.

Today's make-up artists are expected to be able to take a lifecast, and produce small prosthetic effects.

On large-scale productions, when different faces, monsters, creatures or aliens need to be created, the prosthetics are designed and produced by specialist companies. The companies take care of the whole process, from **lifecasting**, sculpting, mould making, art working, to final applications. On some productions the make-up designer may commission the work and have it delivered, to be applied by the make-up production team.

In television, the make-up artists often have to create effects at the last minute and will choose the quickest, easiest ways to deliver what the director wants.

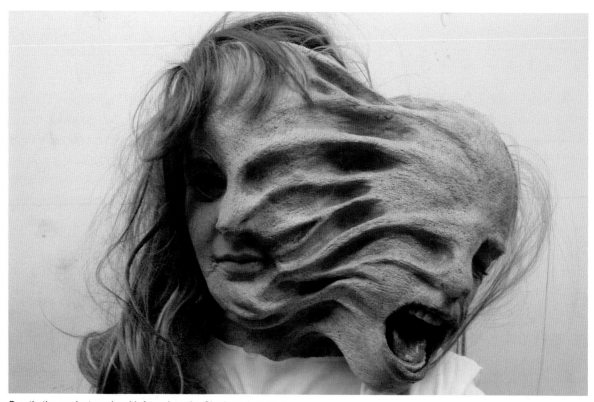

Prosthetics project made with foam latex by Charlotte Jameison

How prosthetics are made

First, if possible, a lifecast is taken of the actor's face or body part. From this, a duplicate positive casting is made with a material such as **plaster**. This is called a face cast or body cast.

Based on this cast a new shape is sculpted (positive); from this, a negative is made of the newly sculpted feature. A positive copy of the sculpture is made in a flexible material such as plastic, latex, silicone, rubber or gelatine. This prosthetic piece is attached to the actor's face or body, and coloured to blend in with the surrounding skin tone.

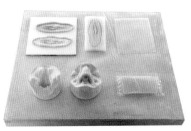

Prosthetics materials

Materials used in casting and modelling

◆ **Plaster** This is the most basic ingredient and the cheapest. There are different types of plaster. Plaster of Paris is soft; dental stones such as Crystacal D, R or lamina are harder and much stronger. Plaster moulds are usually reinforced with fibres or fabrics such as scrim, sacking, hessian, horsehair or even fibreglass. Fibreglass gives a lightweight but very strong mould.

◆ **Alginate** This is used in taking accurate impressions of the face or body parts. It takes between three and seven minutes to set and can be speeded up by using warm water. **Alginate** is affected by temperature. It is better to use cold water to mix it, as the setting time is quicker in hot weather. It is harmless to the skin and sets to a gelatine-like substance. Because it is floppy it needs to be backed with **plaster bandage** to reinforce the shape.

◆ **Gypsona or plaster bandage** This material is used in hospitals for setting broken bones. It is soaked briefly in water, wrung out and then smoothed over the alginate.

◆ **Silicone rubber** This is a room-temperature vulcanising rubber compound, used for making flexible moulds. Silicone rubber work is usually done in specialist workshops as the material is expensive.

◆ **Clay** A good-quality water-based **modelling clay** is used for modelling or sculpting the new feature. It must be kept wet and sealed inside plastic for storage. An oil-based sculpting material called Plastilene is also used. This has the advantage of not drying out, and can be detailed much better with fine textures and pores.

Materials used in making prosthetics

◆ **Gelatine** A powder made from calves' hooves, used to make jelly. It is available as '300-grade technical gelatine'. It is mixed with glycerol and sorbitol and poured into warm moulds. When cool it forms a rubbery compound.

◆ **Liquid latex** A milky liquid which can be painted in layers inside moulds to produce a solid rubber piece. Each painted-in layer should be applied thinly with a brush and allowed to dry before applying the next layer. Allow about four hours for drying between layers – so it is very time-consuming. Latex can also be sloshed around the mould. It is a cheap and easy product to use.

◆ **Foam latex** This is a four- or five-part latex compound, which is whisked to a foam in a food mixer. The foam is poured into cold moulds and cooked in an oven to produce foam latex prosthetic pieces. This is usually done in specialist workshops.

◆ **Cap plastic** In liquid form, as used for making bald caps, plastic can be painted into moulds to make small prosthetic pieces.

Working with pro bondo

Pro bondo is thickened Pros-Aide. Either the Pros-Aide is mixed in an electric mixer slowly for a long period of time, causing the moisture to evaporate, thickening it up, or cabosil/dulling

TOP TIP

There are various types of alginate available on the market. Some are fast setting. Always check manufacturer's instructions before use.

HEALTH & SAFETY

Many prosthetic products may be highly flammable and must be stored correctly according to the manufacturer's instructions. Always follow COSHH regulations.

powder is mixed in to thicken it up. It can be coloured with any water-based pigments. When used in prosthetics, it produces a less flexible appliance than some other products. So it should only be used to make small thin appliances.

Working with silicone

Plat Gel Silicone consists of two or three parts: equal quantities of coloured A and B are mixed together for a harder silicone; and flocking can also be added and it must be coloured with oil based pigments. It is safe to glue on skin, and sets in seven to ten minutes. The addition of a deadener makes the final silicone softer and more flesh-like. Silicone and gelatine are the best products to use for HD realistic character make-ups. However they can be heavy, so the pieces must be kept as thin as possible. When creating a fantasy project with big pieces, foam latex would be the preferred material as it is much lighter and more comfortable for the actor.

CASE PROFILE: KRISTYAN MALLETT, PROSTHETICS MAKE-UP DESIGNER

How long have you been working in the industry?

I have been working in the make-up industry since 1998, starting in theatre, fashion and editorial.

How did you get into the industry?

I always wanted to be a prosthetic make-up artist since I was about seven years old. Watching monster movies and being inspired by great make-up movies such as *American Werewolf in London*, *Legend* and *The Thing*. Throughout school I was engineering every project towards a creative path that had something to do with film or design. I then enrolled in a make-up college as soon as I had the chance. From this I did a few years in fields that were not prosthetic-related. I contacted a make-up effects designer called Nick Dudman, who was at that time doing *The Mummy Returns*, he told me he was doing courses. It was a few years after that conversation that I was able to do his course and so enrolled and it was during the course he offered me a traineeship on *Harry Potter*.

Did you have a lucky break or turning point?

In my career I have had many turning points, one of the most prominent being on *Harry Potter and the Goblet of Fire*. I was running the Silicone Lab. It was the knowledge I gained on this production that opened up doors for me. UK companies hired me to share my knowledge of silicone techniques. If you gain as much knowledge as possible in as many fields in make-up as possible you will always be busy . . . Master those fields and you are likely to be the employer not employee.

What do you enjoy most about the job?

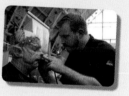

I don't just enjoy but *love* having like-minded people around, watching something great come out of nothing more than an idea. Being in a creative environment is a wonderful place to be.

What do you enjoy least about the job?

Chasing payments from production companies is the thing I hate most. With all the fun of the creativity it sometimes feels awkward to have to get down to business . . . Kind of turns what we do into a real job!

How has the television and film industry changed during your career?

I have noticed that there are more and more people becoming aware that this is a job that they can do and not just a pipe dream. Also over the last five years television budgets have gotten bigger and each episode can be like a short movie so lots more work all around.

What advice would you give to a new make-up artist starting out?

Be passionate, work hard, be humble, remember you are a trainee when you begin so be the best trainee possible and you will climb that ladder.

www.kristyanmallett.com

www.pscomposites.com – supplying prosthetics supplies and services to the industry

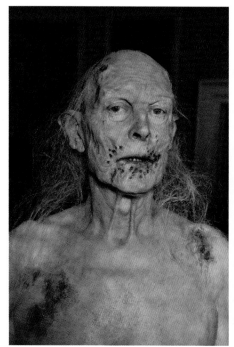

Corpse character – by Kristyan Mallett

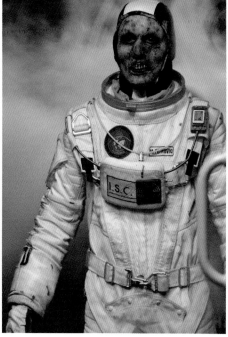

Zombie Astronaut creature – by Kristyan Mallett

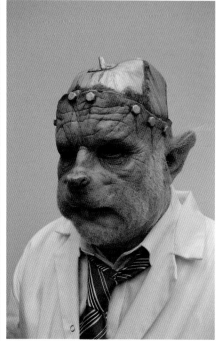

Rat Mad Scientist – by Kristyan Mallett

Mould making

Flat moulds

This type of mould making does not require a lifecast of the actor's facial features. It can be done anywhere: on location or the kitchen table. It is ideal for making wounds, scars, keloid scars, blisters, burns and diseases. They can be made in advance and kept until needed.

Silicone is a popular material for making these types of moulds.

1 On a tile, using wax clay, sculpt your piece. Water-based clay is not suitable for this – because the sculpture will be very thin, it will dry out too quickly. Use a small wire brush to create texture, applying talcum powder where necessary to stop the clay from sticking together. Continue scratching but go lighter and lighter. Use a soft brush to smooth down the wax where necessary.

2 Build a little wax wall to create the **flash** around the sculpt, keeping it about 4 mm away from the sculpt edge.

3 Build a wall around the sculpt to contain the silicone. It can be made with modelling wax or water-based clay.

4 Apply a thin coat of spray wax over the sculpt. A light coat of Vaseline could also be used, but spray wax is better, as it won't affect the sculpt's detail.

5 Mix your silicone, if using Plat Gel. Only use equal parts of A and B with no deadener.

6 Paint a fine layer of silicone over the sculpture, to capture the detail. Your brush must be cleaned in white spirit before the silicone sets and ruins your brush.

7 Slowly pour silicone in the corner, until the sculpt is covered. By pouring the silicone slowly from as high as possible you can reduce the amount of air bubbles in the silicone.

TOP TIP

Whenever you are making a mould and you want it to come apart, always apply a release agent, such as spray wax, or your moulds may not come apart later. If in doubt always spray wax.

8   At the same time pour a thin layer of silicone onto the clean tile. This will give you a sheet of rolling silicone, which will be used later in the filling stage. Let it dry for one hour.

9   Once set, peal the silicone sheet off the tile, remove the silicone mould from the sculpt and clean with soapy water. Sometimes it is necessary to trim the silicone edges, so that the mould sits flat during the filling stage. Once dry, store in a sealed container to protect from dust.

Filling the flat mould   Always spray wax the mould and silicone sheet first, whatever you are putting in it.

Using gelatine

1   Warm both the mould and silicone sheet (not too hot). Melt the gelatine and pour over the warm flat mould. Lay the silicone sheet over the top, spray waxed side down and, using a small rolling pin, roll out the excess gelatine.

2   The harder you press, the thinner the edges will be, but if you press too hard you will lose some of the sculpted shape because the silicone mould is flexible and will squash down.

3   Leave to cool.

4   Remove the silicone sheet and powder the gelatine appliance. If you only need one, you can leave the appliance in the mould ready for application as this will protect the edges.

5   If you need to cast out more than one, gently remove the appliance, powdering as you go and store in an airtight container.

TOP TIP

Some actors may not allow gelatine to be used on them. Gelatine is an animal by-product. If an actor is a vegetarian, using gelatine may be against their ethics and an alternate prosthetic material must be used.

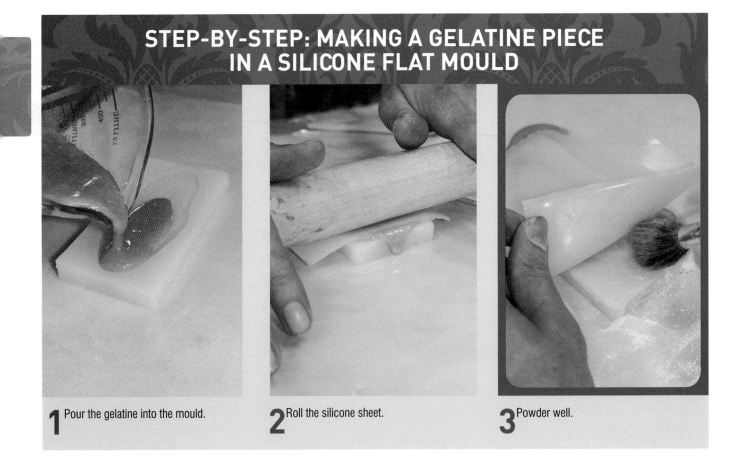

STEP-BY-STEP: MAKING A GELATINE PIECE IN A SILICONE FLAT MOULD

1 Pour the gelatine into the mould.

2 Roll the silicone sheet.

3 Powder well.

Using encapsulated silicone   Encapsulation means, enclosing the soft silicone with the deadener, inside a harder outside skin. Usually cap plastic is used, or Plat Gel A and B only.

1   Apply spray wax to both the mould and silicone sheet.

2   Spray several layers of cap plastic, dissolved in acetone, onto both the mould and silicone sheet. About ten parts of acetone to one part cap plastic. You may need to do several tests to determine the number of layers you need to apply, to give the best thickness of encapsulant. Be careful of the fumes, always wear a fume mask and work in a well-ventilated area.

3   Once dry, mix equal quantities of coloured Plat Gel A and B silicone. If you want the appliance to be softer add some deadener to the mix. The more deadener you add, the softer the appliance will be. The maximum amount is about 200 per cent. About 150 per cent works well – so if you use 20 ml A and 20 ml B you will need 60 ml of deadener.

4   Pour over the flat mould and cover with the silicone sheet. Make sure that the side of the silicone sheet you use is the side with the cap plastic on it, if not the rolling sheet will permanently fix to the silicone appliance. Press down the silicone sheet using a small rolling pin.

5   When the silicone has set, carefully peel off the silicone sheet.

6   Powder the appliance and leave the appliance in the flat mould or remove it if you need to make more. Store any appliances in an airtight container to protect from dust.

> **HEALTH & SAFETY**
>
> Due to the fumes created, always work in a well-ventilated area when working with chemicals. Wear PPE where necessary.

Using pro bondo

1   You don't need to use spray wax with pro bondo as the silicone in the mould it-self acts as a release agent. But if you find the appliances difficult to remove later, apply a very light layer of spray wax to both the mould and rolling silicone sheet. Spread pro bondo carefully into the mould, avoiding trapping any air bubbles. Place the silicone sheet over the mould and press out any excess.

2   Freeze the mould until the pro bondo has set hard.

3   Peel away the silicone rolling sheet and allow the appliance to dry thoroughly, but keep it covered to prevent dust settling on the appliance and don't let the cover touch the piece.

4   When ready to apply, the back of the pro bondo remains tacky.

5   The flat mould is placed into position on the actor and the pro bondo piece sticks to the actor.

6   Peel away the flat mould.

7   Any excess flashing can be removed with IPA, sparingly.

> **ACTIVITY**
>
> **Prosthetic cuts**
>
> Research different forms of cuts, scars and skin diseases and create and make your own scar tray.

Making prosthetic gelatine

When making prosthetic gelatine, as in the following recipe, care should be taken when heating the gelatine as it easily burns, especially if you are using a microwave to prepare it. Very hot gelatine must never be used directly onto a person as it would burn them. Always make sure that any gelatine used is cool enough before applying it to a person's skin.

Tools & equipment

- colouring – cosmetic water-based pigments
- 100 g gelatine
- 200 g glycerine
- 200 g liquid sorbitol
- ½ tablespoon of zinc oxide powder

Ready-made gelatine can also be bought from specialist professional make-up shops and suppliers.

Making the gelatine

1 Mix the liquid sorbitol and glycerine with the gelatine. Heat moderately in a microwave oven, a double boiler saucepan or baby milk warmer. The mixture will clarify and still contain bubbles.

2 In a small bowl, mix the zinc oxide and colourings – light to dark depending on the required skin tone – with a little gelatine, until you are happy with the colour. Add this to the heated mixture. Ideally, this mixture should be made in advance to allow time for the bubbles to rise and disperse. It can be kept (cold) in a plastic bag or container and reheated when needed.

Variations

- Less gelatine makes a softer, weaker appliance.
- More gelatine makes a harder, tougher appliance.
- To make a clear gelatine for blisters, leave out the zinc oxide and colouring.

Colouring

- Always use cosmetic water-based pigments to colour the gelatine. As the appliance is to be glued directly onto a person's skin, things like food colouring can cause staining to the skin.
- Chopped hair or flock can be added to produce a vein texture.

Application of prosthetic piece

Preparing the prosthetic piece for application

Tools & equipment

- acetone
- brushes
- no-colour **face powder**
- Pros-Aide

- **Skin Illustrator palette, or prosthetic colouring, pax paint** – Pros-Aide and cosmetic-grade water-based pigments
- sponges
- witch hazel

Applying the prosthetic piece

1 Cleanse and tone the skin to remove any grease from the actor's face or body where the piece is to be applied. Apply a non-oily barrier cream to the skin. Dry and powder the skin, and remove any excess powder.

2 Position the piece on the actor's skin and powder around it to show the outline.

3 Remove the piece and put a thin layer of Pros-Aide adhesive or Telesis on the underside of the piece, in the middle. Do not apply to the edges yet.

4 Position the piece carefully in the correct place. Once secure, apply more glue under the appliance to the skin, lifting areas of the appliance as you work

outwards. A sponge or brush can be used for the adhesive. Press into place, from the inside outwards. If you fold an edge, lift it with some alcohol on a brush to reposition it.

5   Stick the edges down last, using a modelling tool or small spatula to hold up the edges to prevent them from curling or sticking together.

Alternative method for glueing appliances

1   With the appliance resting in the mould, apply a thin layer of Pros-Aide with a cotton bud over all of the back of the piece, just up to the thin edges near the flashing, but not on the flashing.

2   Allow it to dry, once the Pros-Aide is clear but still tacky, dust with powder, then brush off any excess powder.

3   Prepare the actor's skin – cleanse, tone and use a non-oily barrier cream such as Derma shield. Then dry and powder lightly. Remove any excess powder before application.

4   Place the appliance on the skin, lift half of it up and apply a little IPA to the skin all over the area where the gelatine is to be glued. Lower down the appliance and repeat on the other side.

5   Gently press down the appliance with a powder puff to remove trapped air bubbles.

6   The IPA reactivates the tacky nature of the Pros-Aide sticking the appliance down. The barrier cream will protect the skin from the IPA.

The advantage of using this method is that the glue goes only where you want it and the risk of glue spillage is removed, with no excess glue accidentally attaching the flashing to the actor's skin which would require further cleaning up.

This method can be used with encapsulated silicone but NOT with a pure silicone appliance. Pros-Aide will not stick pure silicone to the skin. If the prosthetic is only made with Plat Gel A and B silicone and no cap plastic, use Telesis or medical spirit gum to stick the appliance to the skin.

The alternative method MUST NOT be used to glue a foam latex appliance, as the IPA will cause the foam to bubble and swell.

Blending the edges of the piece

1   Use witch hazel on a brush for a gelatine appliance, to remove the flash around the piece. Use IPA for a pro bondo appliance, and acetone for an encapsulated plastic or silicone appliance.

2   Continue blending the edges very gently, as it can destroy or weaken the piece if too much product is used. Dry and powder lightly.

3   Any excess powder can be removed with slightly damp cotton wool.

4   Using an orange stipple sponge, apply Pros-Aide lightly over the appliance and over the edge onto the skin. This will seal the appliance and secure it firmly.

5   Allow the Pros-Aide to dry, and then powder with no-colour powder. Pros-Aide will go clear once dry, but will remain very sticky until powdered.

6   Any powder can be removed with slightly damp cotton wool prior to applying any make-up.

HEALTH & SAFETY

When using any form of adhesive product always ensure the actor has been patch tested prior to application.

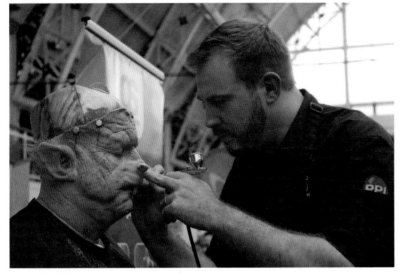

Kristyan Mallett working on his Rat Creature

Artworking the piece

Once the piece has been fixed and sealed, it is ready for colouring.

Study the surrounding skin and note the variations of colour in the actor's natural skin tone. Lessons learned from studying 'Skin Camouflage', Chapter 2, including 'Dot painting' are useful points of reference; also, 'Spatter painting' in 'Body painting', Chapter 5.

Some pieces are translucent and should not be heavily worked on. Thin layers of colour stippled in a random-looking way will help to make the prosthetic feature look realistic. The best tool to use is a sponge with uneven holes in it, and, by tearing holes in a standard wedge sponge, it is easy to stipple colour lightly in layers of different skin tones. A round, natural bristle brush is also good at splattering colour in an uneven pattern, and orange stipple sponges are also used. Some make-up artists use cotton buds: everyone has to find their own way.

There are different ways to achieve a good result. Many make-up artists apply a base coat of reddish colour before stippling skin tones on top. The redness gives the impression of blood under the skin, and this painting method is often used in painting bald caps and in camouflage work in hospitals on skin transplants, for the same reason. Another method is to apply a base colour to the gelatine piece that matches the actor's skin colour, and stipple on top of it in appropriate colours.

Airbrushing is another way of artworking the piece. This is a very useful technique for painting large prosthetics, such as masks or creatures, when the colouring is always done before application.

On small pieces there is not so much work to do, so brush and sponge methods are quick and easy.

When painting prosthetic cuts and wounds, put colour in the cut early. The bright colour will draw the eye to it, distracting attention from the edges.

Another point to remember is that the piece will appear lighter than the skin, so stippling some darker colour will help to fool the camera. Never overdo the colouring; you can't wipe it away but you can easily add more.

Tools & equipment

The following tools and materials should be used for painting pieces:

- baby oil – for removing the products
- brushes – natural bristle (small and large)
- cotton buds
- Pro Clean – for removing the products
- Reel Creations

- Skin Illustrator
- sponges – orange stipple, white wedges with holes torn unevenly
- Sta Color palette – activated with 99 per cent alcohol. Also in liquid form for airbrushing
- Veil camouflage palette

Removing the prosthetic piece

1 Apply cleanser liberally over the edges of the piece. This will start to break down the products and make it easier to remove the piece.

2 Use a small brush dipped in Pro Clean or baby oil to remove the prosthetic piece. Apply the oil to the edges, lift with one hand as you continue loosening it with the brush in your other hand.

3 Once the appliance has been released, use more Pro Clean oil to remove any remaining adhesive from the actor's skin, very gently.

4 Remove make-up in the normal way.

The need for care

Great care should be taken when removing prosthetics. Your understanding of the types of adhesives must include knowledge of the products used to remove them. As more products become available in the field of make-up there is greater choice – but also increased responsibility. Some adhesives are not suitable for use around the eyes, but can be used safely on the chin or nose. This is not because of danger from the adhesive, which should always be safe for use on the skin, but because of danger from the product used to remove the adhesive.

Allowing time

In cases where there are large prosthetics you need to allow as much time to remove them as to apply them. Actors must not be allowed to tear pieces off, as they will damage their skin. Patience and understanding are essential in a make-up artist's job, but are absolutely vital when applying and removing prosthetics.

CASE PROFILE: ANDY DEUBERT, PROSTHETICS MAKE-UP DESIGNER

How long have you been working in the industry?

I was still at college when I got my first job, so that would be nearly 30 years ago.

How did you get into the industry?

An actor who had starred in my diploma movie had a contact in London, which I followed up. By coincidence, there was a director in the building who was looking for a prosthetics make-up artist. I said yes, even though I only knew basic stuff learnt from books. You just need to throw yourself in at the deep end when starting out.

It was a quick learning curve, with many mistakes made along the way, but they were very pleased with the final make-up. The job was an advertisement for Hamlet cigars, and went on to win the Rose Award for best commercial of the year. This was my first lucky break.

Then followed several years of working coast to coast learning how to make foam latex and mechanical and special effects skills. My next break came when I joined the BBC Visual Effects Department, and worked on *Red Dwarf*. I was responsible for sculpting, mould making and fabricating all the foam appliances for the first two series for the character Kryton. Working in the industry can be tough, with very long hours, but the reward of seeing your work on show, sometimes with a credit, more than makes up for it.

How has the industry changed during your career?

A lot has changed over the years with the development of new and improved materials and digital technology. However, the skills required remain very much the same. You still need the patience and talent to work for long periods of time, especially in films, producing hundreds of pieces, some of which may never be seen, and able to use your initiative when something is a rushed job. A knowledge of the latest materials available is invaluable. New silicones are now available for HD natural make-ups and new and improved plastics make the moulds much better and lighter.

CGI [computer-generated imagery] hasn't affected prosthetics work as much as everyone thought, when it first came into practice. Directors and actors would still prefer interaction in front of the camera – it is only when it is physically impossible to achieve the required results that they turn to CGI, or if something needs enhancing.

Gollum from *Lord of the Rings* would have been impossible to create in real life, but they still had the actor Andy Serkis playing him on set and then they replaced him later with CGI. CGI is now used as another tool in the director's kit and opens up the possibility that anything can be done; it is just about the talent of using real physical special effects and CGI together.

What advice would you give to a new make-up artist starting out?

You should work on student films, where everything is done cheaply and you can hone your skills. Never say 'no' or 'can't', say 'I will see what I can do'. Don't specialise to start with, take on anything you can. PRACTICE. Even when you are not working, practice the skills you have learnt – sculpt faces, heads, monsters, and build up a good collection and variety of photos. Finally, contact all the companies and people you would like to work with.

Sectional lifecasting

When making an appliance to fit a specific part of an actor – often the nose – instead of taking an impression of the whole face, many make-up artists like to **sectional lifecast** just the feature itself, because it is quicker and less expensive than casting the entire face.

Taking a cast of the nose

1 About half of the eye socket and cheeks should be covered, as well as the nose, to allow sufficient room for good edges on the final positive.

2 The eyebrows, eyelashes and any facial hair such as moustaches should be coated with Vaseline for protection and to allow ease of separation. The nostrils can be plugged with cotton wool, coated in Vaseline, and the actor can breathe through the mouth.

3 The alginate and plaster bandage are applied in the same way as for a face cast, using smaller quantities of plaster. Allow a few minutes for the plaster bandage to harden before removing the cast from the face. Make sure that the actor's skin is restored to normal.

4 When the cast (negative) has been removed from the face, it can then be filled with plaster. Pour in the freshly mixed plaster (dental stone – Crystacal D or R) and leave it to set.

5 When the plaster has hardened, remove the new plaster cast (positive) from the mould. Correct any minor defects, trim and smooth the surfaces.

Tools & equipment

◆ alginate
◆ cotton wool
◆ dental stone – plaster
◆ plaster bandage
◆ Vaseline

Making a block mould for a nose

For sectional mould making it's better if the final mould has either a square or round shape when finished. Any walling up can be made of clay, metal, lead or damp-proof plastic.

Making the positive mould

1 Take the lifecasted section, and wall up to produce a nice shape. Then mould it by using either alginate or silicone, reinforced with plaster bandage.

2 Once taken off, build a wall around it to contain the mould material and fill with mould material of choice.

3 When the mould is hard, remove the walls. Smooth out any lumps by sanding or scraping, using wet-n-dry sandpaper in water to smooth away any rough features.

4 Cut two or three keys into the mould, away from any area you wish to sculpt on. Keys are small sloping round holes that will allow the finished mould to fit together correctly.

Sculpting the prosthetic nose

1 Sculpt the appliance, using wax or Plastilene on top of the positive mould. Blend the edges down and away from the feature so that the edges will be thin.

2 Detail using the wire brush, talc and plastic sheet.

3 Wall up with clay an overspill or trench around the sculpture, about 6–12 mm thick and 3–4 mm from the edge of the sculpture. This creates an overflow. This overflow or trench is called the flashing.

Making the negative mould This stage consists of building the other half of the mould.

1 Build a box wall of clay around your mould. The wall should be high enough to reach 20 mm above the feature. This is to contain the mould material when making the negative.

2 Using a sponge or brush, blend the outer edge of the walls to seal the edges and to make the walls watertight.

3 Apply spray wax and mix your mould material of choice. Pour it slowly around the modelled piece (not onto it). Keep pouring until the piece is covered and the box mould filled. **DO NOT FORGET TO APPLY A RELEASE AGENT BEFORE YOU DO THIS**. Tap the workbench to bring any air bubbles to the surface. Leave the negative to set in its box.

4 When the mould has set, remove the walls and trim the mould.

5 Leave for two hours, then gently prise the mould apart with a large screwdriver or chisel.

Cleaning the mould

Remove any clay and clean off any remaining wax with white spirit. Wash the mould in warm water using a soft brush in all the cavities. Leave it to dry overnight, when it will be ready to fill with the chosen material.

This mould can be used with all materials except Bondo, to produce your appliance.

Tools & equipment

◆ moulding material
◆ screwdriver or chisel
◆ sponge or brush
◆ spray wax

Filling the mould with your choice of prosthetics material

1 Seal the mould with Vaseline or spray wax.

2 Fill the mould with your choice of product.

3 Close the mould and leave for two hours to set.

Opening the mould

Gently separate the parts of the mould and remove the gelatine piece from the positive mould. First powder it and use a modelling tool to lift it. Then powder it further to stop the edges rolling over as you peel the prosthetic out of the negative mould.

Storing gelatine pieces

Gelatine is good to work with because it is reusable. If the piece is not successful you can melt it and try again. Keep all gelatine pieces in an airtight plastic bag.

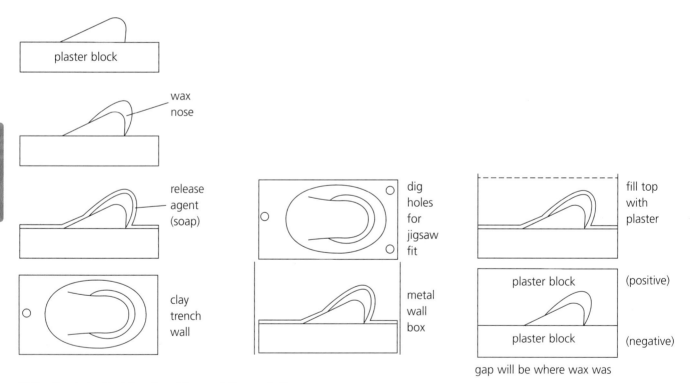

Making the plaster block for a foam latex or gelatine prosthetic nose

Preparing for application, applying the piece, blending the edges, artworking, removal and the need for care can be referred to in the section on flat plate moulds.

Lifecasting and making a larger prosthetic mould and appliance

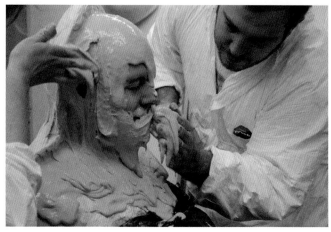

Kristyan Mallett applying alginate for a lifecast

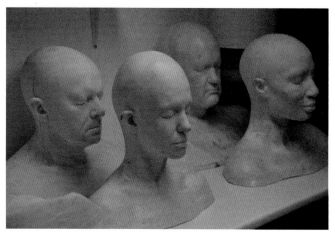

Lifecasts

Caring for the actor

Many people – not just actors – are nervous about having their faces covered in product in order to make a lifecast. Students should practise on one another to understand what it feels like. When lifecasting in film studios it is usual to have the unit nurse present during the procedure. In the classroom there should always be someone at hand with knowledge of first aid methods in case of emergencies. For actors, lifecasting sessions are similar to visiting a dentist. The procedure is out of their control, leaving them vulnerable and helpless. Time must be taken to explain how they will breathe under the cast. Care should be shown in discussing the actor's anxieties before the casting session. It must be made clear that at any time, for whatever reason, the lifecast will be removed immediately if they simply raise an arm in a prearranged signal. The sympathetic, calm manner required by make-up artists in all their work is of prime importance when lifecasting.

Lifecasting application

All tools and materials must be laid out in preparation before the appointed time. The equipment should be neatly arranged and ready-to-hand. Measure the required amount of alginate powder or lifecasting silicone into a bowl. Make sure there are enough strips of plaster bandage in different lengths. You will need enough to cover the face with spare pieces available.

Tools & equipment

- assistants to help with the lifecast and actor
- brushes, soft
- electric mixer
- impression material – either alginate or lifecasting silicone
- mixing bowls
- permanent marker
- petroleum jelly or silicone grease – to cover facial hair, including eyebrows and eyelashes

- plaster bandage – pre-cut in 150 mm and 300 mm strips
- plaster for the positive cast
- scissors
- spatulas and dental tool to prise open the casts
- timer
- tissues and cotton wool

◆ towels, soap, astringent, mild moisturiser
◆ water and cups for measuring
◆ 1 bald cap
◆ 1 large plastic cape

Preparing the actor

1 Seat the actor comfortably and wrap the plastic cape around their shoulders, securing it at the back of the neck. The actor should wear comfortable clothing. Roll neck sweaters are not suitable, as plaster may drip onto the neck.

2 Position the bald cap over the head to protect the hair, making sure that it covers the hairline.

3 Apply petroleum jelly (Vaseline) or cosmetic grade silicone grease to the eyebrows and eyelashes with a thin coating. Do the same with any other facial hair (moustache, beard or sideburns). Alternatively, you could use wax, and then grease on top of the wax to prevent the alginate sticking to it.

Talk to the actor while preparing them for the lifecasting. Make it clear that if they signal you to remove the alginate from their face, you will remove it from the nose, mouth and eyes – in that order. This should help to relieve the claustrophobic sensation they may be feeling. Explain that the alginate will feel very cold at first but will warm up later.

Applying the impression material

Whilst the impression material is being applied, the actor should remain as still as possible and in an upright position in the chair. The face must not be tilted in any direction, either up or down, or from side to side, or the impression will not be accurate.

1 Having prepared the actor, start mixing the alginate by adding cold water to the powder. Using an electric mixer, stir from side-to-side to avoid trapping air in the mix.

2 When the mixture is a creamy paste, apply it to the face. Apply the material with a wooden tool around the nostrils. Then, using your hands, apply the material to the forehead, gently over the eyes and down the face. **Keep the actor's nostrils clear**. If there is a blockage, ask them to expel air sharply through the nose to clear it. Always have a wooden tool standing by to remove any material from around the nostrils too. Use a timer as a guide to how long you have. Gently apply the material to the mouth area. Finally, cover the remaining section over the top of the nose, taking care that the material does not drip over the nostril holes. As the material starts to firm up, smooth down any lumps. Only go on to the next stage, once you are happy the material has set, and will no longer run down over the nose.

3 Try and keep the work area calm, constantly reassure them that everything is fine, and talk to them clearly, explaining every stage as you work. Some calming music playing can often help.

4 Reinforce the material with a plaster bandage. When the material has been smoothly applied, dip the strips of pre-cut plaster bandages into water. Squeeze out excess water before applying the plaster bandage to the impression material. For extra support, a layer of rough hemp can be placed over the wet material before applying the bandage. This is not necessary if you use plenty of plaster bandage.

5 You can now begin placing strips of plaster bandage over the lifecast. Keep inside the edge of the material. Plaster bandage should not directly touch the skin as the alkali in the plaster can cause irritation.

TOP TIP

When casting always make sure that only the required people are present. Any unnecessary noise may distract or stress the person being lifecast.

6   Having covered the face with a layer of the bandage all over the material, you may add extra strips across the face and around the outside of the bandaged area to provide additional support when removing the cast. Keep an eye on the actor, talking reassuringly and watching for the agreed hand signal.

7   When you think the plaster bandages have set (about ten minutes), run your fingers around the edge to make sure the plaster has hardened.

Removing the lifecast

Ask the actor to wriggle their face gently under the lifecast to loosen the impression material. They should lean forward, holding the cast in their hands. As they move their facial muscles, the cast will loosen and fall into their hands.

Alternatively, you can lift the edges of the lifecast, making sure you are lifting the impression material – not just the plaster bandage – and work the lifecast loose.

STEP-BY-STEP: LIFECAST APPLICATION

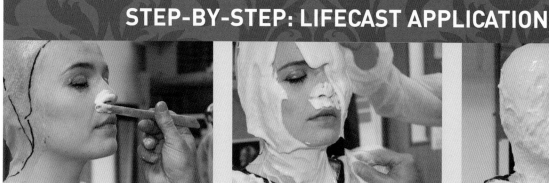

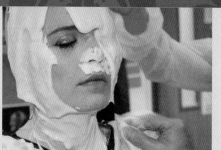

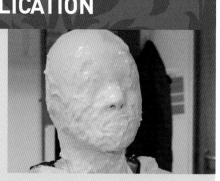

1 Prepare the actor with bald cap and apply Vaseline.

2 Apply alginate.

3 Cover entire face with alginate.

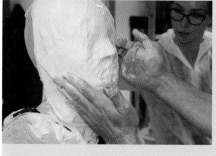

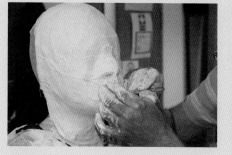

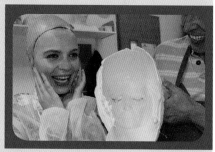

4 Apply plaster bandage.

5 Cover entire face with plaster bandage.

6 Remove the lifecast.

Taking care of the actor and the lifecast

As soon as the lifecast has been removed, the actor's face must be restored to normal. Ask your helper to:

1   Remove any pieces of plaster and impression material from the face with damp cotton wool. The actor can now wash their face with warm water and soap.

2   After drying the face with a clean towel, an astringent may be used to close the skin pores, and then a mild moisturiser gently applied.

Meanwhile, take care of the cast:

1 Cover the outside nose holes with plaster bandage so that the liquid plaster you will use does not leak. Then fill any air bubbles inside with water-based clay.

2 Position the cast gently on a board supported with clay, ensuring that the nose does not get damaged. The outside of the cast, where the nose is, should not touch the table. The weight of the plaster will push the cast down, distorting the nose shape.

3 Mix up your plaster. Half fill a bowl with cold water and sprinkle your plaster over the water. The bowl will almost be full by the time you are ready to mix. When you think you have enough powder in the mix, with one hand, start to stir the mixture. If you need to add more plaster powder, use your other dry hand to add the powder. Then use both hands to mix the plaster, working it through your fingers. When you have a smooth mixture with no lumps, gently pour it into the lifecast. Always pour slowly from a height into the forehead area of the mould first, so that the plaster gently runs down into the nose and fills the mould. Whilst you are pouring, ask an assistant to vibrate the board it is on, to bring any air bubbles to the surface.

4 The cast can now be left to set. With plaster, it first goes hard, then it heats up. Once the plaster has cooled, it is then hard and can be removed.

5 Remove the plaster bandage and impression material.

6 Remove any unwanted lumps of plaster with metal tools. A surf form scraper is good for rounding any outside edges. Then use wet & dry sandpaper with lots of water to finish off. Take care not to damage the detailed parts of the face, you want to leave all the skin texture and details intact.

7 Put the cast somewhere safe.

8 It's also a good idea to take pictures of the actor, to use later, as well as any measurements you need, along with a record of their skin colouring. This will help you in the sculpting stage and the colouring of the final prosthetic appliance.

ACTIVITY

Lifecast project

Plan and design a character that would be used for a lifecast. Your plan should include:

◆ The design of the lifecast.

◆ How to make the lifecast

◆ How to apply the lifecast.

◆ Safe removal of the lifecast.

Include a mood board to show your research with photographs and step-by-step procedures.

Making a positive mould

Never use the original lifecast to make your final mould unless you need it urgently. Always make a copy of the lifecast to make your positive mould.

1 Wall up around the lifecast with clay to produce the desired mould shape.

2 Apply spray wax. If making a positive mould in a form of plaster, use alginate. If making a positive mould in a form of polyester resin or other plastic type of material, use silicone instead as these are affected by the moisture in the alginate and won't set.

3 Cover the desired area in alginate or silicone quite thickly and reinforce heavily with plaster bandage.

4 Take apart and fill with the mould material of choice. Crystacal lamina and fibreglass are recommended because they are safe to use and do not give off toxic fumes. This mould works perfectly well and can be used to produce gelatine, foam and silicone casts – plain and encapsulated.

5 Pour layers of gel coat (thick Crystacal lamina) into the mould. Using a brush, paint the plaster up the sides to form a thick coating.

6 Allow each layer to just dry before adding the next. Reinforce the cast with four layers of fibreglass everywhere and an extra two around the top.

7 It is also useful to fix a wooden handle inside the cast at the back, to use later.

8 Once dry, which takes at least an hour, remove from the alginate, sand the edges, pick off any lumps and using P180 wet and dry sandpaper smooth over the surface of the whole positive mould. The finished mould should have a smooth glassy feel all over. Do not worry if you sand away all the skin texture, you just need a very smooth mould all over

Sculpting the new feature

However skilfully cast, and whatever material it is made from, the piece will only be as good as the shape you create in clay. Sculpting is an art and professional workshops employ people who specialise in sculpting. Whatever your concept, the skill of modelling and sculpting the new feature requires practice.

There are many types of clay and many people prefer Plastilene which is a non-drying, oil-based clay. Types easily obtained are Roma Plastilene and Chavant clay from specialist suppliers. If you use normal clay, it must be kept wet whilst you are working and covered in plastic to keep it moist overnight. Work out your design in advance with sketches or photographs.

Tools & equipment

- bowl of water
- clay or Plastilene
- rough towel, coarse stipple sponge
- sketch or photograph – of the required shape
- spray bottle with water
- various modelling tools – in wood or metal

HEALTH & SAFETY

Be aware that fibreglass dust can be produced when sanding.

HEALTH & SAFETY

Take appropriate health and safety precautions – gloves and goggle masks should be worn when making a mould.

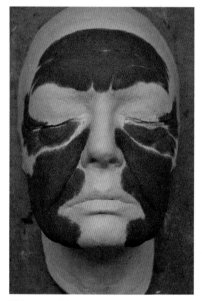

Old age sculpt

Modelling the feature

1 When sculpting, especially if you are not very experienced, it is sometimes a good idea to make a practice sculpture in water-based clay first. Wet clay is much easier and quicker to work with. You can play around with your design and make any changes faster than if you were using wax-based clay.

2 Place the original plaster face cast on a work surface, standing upright against a stand, supported underneath by some lumps of wet clay to hold it in position. It is a good idea to place any artwork designs or reference pictures that you want to use nearby, also fixed vertically next to the plaster face. This makes is easier to

study them whilst you are sculpting. By having the lifecast and reference pictures upright, you can work in a more comfortable position, and you won't find yourself bending over whilst working.

3 Place a small amount of wet clay onto the part of the face that you wish to change. When you have the shape that you want, begin to put in the details. When using wet clay, keep it damp by spraying it with water; clay that is too hard does not produce good results. Remember to sculpt very thin edges, using tools and a wet sponge, smooth away the base of the feature until it blends into the surrounding area of the face cast. Just remember, the more clay you put on, the heavier the final prosthetic will be. So try to use as little clay as possible and keep the sculpture as thin as possible, whilst creating the desired effect.

4 If you need to have a break, sometimes it's a good idea to walk away from your sculpture for a while, or you need to leave a water-based sculpture for any length of time, always spray your sculpture with water and wrap it up well with cling film. Leave the sculpture and lifecast flat down on a table, so that they do not fall over while you are away.

5 When you come back, check your sculpture and make any changes you want to perfect the design. If you are happy with it, you are now ready to begin sculpting the final sculpture in wax on the positive fibreglass mould.

6 Using the practice sculpture as a guide, begin the final sculpture in wax clay on your fibreglass positive mould. You can take measurements from the wet clay sculpture to help you reproduce the same design in the wax. Texture can be added to the wax by gently scratching with a wire brush. Powder with talc, brush off any excess powder and scratch again. Continue doing this, using less pressure each time, until you get the desired effect. A brush can also be used to soften the texture, if you consider it too rough. Try to imitate the texture of the surrounding skin area to which the piece will be applied. Final details can be added by gently pressing through a piece of clear plastic using a small tool or toothpick. You can use this technique to add pores and any fine wrinkles. Finally check that all the edges around the sculpture, where the wax meets the mould, feather down to a very thin layer, and that you don't have any thick ridges. Remember the final prosthetic will need to blend seamlessly onto the person's face, so if you leave any thick edges at this stage they will show as bad joins on the final make-up.

7 At this stage, if you are happy with the wax sculpture, clean off the water-based clay from the original plaster cast and check that the texture of your wax sculpture matches the texture of the person you will be applying to, and make any adjustments accordingly.

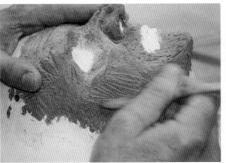
Sculpting in clay.

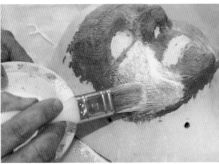
Powdering the sculpt.

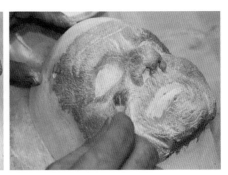
Refining the sculpt.

Casting the mould

Making the negative mould

1 Drill small holes around the sculpt. This is for the bolts that you will use later to hold your moulds together. The holes should be about 3 cm away from the edge of the sculpture and equally spaced about 10 cm apart all the way around.

2 Walling up. Without touching the edge of the sculpture, cover all parts of the mould that remain with thick clay about 1 cm thick. Leave 3–4 mm of mould showing around the sculpt, the clay here can also be a bit thinner and taper down at a slight angle to the mould surface. This will produce the flashing and give you very fine edges on the final prosthetic appliance. Keep the areas around the bolt holes also free of clay, but remember to fill just the small holes with a little wax to prevent any resin or Crystacal filling them up later. It is important that the clay walling up is finished to a very neat and smooth finish, if not, the inside of your final mould will be very rough, making removal of any prosthetic appliance difficult.

3 Spray several light coats of wax all over the sculpt, mould and the walling up.

4 Brush and pour on two–three thick coats of resin or Crystacal lamina, taking care that you apply the coats in a way that fills in all the details of the sculpt and does not damage the texture. Make sure you cover all the bolt holes and the walling up. The thicker the coats, the stronger the mould will be. Take care if you are using polyester resin. If you apply this too thickly it can overheat while setting, which causes cracking and warping. Build up several thin coats instead. Once almost dry, reinforce with four layers of fibreglass, with an extra two layers around the bottom where the drill holes will be.

5 Depending on the moulding material used, wait for it to set properly before opening your mould. Once dry, from the inside drill 6 mm holes for bolts all the way through, then sand down any sharp edges.

6 Before separating, remove all the clay that you can from the walling-up process, as this is binding your mould together. Using a chisel or large screwdriver, gently ease your mould apart. Using wooden tools only, metal might damage your mould, remove all clay from both parts of the finished mould. White spirit and a stiff brush can be used to clean the wax clay off the moulds. Be careful of the fumes – wear a mask or goggles. They can then be washed thoroughly in warm soapy water to remove any remaining chemicals and dried with a clean towel.

7 The moulds should be bolted tightly together and dried well overnight in a warm oven at about 100 degrees centigrade or gas mark 1. This removes any remaining chemicals left inside the mould and improves the quality of the thin edges around the final prosthetic appliance.

8 Once dry, the mould is ready to be filled with your material of choice. This mould can be filled with any material, from gelatine to silicone, foam latex and even encapsulated silicone.

Tools & equipment

- brush
- clay or Plastilene
- file for smoothing new feature
- mould-making material of choice
- spray wax

TOP TIP

Do not forget to use spray wax before you mould your sculpture or your final mould may never come apart.

HEALTH & SAFETY

Remember, if you have been using fibreglass, the dust produced from sanding your mould is toxic if inhaled, and can cause skin irritation. TAKE ALL NECESSARY PRECAUTIONS.

Making the prosthetic piece

The prosthetic piece can be made out of plastic, latex, silicone or gelatine.

There are three latex techniques: painting, slush or foam. The foam latex method will be explained at the end of the chapter.

The painting method

The new feature can be made by painting the inside of the mould with successive layers of liquid latex. Before starting, the latex can be coloured with acrylic paints to give it a flesh tone or other effect. When the latex is dry it will darken in colour.

1 Pour a little latex into the mould and use a brush to paint it evenly into every crevice.

2 Paint the next layer beyond the edge of the piece.

3 Apply about 15 layers, so that the piece will hold its shape. Concentrate the most latex on the middle part of the piece, so that the edges are thin.

4 Leave the casting for six hours, during which time it will become darker in colour.

5 Brushes should be cleaned in pure washing-up liquid to remove any remaining latex, before washing with water.

Tools & equipment

- brushes
- latex
- water-based colouring pigments

The slush method

The slush method uses latex, but without painting it in layers.

1 Pour the latex into the mould and sluice it around, tilting it gently so that the latex runs into the required places.

2 Build up thickness in the middle, but leave the edges thin.

3 Leave the cast overnight to dry.

Colouring the latex

The liquid latex is milky white and can be coloured by adding water-based paints to give it a flesh tone or other effect. Always mix your colour first in a small pot, before adding it to the latex. Because the latex is white, the mix will appear to be much lighter. However, as the latex dries, it will go clearer returning to the original colour you mixed.

Using plastic   This method uses liquid bald cap plastic by painting layers into the mould. The positive mould is not used.

1 Spread a layer of Vaseline inside the mould using a brush, or use spray wax, to provide a release agent. If you forget, depending on the mould material used, the cap plastic may soak into the mould, making it impossible to remove and damaging your mould.

2 Paint in layers of plastic, allowing each layer to dry before painting the next one. The transparent liquid plastic can be coloured by adding an oil-based colouring pigment and flock to create a skin tone or whatever is required.

3 As with the latex feature, more layers should be concentrated in the middle part of the mould, and the edges left thin.

Tools & equipment

- brushes
- liquid bald cap plastic
- oil-based colouring pigments
- Vaseline or spray wax

4 Take care with any fumes produced when working with cap plastic; appropriate protection should be used and work done in a well-ventilated room.

5 Brushes should be cleaned in acetone only, **never** soapy water.

Removing the prosthetic piece from the mould

1 Use talcum powder and a soft brush to lift and peel the edges carefully, powdering with the brush as you go. This stops the material from sticking to itself as you remove it from the mould.

2 When the piece is out of the mould, powder it inside and out. This is to remove any grease from the Vaseline if the prosthetic is plastic. Keep the prosthetic piece on the positive mould to retain its shape until you are ready to use it. Wash and dry the mould thoroughly first.

Caring for the mould

The mould should be washed in soap and water and allowed to dry naturally. You can make as many pieces as you like from the mould, and it will probably be necessary to produce several before you get a good result.

Don't be disappointed if your prosthetic pieces are not as good as expected. This happens a lot at first and will get better with practice.

The face cast can be used for experiments in making all sorts of pieces: eyebags and jowls for ageing, a forehead for monster make-up, a clown's nose, a witch's nose and chin – the possibilities are endless. Each piece must be modelled in clay, and a mould made of each feature. However, if you have used Vaseline or spray wax, the mould should be thoroughly cleaned with soapy water before it can be used with any latex products.

CASE PROFILE: ADRIAN RIGBY, PROSTHETICS MAKE-UP ARTIST

How long have you been working in the industry?

Eighteen years or thereabouts.

How did you get into the industry?

After leaving college in the north-west of England, I struggled to find consistent work there. I did manage to do some bridal, photographic and a couple of low-budget films but nothing really to make a proper living. I knew the bulk of any industry work would be in the south of England. I contacted Nick Dudman, who happened to live fairly close by in the north-west of England and got to show him my basic portfolio in 1999. Then, in early 2001, he invited me to participate on a four-day prosthetics course at his workshop in Kendal, Cumbria. On the last day of the course, he quickly browsed my portfolio again. Little had changed, but based on that, and my work on his course, he offered me a job on the upcoming film *Harry*

Potter & the Chamber of Secrets. With just his word and nothing in writing, I waited five months and moved south. The rest as they say is history …

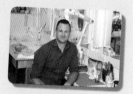

What has been your most significant project(s)?

I always consider myself very lucky to be working and have worked on some great films and television shows but I have to say working on six out of eight of the Harry Potter films has to be the highlight, so far, of my career.

What do you enjoy most about the job?

I love the creativity it allows. Playing a part, no matter how great or small, in helping the actor to become the character they are playing. And working with like-minded people: people that are working from the same page.

the Royal Mail, before embarking on my career as a make-up artist, I was quite used to early morning alarm calls.

What do you enjoy least about the job?

I guess the most common answer to this, and what most people would say, is the early starts and long days. But as I worked for

What advice would you give to a new make-up artist starting out?

Find a way of standing out. I learnt early on that jobs don't come to you. You have to get out there and be proactive.

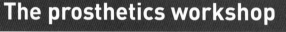

The prosthetics workshop

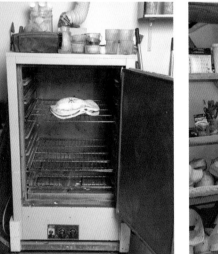

Prosthetics oven

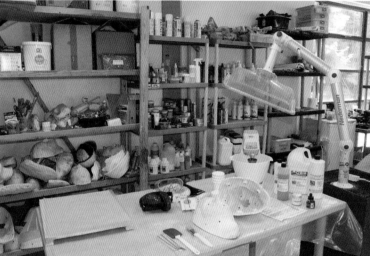

Prosthetics room

The workshop is equipped with an electric food mixer and bowl, weighing scales, a drill and a prosthetics oven for curing the moulds.

An individual mask should be worn. Inhaling plaster dust is also bad for the health, so most of the work in the room should be done wearing a surgical or dentist's mask. For large effects using full heads and bodies, catering mixers and ovens are used.

The temperature and humidity of the workroom affects the foaming process: higher temperatures cause faster setting, lower temperatures make it slower. It is not practical to attempt foaming operations at below 15°C.

Health and safety

The foam latex technician works with highly toxic ingredients. **WARNING: It is dangerous to inhale the products.** To minimise the risks of accidents, follow these rules:

1   Keep all chemicals out of reach of children.

2   Read the instructions before starting and follow the safety rules.

3   Wear safety goggles and gloves.

4   Wash any chemicals from the skin immediately with soap and water.

5   Keep eyewash solution and an eyebath to hand.

HEALTH & SAFETY

You cannot use an oven at home because of the toxic vapours given off during the curing, which would contaminate the oven.

HEALTH & SAFETY

Always check your work area prior to starting. Ensure there is nothing on the floor that could cause a trip hazard. Always clean any spillages immediately to prevent slips.

6   The workshop must be kept clean. The worktops and machinery should be washed down after use.

7   There should be adequate ventilation with extractor fans to get rid of ammonia vapours.

8   Always wash your hands before and after working with foam latex.

9   Read the instruction sheets included with the products, and the labels on the bottles.

10 Never eat or drink in the foam lab or workshop as they will become contaminated.

Foam latex

The advances in technology have affected the prosthetics labs and workshops more than any other area of make-up artistry. To appreciate the time and effort involved, and to progress in this area, students should gain work experience in a professional workshop. The specialist makers of prosthetics are part chemist, part artist and tend to specialise in a particular area such as designing, sculpting, mould making, foam runs, knotting hair and artworking.

A complicated ageing sequence or character change, as it is eventually seen in a film, may have used many prosthetic pieces, and relied on the work of an entire crew of talented people.

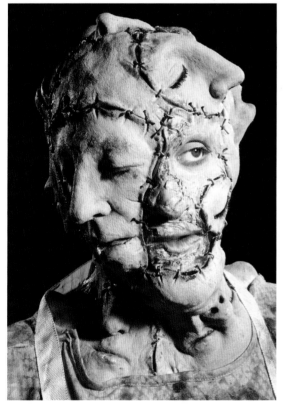

Multi-face foam latex prosthetics project by Lisa Cartlidge – front

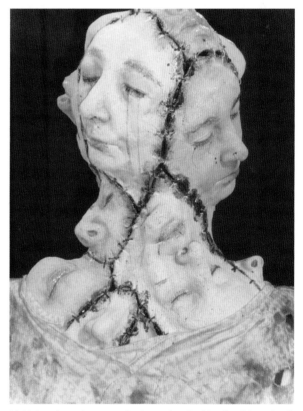

Multi-face foam latex prosthetics project by Lisa Cartlidge – back

Commissioning foam latex pieces

Large prosthetic pieces are often made out of foam latex as this is the lightest material.

Most make-up artists will commission a company to make the prosthetics for the production. In these circumstances the designer will accompany the actor to the workshop for a lifecasting session and discussion about the design requirements. Several visits may be necessary to check on the quality and fit of the piece or pieces on the actor. Here are some aspects to look out for:

1 Make sure that the piece fits exactly when the actor's face is mobile.

2 Check that the edges of the piece are so fine and thin that they blend into the surrounding skin.

3 Check that there are no large air bubbles in the piece.

Don't be afraid to put forward your own ideas to the specialist; you have the visual image in mind as seen by the director. You will be the one applying the prosthetics in the studio and by that time it will be too late to correct any faults. When the foam pieces arrive from the workshop they should have been washed in soap and water to remove chemical smells. The number of duplicate pieces will be whatever you have ordered. With foam latex you need a new piece every day on the shoot.

Foam latex has been used for many years to make prosthetic pieces. There are different companies supplying foam systems, and they all come with precise instructions on their use – with health and safety regulations. Foam latex remains popular because the end result produces light, flexible pieces that stick well to the skin. If the television or film budget can afford the cost it is best to contract the work out to a company, since it cannot be done at home or in the studio. It must be in a controlled workshop environment. Toxic vapours are given off during the curing process, so safety procedures have to be observed – ventilation, safety goggles, gloves and strict cleaning rules. Many make-up artists have no leaning towards this type of work, but they all have to understand the process of how foam pieces are made. After that it is up to the make-up artist to have the skills in artworking and applying the pieces to the actor.

Foam latex ingredients

◆ **Latex base** A high-quality, chemically thickened latex, sterilised with ammonia.

◆ **Foam agent** An emulsion of soaps: when whisked with the latex base, these produce foam.

◆ **Cure agent** A mixture of sulphur and other chemicals that vulcanises the foam latex when it is cured in the oven.

◆ **Gel agent** An acid that turns the latex from a liquid to a semi-solid: it coagulates the foam, preventing it from breaking down.

◆ **Soap release** The release agent which is painted onto the moulds before filling them with foam latex. This makes sure that the foam can be removed easily, without sticking, after the casting has come out of the oven.

HEALTH & SAFETY

Before it has been cured, gel agent is highly toxic.

Filling the moulds and curing the latex

Tools & equipment

- ◆ accurate weighing scales
- ◆ cure agent – 17 g
- ◆ electric oven – to bake the moulds
- ◆ foam agent – 30–45 g
- ◆ gel agent – 4–10 g

- ◆ latex base – 150 g
- ◆ mixer with a large bowl
- ◆ moulds – for filling
- ◆ plastic cups – for measuring the ingredients

- ◆ soap release
- ◆ soft brush – to apply the soap release
- ◆ spatula
- ◆ stopwatch – to time the foam run

Preparation

1   Apply soap release to the plaster moulds and allow to dry.

2   Weigh out the ingredients in plastic cups.

Mixing

1   Add the latex base, foam agent and cure agent to the mixing bowl.

2   The mixing times vary with the different manufacturers of foam latex, and you will need to play around to achieve the desired result. The following times are used as a guide only.

3   Turn on the mixer at high speed for 3–6 minutes, depending on the rise wanted: the greater the rise (volume) the softer the foam.

4   Turn down the mixer to medium speed, to refine the foam and break down the bubbles, for four minutes.

5   Turn the mixer down to a slow speed to refine even more, for a minimum of four minutes.

6   Add the gel agent slowly and mix it into the foam. Mix the two together for at least one minute. It is also possible to add water-based colour at this stage.

7   Stop the mixer and fill the moulds carefully. Make sure that no air is trapped under the foam.

8   Close the moulds together.

9   Leave the foam until it gels. To test for gelling, press the overspill of foam at the side of the mould.

Curing

1   Place the foam-filled moulds into a pre-heated oven at 100°C. Bake them for two to four hours, depending on the size of mould and materials used, until the foam inside the moulds has cured.

2   Remove the moulds from the oven, and let them cool before opening them. Test the texture of the foam with a spatula. It should be springy and sponge-like. When fully cured it will spring back to its shape.

3   Wash the pieces in soapy water, then dry and powder them.

> ### TOP TIP
> Once a mould has been used for latex, it can never be used for making a silicone piece as the chemicals in latex stop the silicone from setting. Gelatine is not affected.

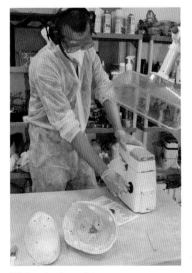
Mixing the foam latex.

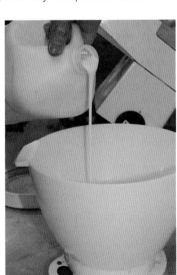
Pouring the foam into the mixer.

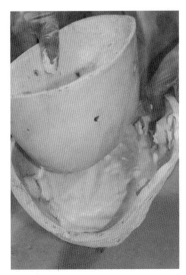
Putting the moulds together.

Keeping records

Foam lab technicians keep a log of their foam runs. This helps them compare temperatures and cooking times with the quality of the results. An accurate record provides continuity and encourages improvements in foam latex work.

As a general guide, if the foam latex gels too quickly add less gelling agent to the mix. If the foam takes too long to gel add more gelling agent

Attaching and artworking the foam pieces

Seal the foam pieces with a thin layer of duo adhesive, dry, then powder them before application. Do not apply the duo to any of the thin edges, as this could damage them; they will be sealed later during the make-up.

The foam pieces are positioned, attached and artworked in the same way as for gelatine pieces, described earlier in the chapter. Pax paints (Pros-Aide and cosmetic-grade water-based pigments) are usually applied in thin layers for a transparent appearance. Freckles and spots can be added to blend with the surrounding skin tone.

Working with silicone

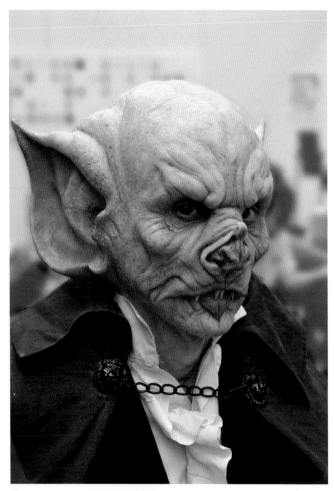

Silicone project by Kristyan Mallett

Silicone is used for HD (High Definition) character make-ups, to make realistic looking skin, as it looks and feels like it. Gelatine can also be used for this. Silicone can also be used for a translucent look.

Filling with silicone

Whether or not you are using plat gel silicone or encapsulated silicone, you must put release agent onto both parts of your mould.

1 Mix 50% IPA with 50 per cent washing-up liquid. Be aware of fumes – wear a mask or safety goggles.

2 Spray several coats onto both parts of the mould. Spraying guarantees you get the mixture into every area.

3 Shake or brush out any excess, then dry thoroughly.

4 When the mould has a good colour and is very dry, apply several coats of spray wax onto both parts of the mould.

As with the flat mould, you can encapsulate your silicone in cap plastic. Use for smaller appliances.

1 Spray several coats of the cap plastic into and on both moulds, including the inside side walls of the negative mould.

2   Mix your silicone with deadener to the desired softness, pour or inject into the mould, clamp tight and bolt together.

3   Allow to set.

If you are using plat gel A and B only as an encapsulant (used for larger appliances):

1   Apply a very thin layer of silicone to both moulds with a sponge, including the inside walls of your negative mould. You need to remove as much excess silicone as possible, especially where the moulds touch each other and around the edges of the sculpted area, or you will get thick edges on the final appliance.

2   Fill as above, with the plat gel silicone with the deadener in it.

To remove the silicone prosthetic, undo any clamps or remove bolts and soak the whole mould in water for at least an hour. The water will seep into the mould and dissolve the washing-up liquid, allowing you to take the mould apart. Keep the positive mould and the silicone appliance in the water. Whilst in the water, position the silicone appliance over the positive mould into its correct position. The mould can now be lifted out of the water with the appliance on, and left to dry. By keeping it in the water, the thin edges of the appliance are protected from ripping. Any excess flashing can now be trimmed, to reduce any weight on the thin edges, but do leave a little flashing, which will keep the thin edges intact. This is removed during application.

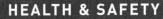

HEALTH & SAFETY

Vinyl gloves should be used when making silicone pieces.

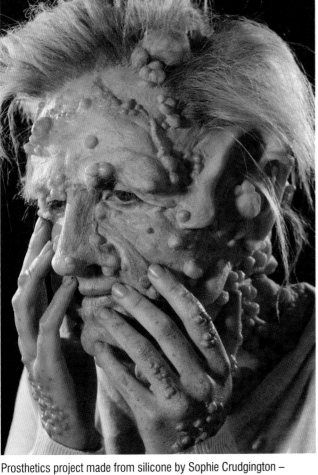

Prosthetics project made from silicone by Sophie Crudgington – front view.

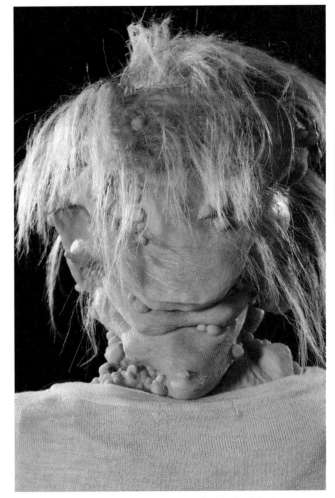

Prosthetics project made from silicone by Sophie Crudgington – back view.

Bald caps

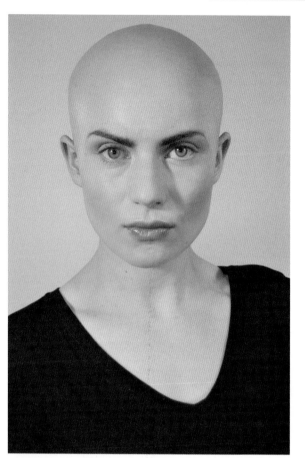

Bald cap

Tools & equipment

- clear adhesive tape
- cling film
- dressmaker's tape measure
- eye pencil
- head block – plastic red head

The purpose of a bald cap is to cover the actor's hair in order to look bald. This could be for ageing, illness, fantasy, creatures, aliens or whatever the story. They are made from plastic or latex. Most make-up artists prefer plastic since it is easy to colour and the edges can be blended with acetone to appear seamless.

Although it might be ages before you are asked for one, every make-up artist should know how to make and apply a bald cap.

Making a bald cap

Using a ready-made bald cap

1 Wrap the actor's hair in cling film.

2 Place the bald cap onto the actor. Check that it is straight and central.

3 Holding it firmly with one hand, draw a line around the hairline, at least 12 mm away from it. Go under the ear and down the back, marking the line on the head block.

4 Trim to the desired shape.

Plastic caps

Bald cap plastic comes in clear liquid form, made of PVC (polyvinyl chloride) and PVA (polyvinyl alcohol) with a plasticiser. Some of the types in use combine acetone as a solvent, with a plasticiser to give elasticity to the product. Cap plastic can be tinted with any colour using oil based colours.

The fumes of the solvents in cap plastic are very strong. The work should be carried out in a well-ventilated room, with open windows and electric fans to blow the fumes away.

The cap is made by painting layers of the plastic onto the solid head block. Unless you are using a metal block, you must first spread Vaseline on the block. Most people use plastic blocks as they are lighter. Each layer of plastic takes ten minutes to dry. Do not apply the next coat until the last one is dry.

Painting the plastic layers onto the head block

1 If there are any grooves in the centre join of the plastic head, file them down and smooth them out with Mortician's wax.

2 Prepare the head block by smearing a thin layer of Vaseline over it, and wipe lightly with a tissue. This acts as a release agent when you remove the cap from the block.

3 Paint the liquid plastic with a large brush – a small house-painting brush is good. Have to hand a jar of acetone to clean the brush after painting each layer.

NOTE: You will need about three layers all over the cap and to the edges; then a further three, with colour, in the middle. Extra layers can be applied to the back to give more strength in attaching the cap to the head.

4 Apply the first layer thinly and quickly. Be methodical and don't paint the same area twice. Work from the top to the edges, keeping it as thin as possible.

5 Leave the layer to dry. You can tell when it is dry because it will change colour. Clean your brush with the acetone.

6 Apply two more layers, each time working slightly inside the outer edges to make them fine for blending when attached to skin. Keep to your method, applying the plastic quickly using gentle strokes. Avoid air bubbles and don't allow any hairs or clogged plastic to come off the brush. While waiting for layers to dry, keep your brush in the acetone to prevent the hairs from sticking together. Dry the brush with a dry cloth before painting the next layer.

Colouring the plastic

1 For the final three layers of plastic you can add some colour – mix the plastic and colouring in a lidded jar, stirring it well to mix. You can use any oil-based colouring products. If the final effect is for a realistic-looking bald head, many make-up artists add a warm colour such as reddish brown or pink as a base for further artworking.

2 Apply the final three layers to the top and back of the head shape. Each layer should finish slightly further from the edge of the previous one, as with the earlier applications.

3 To reinforce the back, apply further layers or place very fine hair lace between the layers of plastic. Leave a small amount of lace free of the edge of the cap. This is what you will use to stick the cap to the skin. Not everyone uses lace, and you will need to find your own method for successful results.

4 When this third or final layer of plastic has been applied, leave the cap to dry overnight.

Taking the bald cap off the block

1 Brush the edges of the plastic with talcum powder. Without tearing the plastic, slip a t-pin or modelling tool between the cap and the block. Gently release the edge all the way around the edge of the cap, powdering the inside as you go.

2 Ease the cap free a little further in, again using the t-pin (pressing down onto the block), and then powder.

3 Once you have enough to hold securely, pull the cap from back to front, to re-move from the block.

4 When the cap is free, powder it inside and out. Clean the block by rubbing it with surgical spirit, and when dry place the cap, inside out, on the block until needed. For long-time storage, keep in a sealed plastic bag.

TOP TIP

The outside of a bald cap is shiny, the inside is matte.

Rubber bald caps

Latex or rubber bald caps are sometimes used if the actor has to move a lot, or for a stunt double. Latex stretches and goes back to its original shape better than plastic. But it is harder to hide the edges: they cannot be safely blended as plastic ones can, so are not as popular.

When making latex rubber caps the head block is stippled with a sponge, and not painted with a brush. After they have been fitted and glued to the actor, the edges are blended with duo adhesive or Bondo, which is cabosil (silica) mixed with Pros-Aide to form a thick paste.

To test a latex bald cap, stretch it out with both hands. On release it should return to its original shape quickly.

Refronting a plastic cap

Old caps can often be reused by putting a new edge around the hairline. This process is called 'refronting'.

1 Put a small smear of Vaseline on the surface of the plastic head block and powder it with talcum or face powder.

2 Put the cap onto the plastic head, pulling the edges out.

3 Using acetone, gently wipe the underneath edges. This sticks the cap down and dissolves the edges. (Acetone is a solvent for bald cap plastic.)

4 Pour some cap plastic into a jar.

5 Place some powder in your chosen colour onto a tissue and sprinkle onto the cap plastic. Stir or shake with lid on.

6 Pour a little of the coloured plastic into a dish. Using a brush 50–75 mm wide, paint on the plastic a little at a time.

Fitting a bald cap

Tools & equipment

- acetone, surgical spirit or witch hazel
- cotton buds
- hair gel, **gafquat** or comb and water
- make-up palette of colours
- plastic cape to protect actor's clothing
- powder puff

- Pros-Aide adhesive – **if the cap is latex**
- scissors
- spirit gum, surgical adhesive, or Pros-Aide
- stipple sponge, powder puff
- tissues
- wooden modelling tool, small round-tip scissors

Preparing the actor

The actor should wear a shirt or top that does not need to be pulled over the head, or be in costume. A plastic cape should be securely tied around their shoulders, seated in a comfortable make-up chair at the right height for the make-up artist, and the fitting can begin.

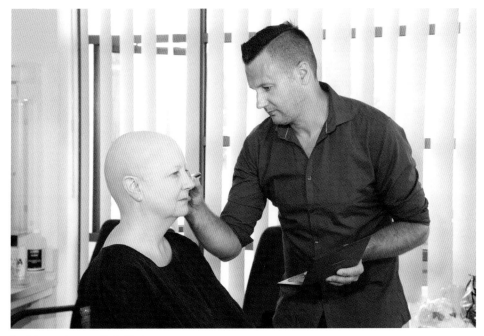

Applying make-up with bald cap

1 Gel the hair back smoothly, or wet and comb instead. If it is long, wrap it around the head, keeping as close as possible to the contour of the head.

2 If the skin is greasy, wipe around the hairline, cleanse and tone, and apply barrier cream.

3 Place the bald cap on the actor's head, starting at the forehead and pulling down to the nape of the neck. Stretch so that it is tight, with no air trapped inside.

4 If the plastic cap has a lot of excess material over the face area, trim it with scissors.

5 Stick the cap at the front of the forehead by pulling the edge up and applying Pros-Aide to the skin beneath. Press the edge down.

6 Anchor the cap at the back by pulling up the cap at the centre of the nape area at the back. Apply Pros-Aide and press down the cap again into position.

7 Draw a circle on the inside area of the ear with your eyebrow pencil, and a line running downwards straight to the bottom of the plastic cap. With your round-tipped scissors, cut up the line to the circle and cut out the circle piece. Repeat on the other ear.

8 Place Pros-Aide from the back to behind each ear. Trim any excess plastic from around the ear area so that it lies flat with no wrinkles. The cap should fit snugly around the ears. Use a wooden modelling tool to press the plastic flat.

9 Next use Pros-Aide to stick the edges of the cap from in front of the ears to the temples and up to the centre forehead anchor point.

10 Once the cap lies flat and feels secure, you can trim any more excess plastic away if necessary. All edges should now be glued down securely.

11 To blend the edges into the skin, use acetone on a cotton bud, holding a tissue below the cotton bud to protect the actor's face.

Do not allow excess acetone to touch the actor's skin, just the edge of the plastic cap. With a latex cap, the edges are blended with a paste such as Bondo or Pros-Aide which seals between the edge and the skin. When blending with acetone or Bondo, always cover the eyes with a powder puff when working on the forehead or temple areas.

12 Once the Pros-Aide is dry, powder gently at the edges.

13 Stipple Pros-Aide all over and slightly onto the skin to add texture and secure the bald cap firmly down. If all the edges are perfect, begin the colouring.

STEP-BY-STEP: APPLYING A BALD CAP

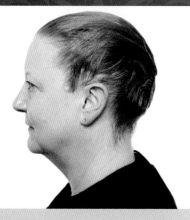

1 Wrap or pincurl the hair close to the head, using gafquat to slick down the front hairline.

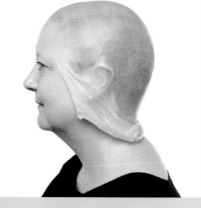

2 Fit the bald cap on the head.

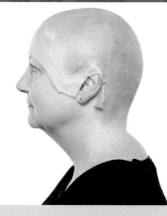

3 Cut a section from the drawn-on ear.

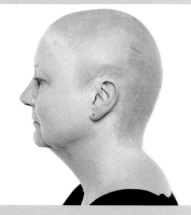

4 Stick down the cap, using adhesive along the edges, and blend the edges with acetone.

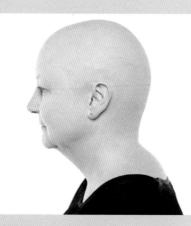

5 Apply camouflage make-up on head.

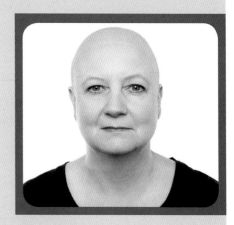

6 Finished look.

Colouring bald caps

Bald caps can be given a natural skin tone colour to look realistic, and this is harder to achieve than fantasy effects using unrealistic colours, where the design can hide the edges if necessary. For a realistic look it helps to stipple pink or red before the foundation colour, in the same way as for prosthetic pieces.

The techniques learned, such as stippling, airbrushing, layering with diluted pax paints, all come into play when artworking bald caps.

Other effects can be achieved by adding hair, e.g. a monk's tonsure, or a wig needing a high forehead for sixteenth century Elizabeth I make-up. Watercolours can be used for fantasy effects, with beading, feathers or sequins stuck on in different designs for bold, exotic or glamorous results.

Removing a bald cap

For removing a bald cap, it is the same as for removing prosthetics, wigs and facial hair, using the appropriate remover for the adhesive. Always use the remover sparingly with the tip of a brush, working gently under the edge of the bald cap to loosen it.

Hold a wad of tissues, a towel or powder puff in the other hand, under the brush. If any adhesive remover drips onto the actor's face, wipe the skin dry immediately. Cover the eyes or ask the actor to close them when working near the eyes.

Once the edges are loosened the cap can easily be removed. When it is off the head you can remove the adhesive from the face, slowly and gently. Sometimes the hair at the back of the neck pulls on the adhesive when the cap is removed, which can be painful. Use scissors to cut the short hairs away if necessary. Cleanse, tone and moisturise the actor's face when you have removed the make-up, in the usual way.

Inserting hair into bald caps

Hair can be laid onto bald caps and prosthetic pieces, but for tight camera close-ups the hair will look more natural if it is inserted into the plastic or latex. For this method you need an adapted sewing needle. Remove the tip at the eye end by rubbing the needle or cutting it off with pliers. The eye of the needle should look fork-like.

Insert the needle into a knotting hook holder. The forked needle can now be used to punch individual hairs or tufts of hair into the bald cap or prosthetic piece.

Take the hair in the left hand and hold the needle in the right hand. Catch hold of the hairs with the forked needle and push them through the plastic or latex from the inside of the cap. Pull the hair through until you have the desired outside length. The ends can be stuck down with adhesive inside the cap, where they will not show.

This technique works well when hair is needed for an ageing character make-up, when you want a few strands of hair across a bald head. It is also a useful technique for prosthetic creature effects.

REVISION QUESTIONS

1 What must you always perform before using prosthetics on your actor/artist?

2 What is the difference between a positive and negative mould?

3 What is the purpose of the flashing when making prosthetic pieces?

4 What would you use to make a bald cap?

5 What are the different types of bald caps available?

13 Character make-up

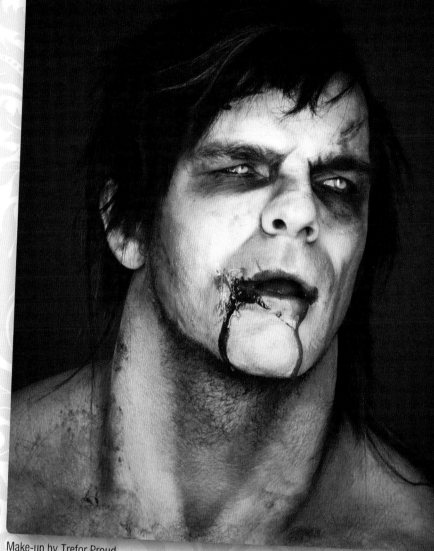

Make-up by Trefor Proud

LEARNING OBJECTIVES

This chapter covers the following:

◆ Research, planning and design for character make-up.

◆ Look-alikes.

◆ Ageing step-by-step procedures.

◆ Ageing for television, film and theatre.

◆ Different methods for creating beards.

◆ Eyebrow blocking.

◆ Portrait project.

KEY TERMS

Analysing the character   Look-alike   Old-age stipple

UNIT TITLE

◆ Prepare to change the performer's appearance

◆ Create and agree original design within hair and/or make-up

◆ Finalise the design within hair and/or make-up

◆ Contribute to design process and acquire resources for hair and/or make-up

INTRODUCTION

This chapter will explain how to create different characters for different areas of the hair and media make-up industry. It will also highlight the importance of research, planning and designing your character before application. Different character transformations are covered, including look-alikes and different types of character ageing for television, film and theatre. You will look at ways to create beards on actors and successful techniques for eyebrow blocking. This chapter also includes a section on portrait projects, which will help to build skills and knowledge of working on a concept, creating a design and executing research. All elements of character work will help prepare you for working in the hair and media make-up industry.

Character make-up

A good character make-up is achieved through preparation, selection and skilful application. Every technique of make-up is drawn on in creating a character; yet the make-up should be limited to what is really necessary for the result to be convincing. A subtle design can often be most effective.

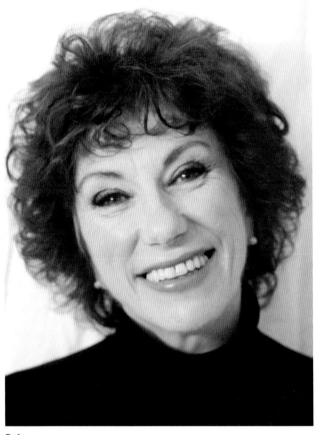

Before

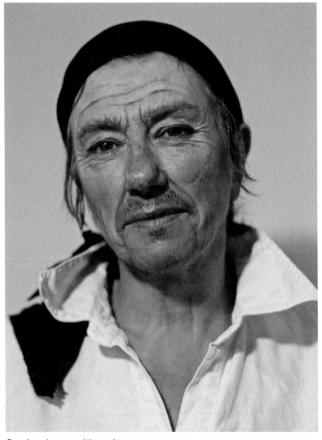

Gender change with ageing

Research, planning and design

The type of production will impose practical constraints:

◆ Whether it is for television, a feature film, theatre, commercial shoot or video.

◆ How much the budget allows for materials and the cost of specialist suppliers.

◆ Length of time allowed for the make-up artist to apply the make-up.

In character work there are three categories:

◆ people in fashion

◆ people no longer in fashion

◆ people ahead of fashion.

Pay attention to the recorded evidence concerning, for example, when it was fashionable to have facial hair or when women wore heavy make-up. Remember that there are always people who are not influenced by fashion: men who have beards and moustaches when others do not, and women who wear no make-up when others do. In period productions the make-up artist should try to create normal-looking people, and not always what was in fashion.

When researching a character there are these factors to consider. Physical appearance is determined by:

1 age

2 temperament

3 social standing

4 race

5 period

6 heredity

7 health.

Other general guidelines in planning a character make-up are:

1 If you don't need it, don't use it.

2 If you do use it, know why you are using it.

3 Try to draw out the character through the use of make-up.

4 Don't work on actors – work with them.

5 Don't stick rigidly to the rules. Instead, draw on all the techniques you know to obtain the maximum effect.

6 For character make-up, mix many different colours and stipple them to give depth and life to the face.

Look-alikes

In recreating a well-known person, the make-up artist aims to achieve as accurate a likeness as possible. It helps if the actor is cast with the likeness in mind, but this is not always the case and adjustments need to be made.

Begin by comparing the face of the actor and the character. **Analysing the character** for differences and similarities, the skin tones, face shape, lips, eye colour, nose shape, eyebrows and hair.

When the character is modern, there will be photographs available for use as reference and details of the person to study; for example, the information that Marilyn Monroe never sunbathed, even though it was fashionable to do so. If the subject is Abraham Lincoln it might be necessary to model a nose for the actor to achieve a likeness. Points of similarity should be emphasised and differences minimised.

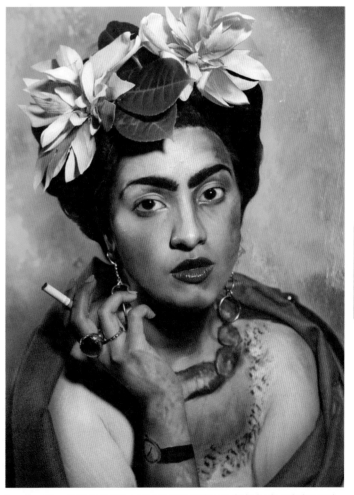

Look-alike of Frida Kahlo achieved with make-up, hair, body painting and costume

In the case of historical figures who pre-date photography we have to rely on paintings or engravings for finding a likeness, and the make-up artist may be asked to adapt the look for present-day audiences. Historical figures such as Winston Churchill, J. F. Kennedy or Charlie Chaplin are within living memory and so well-known that they should look right when played by actors. Archive material is freely available to help with the research and planning of the characters.

Character make-up is as important as the clothes and props. If the likeness has been achieved successfully the actor will be able to perform with greater effectiveness.

ACTIVITY

Anatomy of the face

Research pictures of the bone structure and muscles of the face. Print out images as a reference guide. Analyse the contours of the bone structure and the shape of the facial muscles.

Ageing

Study the faces of older people around you and it will be plain to see the variety of ways in which ageing affects people's appearances. Heredity, race, lifestyle and environment all play a part. Illness and health also play their part: from people looking gaunt and pale to weathered, wrinkly faces. The lines on the face reflect a person's temperament. There are laughter lines, bad-tempered lines and lines caused by stress or illness.

Go back to the beginning and look again at the anatomy of the face. Recall the drawing of drapery folds and the significance of light and shadow. As people get older the flesh becomes looser, and starts to sag downwards. In ageing make-up you need to put shadows where you would put concealer in a beauty make-up: adding bags under the eyes and lines from the nose to mouth. Other techniques are adding grey to eyebrows and hair at the temples, age spots, broken capillaries and adding texture to the skin.

Many people age in the same way as their parents, and for a male actor it is useful to see a photo of his father and for a female actor a photo of her mother which provides an insight into how they will probably age.

When ageing thin faces it is easy to bring out a skull-like effect with shading hollowing out the temples, and drooping eyelids. Plumper faces stay youthful-looking for longer, but you can add a double chin or sagging flesh with highlighting and shading. Hair becomes thicker and coarser in middle age, so you can give a man a dark beard line to take away the smooth, boyish appearance of youth.

Don't overdo the make-up. A woman of 45 will not show extensive signs of ageing if she has looked after her skin and general appearance.

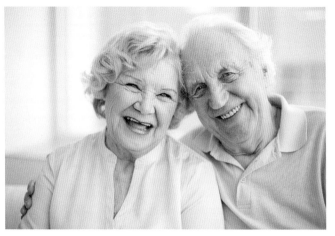

Senior man and woman

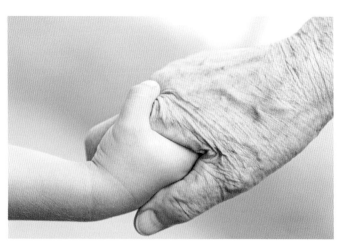

Old woman and child holding hands

Ageing using make-up

Always start by studying the real face of the person you are making up. Study the face, feel the prominences, notice the position and colour of the natural shadows under the eyes and below the jawline. An overhead light will help you to see where these are. When adding the make-up, your aim is to intensify these shadows.

Tools & equipment

- brushes
- cream make-up palette – various colours
- crimson lake pencil or cream make-up
- highlighting and shading cream make-up
- make-up gown
- powder and powder puff or soft powder brush
- stipple sponge

Use some of these techniques for ageing

1 The shading colour must harmonise with the actor's own skin tone. Add a touch of grey to the chosen colour, mixing in a touch of brown and blue from the basic cream palette. For pale, translucent skins, use a touch of mauve or blue.

2 Only use a foundation if it is necessary to change the skin tone. Apply the shading straight onto the bare face, emphasising the places where there are natural shadows. Look for the age lines, checking that these move with the face when you paint them in. Strengthen the circles under the eyes, nose to mouth lines, and crease at the corners of the mouth. Keep the lines clean, don't smudge the face, keep the lines soft at the edges – but not dirty looking.

3 Add highlighting, blending the edges carefully with a clean brush. On more prominent areas add more highlighting. Powder lightly and brush off between layers. Add the lightest highlights and the darkest shadow last.

4 Try adding a speck of grey and green in the hollows of the face.

5 Tone down the lips with a touch of blue (to disguise the youthful red). Don't apply much, unless your intention is to make the actor look ill.

6 If the face is plump and round, emphasise the skin folds; try to make them look as if they have sagged.

7 Whatever the shape of the face, you need to 'break up' the jawline to reduce the firmness of youth. To create the illusion of a double chin, ask the actor to push his or her chin down; then put a shadow in the fold and highlight the bulge where the double chin forms.

8 Using a stipple sponge, stipple dark red and blue in the highlighted area. Draw broken veins on the cheeks with a crimson lake pencil, blending some of them with a fine brush.

9 Apply a little red to the upper eyelids and a broken, blended line to outline the bottom eyelids, to suggest watery eyes.

TOP TIP

People often shrink when they get old. The actor can wear a larger size shirt to create this effect.

TOP TIP

Ivory is a good highlighting colour for ageing.

TOP TIP

The face becomes haggard and drawn in old age creating the illusion of a bigger nose and extended ear lobes.

10 Paint in liver spots with brown make-up.

11 For an ungroomed look, brush cream or white through the eyebrows and brush them down.

12 Age the neck by highlighting the bones and placing shading in the hollows and sockets. Blend the highlighting and shading softly at the edges. There must be no hard lines. Keep checking your work in the mirror, turning the face sideways so that you can see the result.

13 Age the hands; apply highlight to the prominent knuckle bones and along the veins. Shade either side of the veins and between the fingers.

Ageing using stretch and stipple method

When painting with make-up is not enough, there is another technique that can be used to create three-dimensional wrinkles. Products used for this method include a latex-based material called 'old-age stipple' which comes in different colours from neutral to dark skin tones. Another product called 'green marble' is also used, which involves mixing the green marble concentrate with atta gel, which is a clay powder used for face masques.

Old-age stipple is used straight from the bottle. There are six formulas made by W.H. Creations; they are A, B, C, crusty, neutral and dark skin. Most make-up artists use type B old-age stipple or green marble. Whichever product you use, it is the way you stretch the skin that is important. The direction of the stretch decides the way the wrinkles form, and it is important to achieve a natural looking wrinkle in the right place.

Three people are needed when first using this technique: one to stretch the skin, one to stipple the old-age stipple and hold a handheld dryer to dry the area, and a third to powder the area before the skin is released.

Tools & equipment

- barrier cream
- bowl for old-age stipple
- handheld hairdryer
- make-up wrap and tissues
- no-colour powder, powder puff, powder brush
- old-age stipple type B or green marble
- sponge – cut into small pieces for applying the **old-age stipple**

Preparing the actor

1 Place a wrap around the actor's shoulders and tuck a paper tissue around their neck.

2 Apply a small amount of barrier cream to the eye area. Allow this to sink in.

3 Powder to remove all traces of grease.

4 Pour a little old-age stipple into the bowl.

5 Working on one area of the face at a time, pull the skin taut with the fingers, and, with a small piece of sponge, stipple some of the old-age stipple onto the stretched area. Do not overload the sponge. Blend the edges thinly.

6 Use the handheld hairdryer on a cool setting to dry the product. Hold it at a good distance from the actor's face, and make sure it is not too hot or too cold. The skin being stretched should not be released until the area is dried and powdered. When the product has become transparent and shiny it is dry and ready to be powdered.

Areas of the face to stretch

Area of the face	Stretch method
Eye area	Pull skin upwards at eyebrows, with actor's eyes tightly closed. Stipple on eyelids, then: ◆ under eyes: pull skin down towards centre of face ◆ sides of eyes: pull skin at outer corners of the eyes
Forehead	Ask actor to frown and pull hair back at front hairline
Chin area	Tilt chin upwards and stretch skin outwards on both sides of chin
Neck	Pull head backwards to stretch the neck, do underneath the chin and sides of neck
Nose to mouth lines	Pull skin away from centre of face
Upper lip area	Stretch skin left and right
Cheeks	Ask actor to puff out the cheeks and stipple lightly

Wrinkles are formed on the softest parts of the face as indicated above. If you pull the skin vertically the wrinkles will be horizontal; if you stretch horizontally the lines will be vertical.

If you want to age an actor from young to middle-aged, one layer of stipple on the eye areas can be sufficient without having to age the rest of the face. Too many layers can look mask-like, and so much depends on the brief. For an old crone look, many layers may be needed. If the whole face and neck has been done, the hands should be worked on too. Apply to clenched fists on the back of the hands. Old-age spots can help to complete the effect.

Make-up can be applied before the stretch and stipple method. Shading and highlighting are not necessary on top of the product as the wrinkles are three-dimensional and create their own shadows.

TOP TIP

Alcohol-based products such as Skin Illustrator palettes work well to achieve an age spot effect on the hands, as you can make the colours look transparent and you have the freedom to build the depth.

Cut a paintbrush's bristles to a firm stump to help create a stippled liver spot effect.

TOP TIP

Give your actor skincare advice if they are constantly using chemical products on the skin. The skin may become sensitised and will require extra care. Use hypoallergenic products or products that suit the client's skin type.

STEP-BY-STEP: AGEING USING STRETCH AND STIPPLE

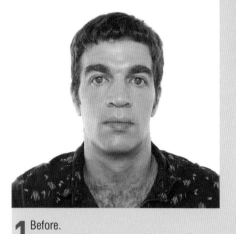

1 Before.

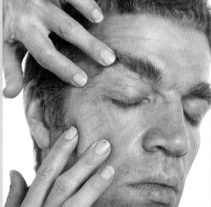

2 Pull skin at outer corners of eye.

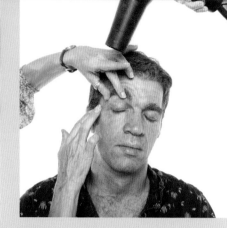

3 Pull skin upwards at eyebrows.

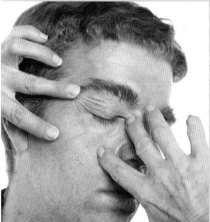

4 Stretch skin.

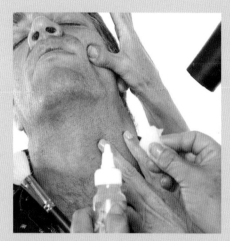

5 Stretch the neck.

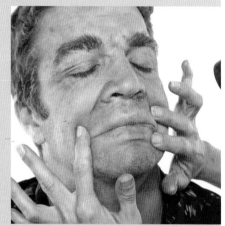

6 Stretch skin left and right.

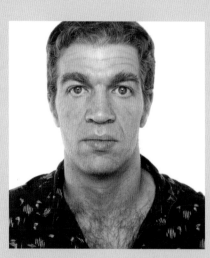

7 The finished look.

Removing the old-age stipple

A pad of cotton wool soaked in warm water will lift the stipple, but do not pull it off in one piece. Oil can also be used to remove it. Take time to remove this type of make-up or you may damage the actor's skin.

Ageing for cinematography and television

In films your work will show every detail. The close-ups are very big on a large screen and the make-up artist's work is more noticeable and therefore open to criticism.

When ageing for film, study the actor's face and let the natural markings, shadows and highlights be your guide. To age the eyebrows, add grey, coarser hairs rather than colouring the natural ones. HD has brought similar needs for television, where details are clearly seen.

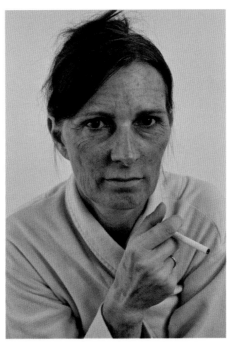

Before ageing   After ageing

Ageing of character 'Gandhi' by Tom Smith

Sir Richard Attenborough was determined to have Tom do the make-up on *Gandhi* in 1980–1981. Tom Smith accepted the job and went to India, not knowing who the actor would be, but expecting to make changes to the actor's face with prosthetics. He took a lab oven, mixing machine and scales but he couldn't take the actual chemicals because Indian customs would not allow them through. They told him he could obtain all the products in Delhi. When he got there, they were delivered in old bottles and boxes, without labels. He experimented with the chemicals in the Delhi hotel garage and modelled some prosthetic pieces.

At this point, Ben Kingsley was cast to play Gandhi. Tom had read the script and made some sketches of five different ages of Mahatma Gandhi's evolution from young man to emaciated old age. (He was 79 when he was assassinated.) The sketches served to remind Tom not to go too far with each change – to hold back, so that there was always something left in reserve.

When Ben Kingsley arrived, Tom tried out some prosthetic pieces on him – but it was decided that the prosthetics interfered with the characterisation: psychologically, it was like putting a mask on him – the make-up was getting in the way of the performance. It was agreed to make up Kingsley without prosthetics. The sense of Gandhi ageing throughout the film was achieved by Tom with painting. His intention was to make it imperceptible, so that through the film the actor as Gandhi grows older without you noticing. As in real life, when you live with someone you are unaware of the ageing process because it is so gradual.

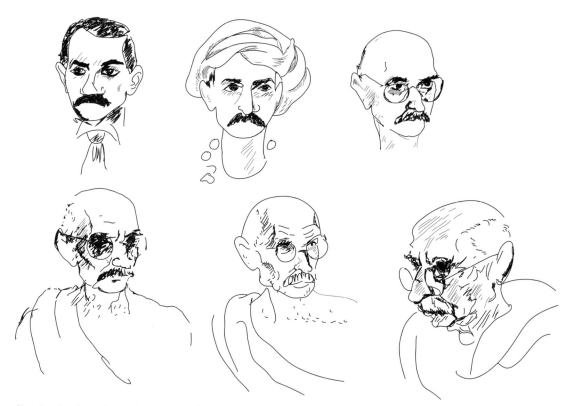

Sketches for the ageing of the character 'Gandhi'

The ageing of the actor, Sir Ben Kingsley, by Tom Smith

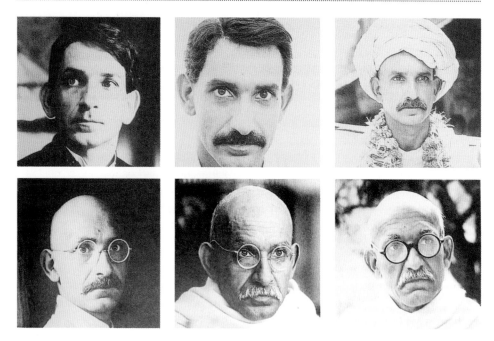

STEP-BY-STEP: AGEING MAKE-UP BY KRISTYAN MALLETT USING PROSTHETICS

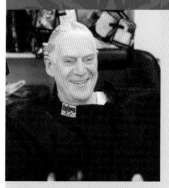

1 Vinyl bald cap application.

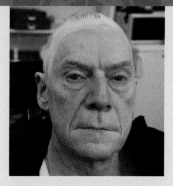

2 Two layers of stretch and stipple around the eyes, upper lip and lower lip.

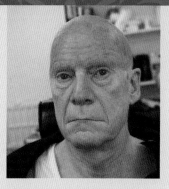

3 Silicone neck piece applied, this piece also has some very fine hairs punched in to it around the upper chest and under chin area.

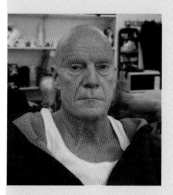

4 Forehead piece, again a silicone piece is put on. This piece has hair punched eyebrows.

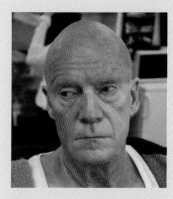

5 Silicone cheek is now applied.

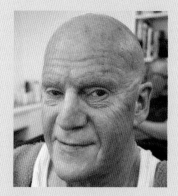

6 The remaining cheek piece is applied.

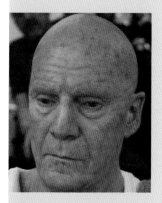

7 After the pieces are stuck down, all the edges are then sealed with a Pros-Aide stipple, then powdered and all the detail fully painted on.

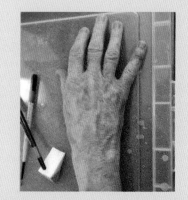

8 Back of hand pieces are then glued on, painted up to a high detailed finish as they are often seen on camera. They are then sealed with green marble to prevent paint being rubbed off.

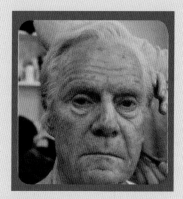

9 After the wig is put on, fake teeth are put in and lenses to help sell the ageing make-up look.

TOP TIP

Always consider what scenes your actor will be performing, this will help you decide what make-up products to use for your stubble application to create the best results. For example, there may be kissing scenes, rainy scenes, etc.

TOP TIP

Always photograph your created look from different angles.

Tools & equipment

- chopped wet hair – 0.5 cm length
- hair lace pieces
- matte spirit gum adhesive
- soft cloth or powder puff
- stiff make-up brush

Tools & equipment

- beard stipple wax
- make-up brush
- tissues
- tweezers
- wet chopped hair – as before

Ageing for theatre

The main consideration is how far away the audience is. For intimate theatre or grand opera, the make-up should be appropriate for the distance from the stage. The skin colour is important, as is the hair, both of which register from a distance. The lines and shapes in ageing for the theatre are more defined, with stronger colours than for television and film.

Beard stubble

Although actors can grow a short stubble by simply not shaving for a few days, it is often necessary to create one. Because filming is seldom in the same order as the storyline, continuity often demands that the actor be both clean-shaven and unshaven in the same day's work.

At a distance the look can be achieved with make-up by stippling bluish-grey or blackish-brown on the actor's natural beardline. This is usually enough for theatre work. For television and film it is necessary to be able to see the hairs sticking out for close-up work.

There are several methods for a realistic-looking one week's growth. It is important to match the stubble growth to the actor's own beard shape, and sparseness or density of growth. The hair should be a blend of colours to look natural; use at least two colours. The hair should be chopped to a length of 0.5 cm whilst wet, making sure the hair is cut to the same length.

Spirit gum and lace method

Apply a thin layer of spirit gum adhesive to the actor's beardline, following the shape carefully. Use the cloth to press onto the adhesive to remove shine. Place a piece of hair lace onto the sticky surface. Use your stiff make-up brush to pick up the chopped wet hair, pressing it into the holes in the lace. Quickly pull the lace off the face, leaving the cut hair behind. The angle that you pull off the lace will affect the direction that the hair stands out from the face.

Beard stipple wax and brush

For close-up work the wax method is good, because, unlike spirit gum adhesive, it does not shine.

Let the chopped wet hair dry on the tissues laid out on the work surface. When the hair is dry, apply beard stipple wax over the actor's beardline. Pick up the dry chopped hair from the tissues with the make-up brush. Using a quick, stippling movement, apply to the wax. This should be done very lightly: too much pressure will flatten the hair. Any hair that is not sticking out should be removed with tweezers. Small areas can be strengthened with dark make-up applied with a small, pointed brush.

Remember to take the growth down onto the neck under the chin as far as the Adam's apple

Removing the stubble

Apply cleaning cream to the beardline and scrape off the hair and wax with a spatula or palette knife. Remove spirit gum with mild mastix remover or surgical spirit.

Finish off with normal cleansing, toning and moisturiser to restore the actor's face to normal.

Eyebrow blocking

Eyebrow wax is useful for blocking out – waxing out – eyebrows, especially for an eighteenth-century period make-up or complete character change for fantasy or alien look. Before applying the wax use a bar of soap to flatten the natural eyebrows. This will prevent the hairs from poking through the wax. You can also use a spirit gum adhesive instead of (or on top of) the soap.

1 Wet the end of the soap bar and use it to flatten the eyebrows firmly to the skin.

2 When the soap has dried, use a modelling tool or spatula to apply a thin layer of eyebrow wax to cover the eyebrows. Make sure it is smooth with no bumps or hard edges.

3 Seal the wax with one or two applications, allowing each layer to dry.

4 Colour the blocked-out eyebrows with make-up and apply foundation colour to the face. Make sure that the eyebrow areas match the foundation colour.

5 Paint in the new eyebrows with brush and make-up. You cannot use pencils on wax.

6 When drawing eyebrows on wax, use a ruler to make sure that they are evenly matched. It is difficult to get both eyebrows the same shape and size when you are not following the natural brow bones.

HEALTH & SAFETY

To avoid cross-infection use a spatula to break off a small piece of soap to use on an individual actor. Dispose of the rest and repeat for further actors.

Tools & equipment

◆ eyebrow wax
◆ isopropyl alcohol (IPA)– to clean the brush after sealer make-up
◆ modelling tool and spatula
◆ sealer
◆ soap and/or spirit gum adhesive

CASE PROFILE: AMANDA WARBURTON, MAKE-UP ARTIST

How long have you been working in the industry?

Twenty-three years! . . . Crikey!

How did you get into the industry?

I worked as a hairdresser for ten years prior to my training course; this proved to be very beneficial as at that time, in films and commercials, make-up artists were being asked to do hair too, which some couldn't do. Through getting names of make-up artists through 'The Knowledge' and contacting them, I was asked to assist and do all the hair! This gave me invaluable experience as well as working with, and learning from, talented and established make-up artists. I also did a stint at the ENO to acquire more knowledge with wigs and worked on several NFS graduation films.

Did you have a lucky break or a turning point?

The first couple of years I mainly focused on stills, photographic, commercials and the music industry. I had an agent for assisting for the latter. Work was sporadic and not always paid well. At that time lots of pop promos were being made. I was assisting on Marcella Detroit's first solo single promo. There were 150 extras and I

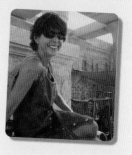

was the only make-up artist working on them! I organised with the third AD which of them would be more featured, and focused specifically on those. To the rest I explained the overall look and asked them to work on each other and themselves! At the end of the day (all went well!) the third AD asked me if I was interested in working in television and film, as his girlfriend was a make-up designer. I met with her and went on to assist her on many jobs, the first being *The Tomorrow People* with Cristian Schmidt, and later included *Jude*, a feature film starring Kate Winslet.

Did you have a lucky break or a turning point?

I've been blessed with working on many lovely things in many lovely places! I think one of them must be *Ancient Egyptians* a drama documentary for CH4/HBO. We filmed in Morocco and Luxor, Egypt. As well as the creativity of recreating the period there were lots of battle scenes and character and casualty make-ups to do.

What do you enjoy most about the job?

I enjoy many aspects of the job, especially the creativity it allows!

How has the fashion industry changed during your career?

For positive reasons, all the new products now available both in fashion and casualty make-up. For negative reasons, 'split days' have been created to save companies money on 'rest day payments' after night shoots. Generally having to work longer hours for not much more money than when I started!

What advice would you give to a new make-up artist starting out?

Pack your personality and sense of humour as well as your kit! Filming involves long hours and can be intense. As well as being good at what you do, you need to be nice to have around! Don't be too pushy and have respect for those who have spent years working and gaining experience; they have a lot of knowledge to share. Always be on time and ready to work. Be constantly flexible! Unplanned changes often happen within the working day.

Clown make-up

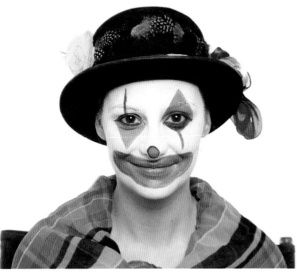

Clown make-up

As well as being fun to do, clown make-ups are good for practising balance and precision. Well-known types are the tramp and the white-faced clown – each face should be individual to the performer.

The tramp clown is usually unshaven, and wears baggy trousers and a battered bowler hat. The eyebrows, eyes and mouth are painted, and he has a bright red bulbous nose. This can be made from half a table tennis ball, painted and stuck on the nose with spirit gum, or by slush moulding for a rubber nose. The mouth is painted red or white, and drawn very large, either turning up to look happy, or down to look sad.

The white-faced clown is more colourful. The outlines should be drawn with black pencil to emphasise the eyebrows, nose, eyes and mouth.

Planning the make-up

Draw the proposed clown design on paper, filling it in with coloured pencils to illustrate the effect.

Clowns can be funny, sad, suspicious, elegant or tragic. Bald caps with crepe hair laid on in bright colours complete the look. White stocking tops pulled over the head to hide the hair or a white bathing hat both make good skull caps. Eye markings are individual, but the black cross over the eyelids is well-known, as are painted teardrops with raised eyebrows.

Pierrot and pierrette

Pierrot has a plain white face. If the actor's eyebrows are too heavy, use soap to plaster them down, and when dry, apply wax or eyebrow plastic on top.

Use white cake make-up to paint the entire face with brush or sponge and water. When dry, powder with white or transparent powder.

The eyebrows should be arched, high up on the face and painted black. The lips should be painted bright red in a cupid's bow. The eyes are defined with black pencil or liquid liner. Two beauty spots complete the look – one on the cheekbone near the eye, the other on the opposite side of the face, nearer the corner of the mouth.

A black skull cap should cover the hair.

For the Pierrette, the girl is made up to look as pretty as possible – she often wears a hat.

Tools & equipment

- additional media – lashes, gems or glitters
- bald cap, bathing hat, stocking tops – black and white
- brushes, sponges
- face charts
- mood boards
- palette of primary-coloured face paints
- primary-coloured pencils or crayons for sketch design
- soft black eyeliner pencil
- water
- white powder, powder puff, powder brush

Portrait project

TOP TIP

Always give your clients advice on how to remove the make-up that you have applied. Explain that by keeping the skin in good condition their make-up application will always have better results.

One of the most exciting projects undertaken by students at Delamar Academy for their End of Year Exhibition, is a Portrait Project. They select a postcard, or download a picture of a portrait painting to recreate on a person – usually a fellow student or family member. The journey from research to final effect is a wonderful learning experience, plus excellent photos for students' portfolios as an end result. Using make-up to copy an artist's painting, which is often oil on canvas, is a challenge. The brush strokes and abstract shapes of light and dark have to be studied in order to develop the picture created by the artist. So much is learned in this project, about shapes of features, skin tones, texture and how to get character into their work.

Researching the project

Art galleries and exhibitions are good sources of research for studying the real paintings, and most of them are available as postcards to take home. Art books, art catalogues and the Internet are also useful for inspiration. It is important to select a subject that is not too difficult to copy because the hair, clothes, accessories and background have to be reproduced for the project. If the painting is of a lady holding a pomegranate, you have to find a pomegranate; if it is a painting of Christ on the Cross, how will you make the cross? Pictures that include animals in the frame are not suitable – where will you find a greyhound or tiger? Backgrounds can be painted in advance on a suitable sized canvas.

Check that you can find the right wig or hairpiece, clothes and jewellery. You might choose to bodypaint a necklace or gloves. Most important of all is to find the right model – someone you can transform into the portrait painting. Skin tone, eye colour, nose and lip shapes must be considered.

Preparation and planning

Find and assemble all the items you will need: the right-looking chair or vase, any flowers or fruit (although perishable goods are best bought on the day), the canvas background frame, the wig or facial hair if needed.

Collect your make-up materials, colours, textures, etc.

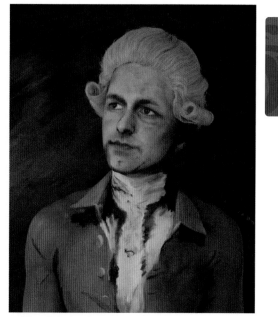
Portrait project with wig and body painting

You need to find or make a costume. You may have to buy or hire it, but try to keep the costs down. If you are using a wig, you need to organise a wig fitting and then block and set it ready to be dressed.

All test make-up must be arranged and done in advance – so that all is ready on the day.

Creating the portrait

On the day, have everything prepared and laid out, ready to go. You should have dressed the wig, painted the canvas, obtained the costume and assembled all accessories.

Make sure that your model is comfortable and allow breaks for coffee and stretching out.

Remember to keep the picture you are copying taped to your workplace, and refer to it frequently.

The materials, tools and techniques that you use are entirely unique to each project.

Photographing the portrait project

When the work is finished, take plenty of time for the photographic session. Check that the framing with the canvas, and your model's pose is the same as the actual painting. Look out for the positioning of the hands, the angle of the shoulders, the shape of the hair and the facial expression.

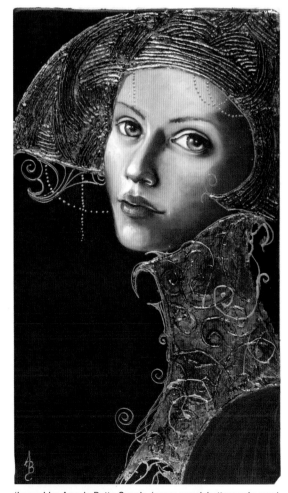

'Isaura' by Angela Betta Casale (www.angelabettacasale.com)

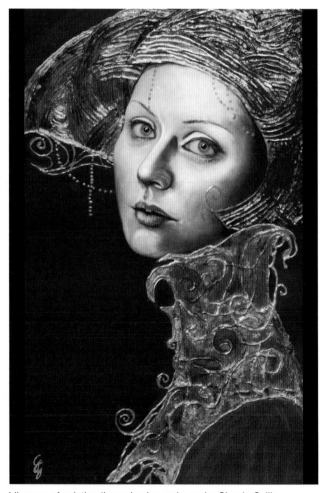

Likeness of painting 'Isaura' using make-up by Giorgio Galliero

Take photographs at the same angle or point of view as the artist did, even if you have to stand on a chair or lie on the floor. Finally, make sure the light source is the same, whether from a window or a floor light. Minor make-up changes can be done at any time during the session.

Keeping a record

Make notes on everything that you did to achieve the likeness, and file them for the future.

Character projects

Make-ups by Oscar and Emmy award winner Trefor Proud, photographer Eric Shwabel

Trefor explains how he achieved the different looks.

Zombie

The zombie make-up was done using four shades of aqua colour, very heavily shaded and highlighted. I then softened the whole effect with a light airbrushing of silver grey. Final touches were baby powder blown off a sheet of paper and then a faint dusting of silver dust. The contact lenses were put in last minute.

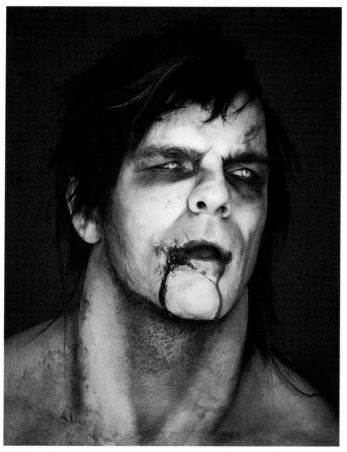

Zombie by Trefor Proud

Lion

The lion was basically done with very strong lines of aqua colour and a minimum of shading. I followed the model's basic muscle structure and emphasized all the major muscle groups. The face was a basic, theatrical lion make-up. The wig was a burnt acrylic wig – basically boiled until it frizzed.

Gold leaf

The gold make-up, though it looks the simplest, was the hardest look to achieve. The model had to be completely shaved smooth. He was then painted with a mixture of 50 per cent honey and 50 per cent water. This all had to be done in a cool dry room with absolutely no draughts. The gold leaf was then lifted out, sheet by sheet, and placed on the model. The reason for no draughts was that the sheets were so thin they could drift away in the slightest breeze and the gold leaf also instantly grabs the nearest surface. Once the model was covered I went in with gold mascara on the eyelashes etc. I waited about 15 minutes and then gently polished the surface with a chamois cloth. This make-up rinses off easily with soap and hot water.

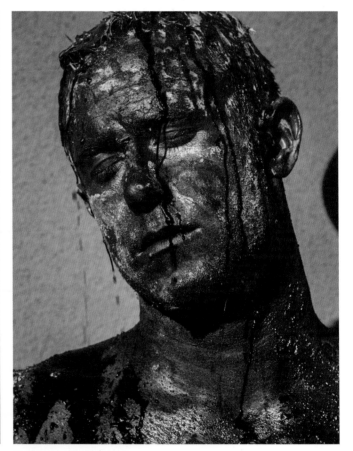

Lion make-up by Trefor Proud

Goldman by Trefor Proud

The section entitled Character projects on pages 287 and 288 was written by Trefor Proud.

CASE PROFILE: ANGIE MUDGE, MAKE-UP DESIGNER

How long have you been working in the industry?

Seventeen years

How did you get into the industry?

I did a three-month intense course in 1997 and said 'yes' to any and every opportunity that was offered to gain as much experience as possible.

Did you have a lucky break or turning point?

I guess so. I was recommended by a friend to design a feature film, which kick started my designing work. That was a turning point.

What has been your most significant project(s)?

A feature called *Stander* that I assisted on was a massive learning experience. We filmed for four months in South Africa. I had two lead actors in hair lace wigs almost every day and I'd had very little experience beforehand with that, so I learned a lot.

What do you enjoy most about the job?

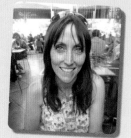

I get the most enjoyment out of a complete transformation. When a look really comes together and works for the character. I enjoy sticking things on like wigs, hair-pieces, facial hair or special effects.

How has the television and film industry changed during your career?

There seems to be less time and money but bigger expectations. The standard of work out there is exceptional at times so people (the viewer as well as the production) expect a high standard even on a tiny budget.

What advice would you give to a new make-up artist starting out?

It's a marathon not a sprint. You have to really want it and be prepared for a hard slog but with great rewards. Go with it. Be available.

REVISION QUESTIONS

1 What test must always be carried out before using ageing products? How far in advance must the test be performed prior to make-up application?

2 What are the purposes of barrier creams?

3 What procedures would you follow if a contra-action occurred during product application?

4 What type of adhesive would be used when applying stubble to the face?

5 What are the differences between a television ageing and theatre ageing look? And what types of products are available?

14 Launching your career

Guest written by Gideon Shawyer

LEARNING OBJECTIVES

This chapter covers the following:

◆ Accreditations, qualifications and competitions.

◆ Building a portfolio.

◆ Work experience.

◆ Marketing yourself.

◆ Social media.

◆ Networking.

◆ Insurance.

◆ Accounts, invoices, tax and contracts.

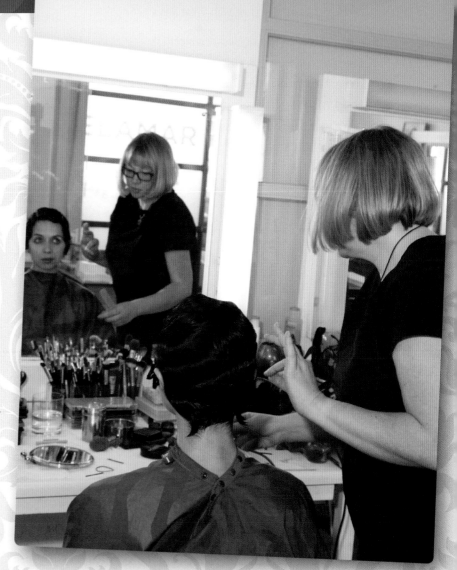

KEY TERM

UNIT TITLE

◆ Manage and market yourself as a freelancer

◆ Facilitate and manage trainees

◆ Agree contracts for hair and/or make-up work

◆ Budget your work and personal expenses

INTRODUCTION

This unit includes invaluable advice to help point you in the right direction during the early stages of your career as a make-up artist; you will cover rates of pay, CVs, contracts, budgets, accounts, tax and invoices. It discusses different accreditations, qualifications and competitions. It will help you to build a professional portfolio and understand what marketing strategies you may use. There are various different social media outlets that will help you as a make-up artist to communicate with the industry, including Facebook and Twitter. The importance of work experience and continuing to build your skills throughout your career are also discussed. Your training in basic hair or beauty will help as a starting point on your career path to becoming a make-up artist and this unit will help you understand how to climb the ladder and build on those skills. With additional training such as hair and media make-up courses and lots of hard work, you will be on your way to an exciting and successful career.

Launching your career

Whether you are self-taught or go to a school, college, an academy or a university you will need to take responsibility for launching your career yourself. The better academies will recommend their graduates for trainee or make-up artist roles, but it is still your responsibility to make contacts and find work in the industry.

As some of you may have purchased this book before choosing a make-up school, you should look at where best to train. Do your research: look at different schools, ideally talk to the students and graduates, and go to the one that you think is best for you. Some schools have a better reputation due to their alumni and tutors, and these contacts can be used by more recent graduates to get their first jobs. However, you need to find the institution that will support your training needs and help you to achieve your career aspirations.

Accreditations, qualifications and competitions

Accreditations and qualifications

Some colleges and courses carry an accreditation from an industry body. This demonstrates that the school, college or academy has been approved to teach their courses. Some colleges have also linked up with each other to form a college group. With all of these accreditations it is important to understand what benefit that accreditation will bring. If there is a qualification attached to the course, such as an NVQ, it shows the range of skills taught; however, as there are so many schools teaching NVQs it is not the case that they all teach them to the same standard. You should look at the school individually as well as the qualification.

Competitions

There are many competitions that can help develop your reputation and skills, as they are generally judged by experienced professionals, and it is a way to differentiate yourself from other make-up artists. Some competitions can be expensive, so you need to bear this in mind when entering. You may also need to consider the time and cost of the model, costume, props and make-up for your design. Whilst it is the make-up that is judged, the rest of the look will also have an effect.

TOP TIP

Research make-up artists that inspire you. Where did they train? What have they worked on since? Who has assisted them?

HEALTH & SAFETY

When entering competitions, be aware it is not just your skill that will be judged but your ability to follow health and safety standards and work safely.

Building a portfolio

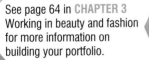

See page 64 in **CHAPTER 3** Working in beauty and fashion for more information on building your portfolio.

When you first start doing work or work experience you need to have a folder of photos of your work, called a portfolio. Your portfolio does not necessarily have to be a physical collection of glossy prints, but you need to be able to show examples of your work – for instance on an ebook, website or tablet. This could be work you produced in college, student films or projects that you have created in your own time. At some academies and training institutions, such as Delamar Academy, students do not need a portfolio for their first projects as the academy has a sufficient reputation that producers will trust students have been well-trained. However, when students/graduates move onto more specific and better-paid work, which might involve attending interviews, they are recommended for, students/graduates will need to take their portfolio.

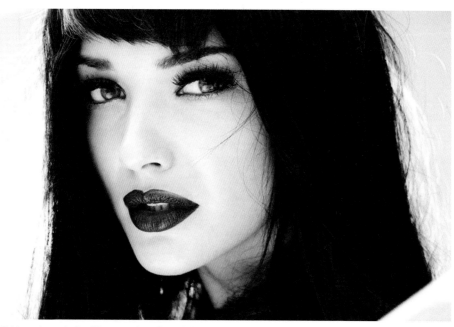

ELLE Magazine – India; Photographer: Suresh Natarajan; Make-up Artist: Namrata Soni; Model: Amy Jackson

Your portfolio is an aid to your curriculum vitae (CV) and as such it should be tailored for the type of work that you are looking to get. For example, if you are going to an interview for an editorial piece, you must not bring your best prosthetics or period make-ups. They might be impressive, but it is not what the interviewer wants to see to establish whether you are right for the shoot. Do not have too many pictures – particularly of the same make-up project. You should limit your CV to one or two pages and also limit the number of photos in your portfolio to your best work, rather than numerous photos to pad it out.

If you are looking to work in body art, you need to have photos of body art (as opposed to face painting). This is partly to show your skills and creativity, but also to show you are used to working on a large area and can plan your time accordingly.

Do not use 'selfie' make-up as examples of your work in your portfolio, whether it be for beauty, fashion or special effects. While being able to create a good bruise on your arm is impressive, you should create the effect on someone else. The interviewer would expect you to be able to do your own make-up; therefore, they are more interested to see that you can do make-up on other people.

Your photographs should show the complete make-up look and costume. If it is a wedding make-up the model should be in a wedding dress. If the photograph is of a car accident victim, the model should have the bruises or wounds that are typical for that type of accident, as well as beauty, party or dirty make-up depending on the character portrayed.

Wedding portfolio

If you are looking for work as a wedding make-up artist, you need photos of brides whose make-up you have previously done. This does not need to be a paid job, and can be a friend's wedding, but brides that look like models will appear more professional in your portfolio. Get permission to use the pictures in your portfolio, and if she (or he) is willing, also take a 'before' picture. This is especially useful if there is camouflage make-up involved.

Fashion portfolio

A fashion portfolio is different from other portfolios for several reasons, first because the photos need to be well lit and professionally taken, and second they can be airbrushed. A full fashion portfolio should have at least ten pictures, with at least six looks you are really proud of. The majority of the pictures should demonstrate you know how to apply a good base as, when assisting, this is what the make-up artist (or their agent) wants to see. Once you are happy you have the base photos, include others to specifically show your creativity.

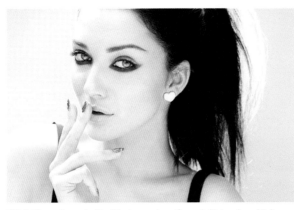

ELLE Magazine – India; Photographer: Suresh Natarajan; Make-up Artist: Namrata Soni; Model: Amy Jackson

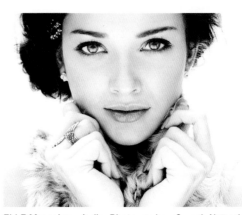

ELLE Magazine – India; Photographer: Suresh Natarajan; Make-up Artist: Namrata Soni; Model: Amy Jackson

When you are building up your portfolio you might do **time for print (TFP)** work, which is an arrangement between a model and/or make-up artist and a photographer. The photographer agrees to provide the model and/or make-up artist with an agreed number of pictures of the best photographs from the session. You might have to do quite a lot of shoots to build up your portfolio as some will not go as well as hoped – whether due to you, the photographer or the model. When doing a TFP job, you should make sure it is not work that should be paid for because this devalues your work (and the work of other make-up artists) and can have minimum wage implications. It may reduce your ability to charge the correct rate for similar work if you have previously done it for free. It can also be difficult to get the pictures from the photographer.

Contact model agents and offer to work with their new faces on **test shoots**, this is a good way to meet photographers. Always expect to do the work experience for free and if the agent or photographer gives you anything this is a bonus. It is not unheard of for agents to be sent cakes by an assistant (or someone wanting to be an assistant). Again, this can be expensive so don't feel you have to send cakes to everyone you want to work for.

Prosthetics or special effects portfolio

In a first prosthetics portfolio you will want to display a wide range of skills, even if you have not created a lot of pieces. Take pictures of different stages of the development to show you possess those skills. Make sure you appear in some of the pictures to demonstrate that it is your work. People passing off other people's work as their own is an issue in the industry, so these photos will remove any doubt. The photos should show enough detail to showcase your level of skill. If you have an interview think about what they want you to do. If it's sculpting then consider bringing the piece you sculpted so they can see it in more detail.

Make-up and hair portfolio

The make-up and hair portfolio will often show a wide range of skills from different periods, using different techniques. If you have enough good photos, tailor this portfolio depending on the type of work you are trying to get. If not, use your best photographs that show a range of skills.

Work experience

Student films/fashion shows

Delamar Academy runs an agency that receives requests for make-up artists for student films on a regular basis. Generally there is a lack of students that are available rather than a lack of films for them to work on. Some schools and colleges will do the same. For those who are self-taught there is work experience that can be found on the Internet or by contacting film schools and fashion schools directly.

When doing work experience it is important to take it seriously and be professional, as this is the start of the next stage of your career. As the saying goes: 'today's runner is tomorrow's producer'. You will have more freedom to be more creative than you will have at any other time in your career, until you are a designer. It is also important to know your worth. When you have worked with someone for expenses or below your usual daily rate, it is important to ask for a rate that you think you deserve the next time you work for them.

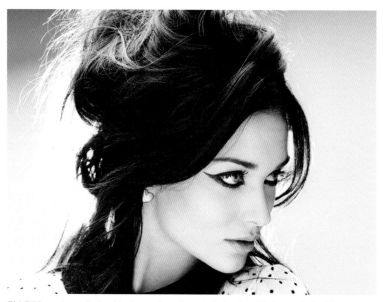

ELLE Magazine – India; Photographer: Suresh Natarajan; Make-up Artist: Namrata Soni; Model: Amy Jackson

Working for brands

Working for make-up brands is a brilliant way to keep practising and also to build up a make-up kit. Most of the brands will give free (or heavily discounted) products to their staff. The knowledge of different brands is also incredibly useful and is becoming more so as products become more advanced. Many of the fashion shows are sponsored by brands, so it will be their teams that perform at the show.

> "Always know a little about the brand and the products, and have some idea about the business side, as you will most likely be working in a retail environment. Having knowledge of what will be expected from you in the sales environment, along with your professional training, will perhaps make you the stronger candidate.
>
> *Jane Richardson, International Lead Make-up Artist for Nars*

HEALTH & SAFETY

As a trainee be aware there are health and safety laws in place to safeguard your health. There are laws as to how many hours you can work in a day, with a rest (known as 'turnaround time' in the film industry) in-between each working day.

Most trainee make-up artists will also need to earn money whilst completing work experience. Working in a store part-time or on a flexible contract can help a trainee make-up artist to balance training and earning money.

Negotiating a rate

All make-up artists need to learn how to discuss money. For example, trainee make-up artists need to discuss the expenses required for materials on a job, and designers will need to negotiate assistants' daily rates. This is essential throughout a make-up artist's career. Some people find it difficult but it is an invaluable skill to learn. Pay negotiation can be difficult as the producer will be reluctant to disclose their budget. Likewise the make-up artist will not want to disclose their daily rate until they know the producer's budget, in case they can negotiate a more attractive rate. Game theory suggests that whoever says the first figure (the producer or the make-up artist) generally loses their bargaining power.

An agent has a slight advantage as they can ask the producer to disclose their budget on the pretence that the agent can source suitable make-up artists available within the producer's budget.

The main considerations when setting your budget are:

◆ What is the producer willing to pay?

◆ What rate am I prepared to do the work for?

The first question is quite hard to know, but the budget will give an idea. The second question will be based on the hours, the travel time, the make-up involved and many other details. The market rate should also be considered; however, on the larger jobs there is generally a wage structure for each level within the team. These general levels are outlined in the following table; however, these can change depending on the production. The show plot person will mainly work during the show, and be less involved in setting/maintaining wigs. Swings are temporary cover for people on leave.

Typical job roles in television and film	Typical job roles in theatre
Designer	Designer
Head of department	Supervisor
Supervisor	Head of department
Make-up artist	Deputy
Assistant	Assistant
Junior	Show plot person
Trainee	Swing
Work experience	Trainee
	Work experience

Whilst it is possible to undercut fellow professionals, it can then become harder to increase your rate later on. It can also become harder to work with those make-up artists that have been undercut.

If you have been previously working as a trainee (at a trainee rate) and you feel you are now experienced enough to work as an assistant, you can apply for an assistant role, at an assistant's rate. If you are recommended for a job, the make-up artist or agent that recommends you will often have said what level they think you are capable of working at. It is possible that there will not be a budget for you to work at a higher-level rate. You can then choose to work for the rate offered or you can turn the job down; in which case you can say that you cannot afford to work for a lower rate anymore, but you can recommend someone else. You will be surprised how many times sufficient budget is found. However, if they choose to take the person you recommend (who is below your level of experience) then you can be satisfied that it was a job that you are too experienced to do.

TOP TIP

To check up-to-date recommended day rates visit the BECTU website (www.bectu.org.uk).

How to market yourself

On every job, you are constantly showing a version of yourself and other people will be making opinions based upon how you look, act, sound and what you do. The various forms of marketing will simply be based on the version you show in different mediums.

Social media

Social media is a relatively new phenomenon. Thirty years ago, when a make-up artist was starting in the industry, they would use the *Yellow Pages*, *The Knowledge* or *Kays* to find make-up designers' contact details and either use the telephone or write a letter to enquire about work. Now you can create a website or use social media to advertise your views or your skills cheaper and easier than ever before. However, so can everyone else, which means you now have to work harder to get designers' attention.

Most make-up artists use platforms such as Twitter, Facebook, Pinterest and Instagram. As the portfolio is very visual, Facebook, Pinterest and Instagram can serve very well as a low-cost alternative to creating a website. Facebook is also used a lot for forming groups to allow easy networking. If you search Facebook there are several groups for make-up artists in your area or national and international networks to join.

Social media is very good for either recommending people or getting last-minute jobs out to a lot of people (through a network of tweeting or sharing that occurs).

TOP TIP

Whilst social media can be a great networking tool, it is easy for someone to pretend they are more experienced or knowledgeable than they are. Any advice should be corroborated by trusted sources.

TOP TIP

Using social media

◆ Be positive, professional, mature, respectful and informative.

◆ Do not spam people.

◆ Do not use social media constantly.

◆ Use social media as a platform to post images of your work or visual inspirations.

◆ Many heads of department and supervisors will look you up online before they call, make sure they will not be put off calling you.

◆ Find and follow designers, make-up academies and companies who can inform, enhance and develop your career and knowledge of your trade.

◆ Use social media to get informed about your industry – all the information is at your fingertips.

Matt Gallagher, thecallsheet

The great benefit with social media is that the user can help other users easily. Academies try to promote newly established make-up artists and use social media to talk to other less-experienced artists about how they can break into the industry.

More recently a number of websites have been created for networking such as *Mandy* and *Starnow*. There are similar sites for the film and television industry such as *thecallsheet*. These sites are generally free to join, but have a monthly fee to get all of the site's functions.

Blogging

Blogging is a relatively new but widespread phenomenon, where a make-up artist can give their opinion on products or show demonstrations. With an increased following, the successful blogger will often get free material or invites to events.

Websites

A website is still the best way to promote yourself in order to get work that is not through recommendations. Make sure your website is kept up-to-date with your best photographs. As with your portfolio, your website should showcase your creativity and accurately represent you.

Try not to change your website too often as the user's Internet browser will often save pictures and text from different versions leaving a cluttered display. Users will need to clear their browsing history to correct it, but many users will simply leave the site.

Networking events

As with all marketing, if you decide to attend a networking event you need to make it worthwhile. Networking events will be of limited benefit if you are too shy to talk to anyone. As with everything, preparation is key. Research the make-up artists who are due to speak or companies that will be there. Who do you want to speak to? What do you want to say? If you want to show them your portfolio, where are the pictures that are most relevant?

In the make-up industry the main networking event worldwide is the International Make-up Artist Trade Show (IMATS). IMATS holds events in Los Angeles, New York, London, Vancouver, Sydney and Toronto. In the UK, the United Make-up Expo is also an important event to attend. It is smaller, which means there is more time to talk to make-up artists; however, it does not attract as many of the bigger make-up brands. As a trainee make-up artist it is important to attend both events.

The Make-up Show has events in Los Angeles, New York, Chicago, Dallas and Orlando. Another worldwide event is Professional Beauty, which currently focuses more on beauty therapy than make-up. There are also niche events such as those organised by brands (for example, Charles Fox) or trade unions (such as the Broadcasting, Entertainment, Cinematograph and Theatre Union [BECTU], www.bectu.org.uk) or for a specific area (such as the Afro Hair Show). The bigger shows are likely to have more to see, but the smaller shows may have less make-up artists looking for work and contacts.

ACTIVITY

Video promotion

In small groups, plan a short video piece that will be suitable for a show reel on your website, this could be a backstage catwalk show, casualty scene, etc. Film the event. Remember to be professional. Follow health and safety rules. Keep it short and eye-catching.

TOP TIP

As with all marketing, you need to have good pictures and make sure everything is spelt correctly and is grammatically correct.

TOP TIP

Make use of the exhibitions at networking events. Before you go, research the exhibitors and decide which ones you want to speak to and what to say.

TOP TIP

Ensure you have enough business cards to give out to potential clients and employers. You don't want to run out just before you have a chance encounter with another make-up artist.

Business cards

Your business cards should be very personal to you. Like your website, there are various companies available who can design your business card depending on your budget and how creative you want to be. Make sure the details are clear (and correct) and that you carry the cards around with you. There is no point in getting business cards made if you cannot use them when you need them.

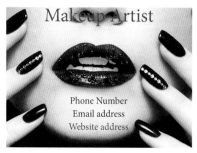

Example business card

Adverts

It may be helpful to advertise beyond your current network of friends and friends of friends. Once your pictures and business cards are ready, you should research suitable opportunities to advertise in magazines or shops, or consider using direct mailshots. With each form of advertising it is important to consider the cost and whether the reader of the advert is within the profile you are aiming your advertising at.

ACTIVITY

Design an advert

Design an advert that will promote you as a make-up artist. Remember to include your contact details, images of your work and a few written words. Remember you are promoting yourself and make it professional.

CVs and contacts

There are several different designs for CVs and, like other marketing tools, you can be as creative and as minimalist as you want.

◆ Make sure spelling is correct.

◆ Make sure any change of font is intentional and consistent.

◆ Put the most relevant information at the top.

◆ If you only have a page of relevant information fit it in one page.

◆ If you have two pages of relevant information you can use two pages, but no more.

Covering letters

There is not a standard covering letter used within the media industry, and trying to use one can make your letter seem formulaic. Plan the structure of your cover letter, using different paragraphs for each topic.

You should tailor the letter specifically to the person you are writing to. Your letter must explain:

◆ Why you want to work for them/on that project.

◆ The skills you have that would be helpful.

TOP TIP

Triple check the grammar and spelling in your cover letter and CV.

How to contact make-up artists (MUAs)

When making contact with other make-up artists it is important to remember:

◆ Make-up artists may be casual, friendly people but they are not your friends. Do not make a friend request on social media sites (although you obviously should accept one).

◆ If you want to contact a make-up artist you should find out their professional contact details (email address, possibly from their website).

◆ You should be professional and to the point.

◆ If calling a make-up artist, plan what you want to say. Do not take up too much of their time.

Insurance

Whether or not you have a legal contract you should at least have third party insurance. It is a legal requirement in many parts of the industry. This is to provide insurance cover for using make-up or any other product that could cause an allergic reaction for a model you are working on.

TOP TIP

Be aware there are various different insurances available on the market. BECTU includes insurance as part of its membership fees. The National Association for Screen Make-up Artists and Hairdressers [NASMAH] also have agreed a group rate for film and television. The Guild, British Association of Beauty Therapy and Cosmetology (BABTAC) or Association of Beauty Therapists (ABT) are recommended for beauty make-up. Other insurances are available from independent companies.

Your first job

Before beginning a first job, you may have spoken to the designer, head of crowd, manager or head of department and agreed possible work and dates. As the trainee, you may have months to prepare or you might be given less than a day's notice. Do not be surprised or annoyed at the lack of prior notice, being flexible is part of a make-up artist's job and you will get used to adapting to tight schedules.

Whether a job is paid or unpaid, you should treat the work the same. A trainee will have less responsibility than the rest of the team, so enjoy the experience. Your actual role will vary according to what the Designer, Supervisor or Head of Crowd likes their trainees to do. As with all jobs, there are some golden rules:

◆ Do not be late.

◆ Listen. If you do not understand, ask.

◆ If you see something needs doing offer to do it. Show you are keen.

◆ If you have started work before breakfast was available, offer to get it for the team.

◆ Be friendly and polite – but not so friendly with other teams that you come across as neglecting your work.

◆ Do not leave until any tidying and cleaning is complete.

It is important to think about contingency plans. For example, your car may break down, or bad traffic may make you late. You may fall behind the agreed timescale for a job. The important thing is not to panic. If you need to adjust your time, or someone else's expectations, then let everyone involved know as early as possible.

Business skills

Book-keeping/accountancy

When you have started earning money you will need to start paying tax. It is good practice to start doing your own book-keeping. This will mean accountancy fees are lower (because you would have done a lot of the work already) and you will be able to keep track of your outgoings and expenses.

DAILY TAKINGS

DATE of invoice	INVOICE NUMBER	FROM WHOM	SERVICE	AMOUNT	CASH	CHQ/ CARD/ BANK	DATE PAID
07/04/2016	123	Spike	Photo shoot	200.00	*		29/10/2016
11/04/2016	124	JCM Proms	Calendar	420.00		*	22/06/2016
12/04/2016	125	Hilary Carty	False nails	25.00	*		12/04/2016
28/04/2016	126	GTV	Filming	1080.00		*	
12/05/2016	127	Marcella Smith	Bridal services	175.00		*	15/08/2016

EXPENSES

DATE	Receipt number	Supplier	Goods and services	AMOUNT	CASH	CHQ/ CARD/ BANK
06/04/2016	1	Telephone co	Phone bill	40.00		*
07/04/2016	2	IMPS	Insurance	22.00		*
09/04/2016	3	Chemist	Nail varnish	4.00	*	
11/04/2016	4	B&P	Petrol	80.00		*
11/04/2016	5	Ma mag	Subscription	42.00		*
	6					
	7					

Example freelance accounts

You may want to open a separate bank account or use a separate credit card for work purchases. You should save all of your receipts for anything you bought for work purposes, such as products, equipment and work-related telephone calls, as this will reduce your tax bill.

It is important to consult an accountant for up-to-date tax advice. You can break down your expenses into as much detail as you want, but the following is a list of typical categories of expenses:

◆ Product supplies – make-up, tissues, wet wipes, etc.

◆ Postage, printing and packaging – could also include stationery, business cards, etc.

◆ Repairs and servicing of equipment.

◆ Equipment hire.

◆ Insurance and licences.

◆ Office equipment – where it is bought for work purposes.

◆ Event costs – e.g. IMATS, United Make-up Artists Expo (UMAe) tickets, etc.

◆ Uniforms.

- Reference books and magazines.

- Advertising – websites, magazine adverts, etc.

- Professional fees – accountant, web designer, agent, etc.

- Travel – the proportion of (petrol and car maintenance) costs that are reclaimed should be backed up by a log of personal/business driving. Fares are reclaimable if for work purposes.

- Subsistence – food/necessities on business trips that are not covered with 'per diems'.

- Telephone.

- Bank charges on your business account.

- Office – Internet costs can be claimed if it is for work purposes, but you must be able to justify the portion you are reclaiming. If you do not work from home, all rent and rates from your business address can be claimed (as it is 100 per cent business expenses).

- Tools and equipment – e.g. make-up brushes, airbrush compressor, etc.

When recording accounts, add a column and detail for 'drawings' (personal expenses or money transferred to a personal account) as this gives you a full picture of what you are spending money on. Once you have details of how much you spend each month (and on what) you will know what you should be charging in order to make a profit. Keeping records will also allow you to work out where you can save money.

By law you are required to keep any remittance advice slips, purchase orders, cheque book stubs, cancelled cheques, bank paying-in books, bank statements, delivery notes, till rolls, and copies of payments made or received using an online banking system.

Cash flow forecasting

When you have calculated how much you spend in a given week or month, you should be able to forecast how much you will spend in future weeks or months. You need enough available funds at all times to ensure the smooth running of your business. This is important to ensure you do not end up trying to get to a job without enough money to buy petrol, materials, etc. Even profitable businesses can go bust simply because they run out of cash.

In order to create a cash flow forecast you should include the cash in your business bank account:

Plus

- Money you expect to receive (be realistic about when people will pay you).

- Any interest you expect to get from savings.

Minus

- Expenses such as petrol, make-up materials, etc.

- Interest to be paid.

- Credit card bills and other expenses (you may have bought the goods but not yet paid for them).

- General living costs (food, mortgage, telephone bill, etc.).

> **TOP TIP**
>
> You cannot claim expenses on travel to your regular workplace.

> **TOP TIP**
>
> A 'per diem' (literally 'per day') is a daily allowance to cover expenses whilst working away from home.

Note: See Guidelines and Explanation contained in this file, for instructions on the completion of this cash flow projection.
Checking: See cell A55 for checks that spreadsheet is calculating correctly.

Monthly cash flow projection
Enter company name here
Enter date here

	Pre-Startup	Month 1	Month 2	Month 3	Month 4	Month 5	Month 6	Month 7	Month 8	Month 9	Month 10	Month 11	Month 12	TOTAL
1. CASH ON THE PREMISES [Beginning of month]		-	-	-	-	-	-	-	-	-	-	-	-	
2. INCOME														
(a) Cash sales														-
(b) Collections from credit accounts														-
(c) Loan or other cash injection														-
3. TOTAL CASH RECEIPTS [2a + 2b + 2c = 3]	-	-	-	-	-	-	-	-	-	-	-	-	-	-
4. TOTAL CASH AVAILABLE [Before cash out] (1 + 3)	-	-	-	-	-	-	-	-	-	-	-	-	-	
5. OUTGOINGS														
(a) Purchases (merchandise)														-
(b) Gross wages (excludes withdrawals)														-
(c) Payroll expenses (taxes, etc.)														-
(d) Outside services														-
(e) Supplies (office and operating)														-
(f) Repairs and maintenance														-
(g) Advertising														-
(h) Travel expenses (including deliveries)														-
(i) Accounting and legal														-
(j) Rent														-
(k) Telephone														-
(l) Utilities														-
(m) Insurance														-
(n) Taxes (real estate, etc.)														-
(o) Interest														-
(p) Other expenses [specify each]														-
														-
														-
(q) Miscellaneous [unspecified]														-
(r) Subtotal	-	-	-	-	-	-	-	-	-	-	-	-	-	-
(s) Loan principal payment														-
(t) Capital purchases [specify]														-
(u) Other start-up costs														
(v) Reserve and/or escrow [specify]														-
(w) Owner's withdrawal														-
6. TOTAL CASH PAID OUT [Total from 5a to 5w]	-	-	-	-	-	-	-	-	-	-	-	-	-	
7. CASH POSITION [End of month] (4 minus 6)	-	-	-	-	-	-	-	-	-	-	-	-	-	
ESSENTIAL OPERATING DATA [Non-cash flow information]														
A. Sales volume [pounds sterling]														-
B. Accounts receivable [end of month]														
C. Bad debt [end of month]														-
D. Stock on hand [end of month]														
E. Accounts payable [end of month]														
F. Depreciation														-
CHECKING (calculation verification) [See Guidelines worksheet for details]														
CHECK #1	Verified													
CHECK #2	Verified													
CHECK #3	Verified													
CHECK #4	Verified													

Cash flow projection worksheet

You may want to have separate business and personal expenses, but that is over-complicating things at this stage. The total should equal what you expect to be in your bank account at the end of the period.

Invoices

When you start doing paid work you should also set up a system to make sure your invoices for completed work have been paid. If you are not paid within your payment terms (as written on your invoice) you should have a schedule for chasing payments. Your invoice should include:

1 Your name, address and contact details (or the business name and address).

2 The name and address of the company you are invoicing.

3 Contact name at the company you are invoicing (if you have it).

4 The invoice date.

5 The date (or dates) the work was carried out.

6 Detail of the service provided.

7 The total amount on the invoice.

8 The payment terms for the invoice (e.g. pay within 28 days of invoice date).

9 Details of how to pay the invoice (your bank details etc.).

10 If you are value-added tax (VAT) registered you must also include the amount of VAT charged and your VAT registration number.

11 If you are a registered limited company you must also include your company and the company's registered address.

You might also include:

1 A unique invoice reference that applies to that invoice only.

2 Purchase order number (if applicable – the customer will give you this).

INVOICE

[Your name]
[Your address]

To:
[Company contact name]
[Company name]
[Company address]

[Date]

Invoice number	
Company number	
VAT number	

Please pay by BACS to:

Account details available on request.

Example invoice

Tax

When you start earning money as a freelance make-up artist you will be officially self-employed and will need to register with Her Majesty's Revenue and Customs (HMRC).

In order to work as a contractor (such as a freelance make-up artist) you must ensure you satisfy the tax rules known as IR35. This includes a number of variables that establish whether you are employed or self-employed such as:

1   Do you have control over your own hours and days worked and are you directly supervised?

2   Do you use your own tools and equipment?

3   Can you find a replacement that can do your job if you cannot do it?

4   Do you bear the financial risk of receiving a regular salary/ employment from one employer or number of employers?

If you are unsure you should contact an accountant or HMRC.

Registering for self-assessment can take a few months to complete, so you should ensure you do it before the July of the year you will be paying tax on. You will automatically be registered for schedule 2 and 4 national insurance (which is currently separate to income tax).

When you pay your tax as a self-employed person for the first time the government will assume constant income for the next year and so you will have to pay an extra 50 per cent. For example if you made a profit of £15,000 between April 2015 and March 2016, in January 2017 you will be expected to pay tax on that profit plus the expected profit (£7500) between April 2016 and September 2016.

Agreeing contracts

Agreeing contracts is quite a large area of discussion. The simplest route is to speak to a lawyer about a standard contract, which can be for anything from a wedding (at which you are to be a make-up artist) to your employees in your new company.

If you are creating a non-standard contract or writing your own terms and conditions it is important to ensure you are aware of current legislation you must adhere to, such as the Supply of Goods and Services Act 1982, which entitles a customer to a 'cool-down period' if they change their mind on a product they have bought or a service they have booked. A contract does not have to be written but it does need to be able to be proven. This could be through the status quo, but verbal contracts are often hard to prove.

As a trainee you are unlikely to be able to negotiate your contract, but as the designer you possibly would. If you are providing a service (such as a wedding make-up artist) you would be expected to create a standard contract. There are many make-up artists within the industry who do not use a contract; this comes down to personal preference and your risk tolerance, but, as well as preparing for the unexpected, a contract makes your service look more professional.

The head terms that need to be negotiated include:

1   Price.

2   What is included in the service (such as number of models).

3   Expenses to be included (make-up, travel, etc.).

4   Time allowed (including start time).

5   Outcomes expected.

6   Payment terms.

TOP TIP

Visit www.hmrc.gov.uk/ for more information on tax.

Managing your team

Working as a designer/supervisor

When you start your career as a make-up artist you will go for interviews with producers in order to be considered for a project. If they are organised you will have a script and will be expected to bring mood boards of how you envisage the project will look. If the project involves too much work for one person you will be expected to manage a team of make-up artists. This can sound daunting but it does not need to be.

You will need to add other make-up artists and their kit to your budget. You will also need to look at all of the production days to decide which days (such as crowd days) you will need extra artists.

Managing trainees/other make-up artists

When you start managing trainees and other make-up artists it is important to get the level and amount of communication right. If you do not tell your team things they need to know, they will not be able to do everything as you want. Equally, if you give them too much information you can overwhelm them. It is helpful to give a staff member responsibility for certain areas; this could be maintaining the continuity file or supplies for the make-up bus or correspondences with make-up artists required for future days ('the dailies'). This can allow you to oversee them while also being able to do other things.

Managing a team on set is similar to managing a team anywhere else and the morale of the team is key to their performance.

Delamar graduate, Ria Biggerstaff, designed her first feature film less than two years after completing her media make-up course:

> "
> My first role as a make-up designer, on an established feature film, was an eye-opening experience. I received an interview for *Kids in Love* on the back of a recommendation from a line producer I'd previously worked with (which shows the importance of being nice and professional to everyone around you). As well as designing, I was also personal make-up artist to supermodel Cara Delevingne and Bafta-winning actor Will Poulter. It is important to find a good balance with these roles; not neglecting one for the other. And if you can't find that balance, delegate your work. Do one job well, rather than two jobs badly.
>
> On all interviews, I'd recommend you to be professional, knowledgeable and confident; find a connection with the interviewer and be yourself. Don't lie about your abilities or experiences, as you will be found out somewhere down the line. When crewing up, I knew I would need a strong support team around me. A team, who would work well with each other, would be focused and dedicated to the job and respect me as a designer.
>
> *Ria Biggerstaff*

TOP TIP

Always work to the best of your ability as you never know who might be recommending you (or not recommending you) as a result.

Running a salon

Faith Bailey, started her own salon called Perch and Preen:

> The original idea for Perch and Preen came out of the realisation that the traditional appointments system doesn't work for everyone. My vision was for a fresh, funky environment offering a great mix of affordable treatments to encourage local women to adopt the European approach – that basic good grooming is a necessity not a luxury!
>
> The motivation behind the business was always flexibility – my business fits around me and my family, not the other way around. All successful business plans begin with a strong idea. My start-up finance was just £2000 of savings, which paid for my first month's rent and some minimal fixtures and fittings that I have added to gradually. Don't be daunted by thoughts of huge investment, if you have a clear idea of what you want to do, research it thoroughly and start with what you know you can afford. My business is proof that with determination and vision, anything is possible.
>
> *Faith Bailey, owner of Perch and Preen*

Other businesses

Delamar graduate Cate Hall created the app 'Continuity Pro':

> Since graduating I have been very fortunate and worked mainly as a hair and make-up designer for feature films. I started designing very low budget productions, and gradually over the years the size and budget of my productions has increased. It was my experience managing small budgets that prompted me to design and release the Continuity Pro apps. With the Continuity Pro app, project information (title, character names, scene descriptions, etc.), make-up notes and photographs can be entered directly at the time of shooting, rather than hurriedly at the make-up truck at the end of a long day. All projects have the option of password protection and can be synced with other tablets. Ideally everyone on the team would have the app on a tablet (or at least one on each set and one in the make-up bus) allowing everyone the same access to the same photos.
>
> *Cate Hall*

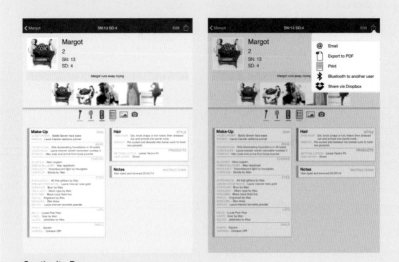

Continuity Pro

Make-up artists require a system to ensure there are pictures of all make-ups in case they are needed for continuity purposes. Traditionally, since the advent of digital cameras, film departments have spent time at the end of a long shooting day, printing, cutting and sticking photos into a folder before writing notes out by hand. The cost of ink and paper is enormous, and it was this cost that prompted me to search for a continuity app for the iPad. When I didn't find one, I saw the opportunity to make one myself.

I found a developer by chance (a friend's neighbour) and gave him my design on four sheets of A4 paper plus a list of 'must have' features such as password protection and PDF generation. I then invested some savings and started the long process of testing many prototypes before the Continuity Pro apps for make-up, costume and art department were released in summer 2012.

The hardest part of the journey has been branching out into an industry I don't have experience of or understand. Learning to respond to people's support requests specifically and technically and creating a rigorous testing process by myself. We started off with quite a simple model which was a little unstable as it tried to cope with so many photographs, and have gradually improved it to the point where it is now a tool I'm very proud of.

Running a business alongside being a full-time working make-up designer is a real challenge. But using the app on every job I do is so rewarding, as it assures me of its efficiency and convenience. Being able to record continuity right then and there on set leaves little room for mistakes.

My apps are now selling worldwide and are being used on productions such as *House of Cards*, *Game of Thrones*, *Two Broke Girls* and *Terms of Engagement*. I have over 1000 users and frequently receive emails full of thanks and compliments. I've revamped the website at www.continuitypro.com and created free downloadable user guides, so I rarely receive support requests at all any more. I'm currently negotiating with investors so that I can take on a full-time employee and expand the app further.

Cate Hall, creator of Continuity Pro

Agencies and organisations

Within the industry there are several agencies that operate at different levels. As agents generally work on commission you will not be able to get an agent until your skills and reputation have reached the level where you are designing mid- or big-budget features or commercials.

Fashion agencies

Within the fashion industry the days of needing a physical portfolio are gone. While some will prefer the physical portfolio, the vast majority are happy with e-books and websites, so you should focus on that. Agents are very busy people (if they are any good) so email them rather than call. It is easy to find their contact details, so send your CV with your website information.

If you assist a make-up artist who is with an agency, you can become an approved assistant for the agency's make-up artists. A similar process takes place in the film industry, where make-up artists will recommend good assistants to each other.

TOP TIP

When you are working regularly and have built your own reputation you might decide you need a diary service. A diary service effectively answers the telephone and puts jobs in your diary. Some have apps where you can accept or decline job invites. As you will not be able to answer the telephone when you are on set; the diary service will answer the telephone for you and accept/reject the job on your behalf.

Unions

In the UK you can join a union when you are still a student. In the USA you have to qualify through industry experience. BECTU represents anyone who works in media and entertainment sectors, including hair and make-up artists. The union is an organisation of workers who come together to improve the integrity of the industry. A union can help its members when negotiating details such as daily rates or maximum hours. BECTU negotiates pay levels with many employers and advises freelancers on rates through the rate cards that are published on its website. It also advises and supports members on the issue of unpaid work, which is often expected of new entrants in many departments within the industry.

The strength of any union is the members' ability to unite together over common issues of concern, so where conditions are deemed unacceptable to the group the union can negotiate a better deal on behalf of its members. The unions in the USA, for example, have a lot more influence in the industry than those in the UK. This stops union films from hiring one person to do everything (make-up and hair, for example), whereas in the UK make-up artists will generally be expected to be able to do both unless the film or television production has separate teams. A US artist would also not generally be in a television or film union as well as a theatre union, whereas in the UK an artist would move between the theatre and period dramas fairly often.

In recent years, BECTU has made progress in its efforts to end the practice of unpaid prep and wrap hours that affects certain departments in both film and television. The prep and wrap hours are the time before and after the camera starts rolling (which can be the majority of a make-up artist's day). It is expected that new agreements under negotiation with the Producers' Alliance for Cinema and Television (PACT) will significantly reduce this practice. BECTU also provides useful services such as insurance and legal representation.

CASE PROFILE: OLIVER HICKEY, FILM AND TV CAMERA OPERATOR

What do you enjoy most about the job?

The variety of the job is the best thing – no two jobs or days seem to be the same, so boredom is not an issue.

What do you enjoy least about the job?

The hours can play havoc with social and domestic lives – you need an understanding partner.

How has the television and film industry changed during your career?

Technology has advanced massively. Advancements in cameras and lighting have made cameras cheaper, better and with 4k resolution and upwards images, that work is very much finer now.

What advice would you give to a new make-up artist starting out?

Take as much work as possible and learn as much as you can. Absorb all advice you're given, suck it all up and you will learn from good and bad times.

REVISION QUESTIONS

1 Which events are in your local area and how should you prepare before going to them?

2 What platforms (such as social media) can you use to market your skills?

3 What information do you need to create a cash flow forecast?

4 How many pictures should you have for a full fashion portfolio?

5 What does TFP stand for?

6 Who inspires you and what work have they done that you found particularly inspirational?

7 What are the most important character traits you want to portray as a make-up artist?

8 What experiences have you had (both as a make-up artist and elsewhere) that you think bring transferable skills to your next role?

Epilogue

Make-up artist Tom Smith first worked with Richard Attenborough when Attenborough was acting in the film *Dock Brief* in 1962. Tom gave him a nose which was so successful that no one could see that it was false. Attenborough strolled around the studios and was amazed to find his changed nose made him unrecognisable. Tom insisted that it was a lucky accident. He had taken a cast of Attenborough's own nose at a board meeting and cast it that night using cap plastic, cake make-up and water, leaving it to set in a warm oven overnight. It was so successful that Tom couldn't find the edges to peel it off, and had to cut it down the middle with scissors.

Perhaps it was this early experience that made Sir Richard Attenborough, as he by now was, determined to have Tom do the make-up on *Gandhi* in 1980–1981, more than 20 years later. At the time, Tom was working on *Raiders of the Lost Ark* for Steven Spielberg, and he found himself deluged with photos of Gandhi, Nehru and other characters of the period.

TOM SMITH BIOGRAPHY

Tom was an amazing artist, who worked on iconic films such as: *Repulsion*, *Sleuth* and *The Shining*, as well as *Raiders of the Lost Ark* and *Gandhi*. He was able to elevate make-up to something beyond the application of **panstick** to an actor's face.

Tom worked with Roman Polanski on four occasions and loved the freedom Polanski gave during the film-making process, effectively allowing Tom licence to create special effects such as the latex wall in the famous scene in *Repulsion* as Catherine Deneuve's character descends into madness, arms grabbing at her from the wall.

On the release of *The Shining*, celebrated American make-up artist, Dick Smith wrote to Tom expressing his admiration for the special effects make-up and referred to the 'old woman in the bath' scene as 'The best "rot" I've ever seen!' It was a taxing experience working with Stanley Kubrick but was undoubtedly one that stretched Tom's great ability to produce some phenomenal work.

Tom loved working on *Raiders of the Lost Ark* and on *The Temple of Doom* and, not unlike with Polanski, was impressed with the freedom afforded to him by the director, Steven Spielberg. So impressed was Spielberg with Tom's creative ability, that he invited him to come to California for six months to work on ideas. At the time, however, Tom had just been contracted as chief make-up designer on *Gandhi*, for which he received an Academy Award nomination for Best Make-up.

Tom's work on *Gandhi* was probably one of his greatest achievements in 40 years in the British film industry. He largely rejected the use of prosthetics, although he had been to some extent formative in their development within the industry – witness his incredible use of prosthetics on Michael Caine in *Sleuth* to create the character of Inspector Doppler. *Gandhi* brought Tom full circle and allowed him full rein as an artist to create the ageing process on Ben Kingsley with pure make-up. Early morning each day, in the make-up chair Ben and Tom would chat and take tea while Tom worked his magic. Finally Ben Kingsley would say 'He's arrived – Gandhi is here'.

It was wonderful to be there when Tom, my father, received the BAFTA 'Special Award' in 1992 for lifetime achievement in the British film industry.

Written by Gareth Devonald Smith

The make-up artist's attitude

When Tom was doing the make-up on *Macbeth* in 1968, director Roman Polanski asked him, 'How many awards have you got, Tom?'

'None', replied Tom.

'BAFTAs, Oscars – you must have won some?' said Polanski.

'No', said Tom, 'nominations, yes, but winning, no. You see, if you can notice the make-up, you've failed. You've destroyed the illusion.'

'I see', said Polanski, 'you're in the kitchen.'

When an actor has thought through, developed and rehearsed his or her part; when the director has given assistance and constructive criticism concerning how the role fits within the film or play; when they are in accord, the lighting is arranged and the costumes are ready, then the only remaining contribution to a good, or even a great performance, is the visual appearance of the performer.

This is in the hands of the make-up artist.

If the make-up is true, in combination with the feelings of the actor it will afford the audience a true appreciation of the production.

Glossary

Acetone A liquid solvent which melts plastic. It can be used for cleaning the hair lace on postiche but should never be used directly on the skin. Commonly it is used as an ingredient in nail varnish. It is available from chemists. Can also be used for thinning the edges of bald caps if they are made of plastic.

Adhesive A means of sticking different surfaces together. Various types are available for use with wig hair laces, eyelashes, prosthetics and so on. Adhesives are available from theatrical suppliers and chemists.

Alginate A dental impression material used in lifecasting. It is available from dental suppliers.

Analysing the character The technique of determining the make-up requirements of an actor, according to the script.

Appliances Prosthetic pieces which are applied to the actor's face or body.

Aquacolour A water-based cake make-up which is grease-free and is applied with a damp sponge or brush. It is used for body make-up and fantasy painting.

Blending The technique of graduating the intensity of the colour from its strongest tone to its lightest until it disappears into the natural skin tone.

Block A head-shaped template for use in wig work, or a beard-shaped one for facial hair work. It can be malleable, wooden or plastic. The plastic version is used for making bald caps and when coloured red are called 'red heads'.

Blocking pins Pins used to attach wigs to blocks. They are available from hairdressing suppliers.

Breaking down The technique of applying make-up to achieve a natural weathered or discoloured effect according to the action and location, such as for a coal mine, desert, fight scene or the aftermath of an earthquake.

Breaking down the script The technique of going through a script systematically in order to organise crowd scenes, location, continuity needs and changes of make-up and hairstyles.

Camouflage make-up High density creams used for covering scars and other remedial work, available from chemist and theatrical make-up suppliers.

Castor oil An oil used with make-up for colouring prosthetic pieces.

Chamois leather Traditionally used to cool down actors by dampening the leather, sprinkling with cologne and swinging it in the air until ice-cold. It is then applied to forehead, back of neck and inside of wrists.

Chinese brushes Long, pointed brushes for watercolour painting to produce various effects, including marbling.

Compressed powders Powders in a variety of colours, shiny or matt, used as colouring for eyelids (eyeshadows) or for the cheeks (blushers or rouge). They are also used for colouring eyebrows. Available from make-up suppliers. Also available in body powders.

Contact lenses Lenses used for special effects in films or television production to change the eye colour. They must be supplied and fitted by a qualified optician.

Continuity The technique of achieving a seamless sequence in productions (which are usually filmed out of order) by making sure the make-up and hair 'match' the preceding and following shots.

Double knotting The technique of using two knots together when knotting hair onto a foundation net.

Drawing mats Mats used in postiche work for drawing hair.

Dressing out a wig The technique of styling the hair with tools such as rollers, tongs, a hairdryer and brushes to produce the finished effect.

False eyelashes Lashes used for extra emphasis on the eyes, available in different lengths and thicknesses. They are trimmed, then applied with a latex adhesive.

Face powder Powder used over the foundation to set it and to reduce shine. An all-purpose translucent loose powder is enough to suit all occasions, though many colours are available. Face powder in compact form (compressed face powder) can be applied directly to the skin without a base, or used on top of the foundation base to give a matt finish.

Fantasy make-up A make-up that does not look natural. It might be bizarre or stylised, such as for a witch or a statue.

Flash The edge of a prosthetic piece made of gelatine or foam latex. The flash is sculpted prior to casting to provide an overflow for the foam or gelatine.

Foundation (face) The make-up base used to achieve a complexion in the desired colour.

Foundation (wigs) The base, made out of net into which hair is knotted to make a wig.

Gafquat Used to hold down hair under bald caps and wigs. It is a water soluble copolymer.

Gelatine A material used for directly applied casualty effects and for making prosthetic pieces.

Glycerine A material mixed with water and used to simulate perspiration and tears. A spoonful of glycerine mixed with a bottle of rosewater is a good refresher or toner for dry skins. Glycerine is available from chemists.

Hackle A tool used in combing and mixing loose hair. Constructed of metal spikes set in a wooden block, it is rather like a miniature bed of nails.

Hair, human Hair used for making fine wigs, toupees and other hairpieces.

Hair, synthetic Hair generally used for stylised wigs and normally made into weft for wigs, beards and moustaches.

Hair, yak Course yak hair is used for laying on directly applied hair for beards and moustaches.

Hair lace A net-like material, also called ventilating net, into which hair is knotted for many types of postiche.

Highlighting The technique of using a light colour to make a feature more obvious.

Isopropyl Alcohol (known as IPA) A clear cleaning agent used for washing and sterilising make-up brushes and equipment. Also used as an activator for skin illustrator palettes.

Karo syrup A type of syrup used in the manufacture of artificial blood. It is available from specialist grocers.

Knotting hooks Hooks attached to needles, used for inserting hair into gauze when making postiche.

Latex A natural rubber in milky-white foam, available in varying densities. It is used for creating wrinkles in ageing make-up; in casualty effects, for peeling skin and the like; and in making bald caps and filling moulds in prosthetic work.

Laying a beard The technique of making a beard by applying loose hair directly onto the face.

Laying on hair The technique of sticking loose hair directly onto the face and then dressing it with tongs.

Lifecasting The technique of taking an impression of the actor's face or body and casting it in stone.

Lifecasting, sectional The technique of taking an impression of a section or piece of the actor's face or body and casting it into stone.

Look-alike The character make-up required to make the actor look like someone else.

Look book (designer) This may be a mood book or board that designers use to portray their ideas of the look/theme.

Luminous make-up Fluorescent make-up for fantasy make-up effects for use under ultraviolet lights. It is available from theatrical make-up suppliers as a cream, a liquid or a gel.

Modelling clay Clay used for sculpting features in prosthetic work. It is available from pottery and artists' suppliers.

Modelling tools Tools used for building and modelling in clay, plastic and wax. Sculpting tools and dentists' tools are useful to the make-up artist.

Modelling with wax The technique of building up a natural feature and changing its shape using wax directly applied to the face and body.

Mortician's wax Wax used for modelling directly onto the face, when blocking out eyebrows, changing the shape of the nose and so on.

Moustache wax A colour wax used to curl the ends of moustaches.

Old-age stipple A latex product used for wrinkled ageing effects. It can be obtained in different flesh colours from theatrical make-up suppliers.

Pancake A cake make-up which is grease-free. It was first made by Max Factor.

Panstick A cream stick make-up base, also available in paintbox-style containers, obtained from theatrical make-up shops.

Pencils Wooden pencils with soft grease lead, used for colouring eyebrows and outlining eyes and lips.

Plaster A material used for making positive and negative moulds in prosthetic work. It is available from dental or artists' suppliers.

Plaster bandage Bandage used to reinforce the impression when lifecasting.

Plastic A material used in liquid form to paint layers when making bald caps and prosthetic pieces. Glatzan is a well-known make available from theatrical make-up shops. Plastic should never be used directly on the skin.

Plastic scar material A material in tube form used for modelling scars and the like directly onto the skin. Although especially formulated for use on the skin, this material should always be tested on the back of the actor's hand first, in case of irritation.

Plastic spray An artificial latex spray used for setting facial hair when making hair on the block. It is not for facial use.

Plastilene A material used for modelling in prosthetic work. Although not as good as clay, unlike clay it does not need wetting. It is available from artists' suppliers.

Portfolio A collection of professional images that is developed to showcase work. This may be leather bound or electronic.

Powder brush A soft brush used for removing excess powder from the face.

Pro bondo Thickened Pros-Aide used for making small prosthetics pieces.

Pros-Aide A waterproof adhesive used in the medical, prosthetic and special effects make-up industries.

Rubber-mask greasepaint A caster oil-based product, available in various colours, used for painting on top of latex.

Sealer A material used on top of wax, nose putty and prosthetic pieces before applying make-up.

Section life casting When making an appliance to fit specific part of the actor, often the nose, instead of taking an impression of the whole face, many make-up artists like to sectional life cast just the feature itself as it is quicker and less expensive than casting the entire face.

Shading The technique of using a darker colour to make a feature less obvious.

Silicone Used for filling moulds and making pieces for prosthetics work.

Skin illustrator palettes Palettes used for special effects, prosthetics and camouflage work.

Spirit gum The adhesive most commonly used in attaching wigs, beards, moustaches, bald caps and the like. It is available from theatrical make-up shops.

Standing by Staying near the actors on the set, ready to retouch the make-up when necessary.

Stippling The technique of using an open-pored sponge and applying make-up with a dabbing movement in order to provide a textured effect.

Straight make-up The technique of defining and correcting a face with make-up.

Stubble paste Wax in stick form, used on the face before applying chopped-up hair to create a beard stubble.

Swing job A position in the theatre for professional freelancers to provide job cover for members of the department who are absent due to illness or holiday.

Test shoots (photography) Photographs taken by the photographer, model and make-up artist working together unpaid to produce pictures of their portfolio.

Test shots (cinematography) The filming and viewing on a screen of the lighting, hair, make-up and costumes to try them out.

TFP (Time for Print) Photoshoots where a photographer, a model, a make-up artist and possibly a designer agree to do the photoshoot without being paid on the basis that the photographer will give them a copy of the photo for their portfolio.

Tong heater An electronic heater for heating iron tongs used in dressing postiche.

Tongs Iron tools heated up to dress hair.

Toning down a colour Toning down a colour is often asked for by the make-up designer or director and can be done in various ways by neutralising, or adding a touch of grey – and in certain cases taking away some of the colour with a cotton bud, for example over bright blusher or eyeshadow. Finish by powdering the area which also helps to tone it down. It is always best to take the actor off set when possible.

Toning down a period look The technique of making a look more modern.

Tooth enamel A material used for painting the teeth. It is available in white, cream, nicotine, yellow, black, gold and silver from theatrical make-up shops.

Watercolour brushes Brushes used for applying sealer, collodion, spirit gum, acrylic paints, latex and cap plastic. They should be cleaned in the appropriate solvent immediately after use.

Waterproofing the make-up The technique of protecting the make-up for filming in water.

Waxing out The technique of using a layer of wax to cover a feature such as the eyebrows before applying make-up.

Wig stand A stand used to hold a wig or moustache block while dressing postiche. Stands are available either freestanding or as a shorter version that clamps to a workbench or table.

Witch hazel A material used for blending the edges of gelatine pieces. A spoonful mixed in a bottle of rosewater makes a good refresher or toner for greasy skin. Witch hazel is available from chemists.

Index